The Complete Book of Sailboat Buying

Volume II

Belvoir Publications Inc.
1111 East Putnam Avenue
Riverside, Connecticut 06878

ISBN: 0-9615196-7-3

Contents

Introduction

Every sailor has a sailboat waiting for him somewhere. The trick is, of course, to know her when you see her, for she is an elusive genie that may take on many forms. For one person, she may be a nimble, trailerable daysailer; for another person, a rugged and heavy displacement cruiser; for yet another, a sleek and demanding racer.

It's even likely that "The Right Boat" will change forms several times within a sailor's lifetime—metamorphosing from a racing boat for his teens and twenties, to a cruiser for his later years. Indeed, many boatowners learn one lesson from their experiences after owning several sailboats: there is no one, true perfect yacht *for all time*, but merely, the best yacht *for the times at hand*.

In Volume 1 of **The Complete Book of Practical Sailboat Buying**, we have outlined, in concept, the many and various things to consider when preparing to buy a boat. In this second volume, we apply the same concepts in scrutinizing a series of production sailboats in the range of length from 19 feet all the way up to 42 feet, with prices to match virtually any sailor's budget.

Although we focus on 44 models, there are actually perhaps two dozen more that are glimpsed in passing or mentioned in some detail. These evaluations are drawn from the pages of *The Practical Sailor*; each represents a boat that had achieved at least modest popularity and was still in production at the time of the original evaluation. Prices, features, options and even construction methods may have changed in the time since the original evaluation was published. (For a list of the original dates of publication, please see page 362.)

Unfortunately, the boatbuilding industry has seen hard times in recent years, and some of these boats can no longer be bought new. However, they may be found in some abundance on the used-boat market. The companies listed within this book as still in operation are the "survivors." Interestingly, the list does much to scotch the myth that only the "good" boatbuilders were the ones who failed to make it, leaving us only cheap and poorly built boats as a legacy. In fact, it was a collection of good and bad boats that went out of production, and it is still a collection of good and bad boats that remain.

It will be easy to recognize a number of concerns that we raise in virtually every evaluation. For one thing, we try to point it out sharply whenever a boat is really not fit for offshore sailing. This is not because we think offshore sailing is the highest, purest art of the sailor, but because it has very particular design requirements for safety that need not be applied to a coastal or inland sailboat. It can come down to a one-shot chance of survival, when a heavy wave catches the boat from astern and demonstrates whether the drop boards will stay in place, whether the cockpit will empty quickly enough, and whether the boat can be controlled at all during the episode. If the design is unsuited, the boat may sink. It's as simple as that.

Other matters are not so stark, but are important in every boat. For instance, in many evaluations we try to assess the likelihood of expensive repairs when the given configuration of keel and rudder suffers the inevitable brush with a sandy bottom, or even firmer terror. We speak up when we think a hull to deck joint might be the hands-down loser in a tussle with a dock. We even turn our noses up sometimes—when a designer chooses to situate the potty between the V-berths, for instance.

We believe these are the items one ought to be stealing glances at when the yacht broker launches off into a detailed explanation of the workings of the autopilot or loran receiver. It's all too common for boats to be sold on the basis of whizzbangs and doodads, overlooking serious flaws in basic design.

Of course, many a sailboat represents a dream of passages to Tahiti or races won by half a boat length. It's no sin to dream, of course, but it can be frustrating if there's no way to attain one's dreams. In its way, this book strives to make the sailor's dreams achievable.

There really *is* a boat waiting for you, and she may be just around the corner, in the pages ahead. Go for it!

The Editors
Newport, 1987

The Practical Sailor's Evaluations of 44 Popular Sailboats

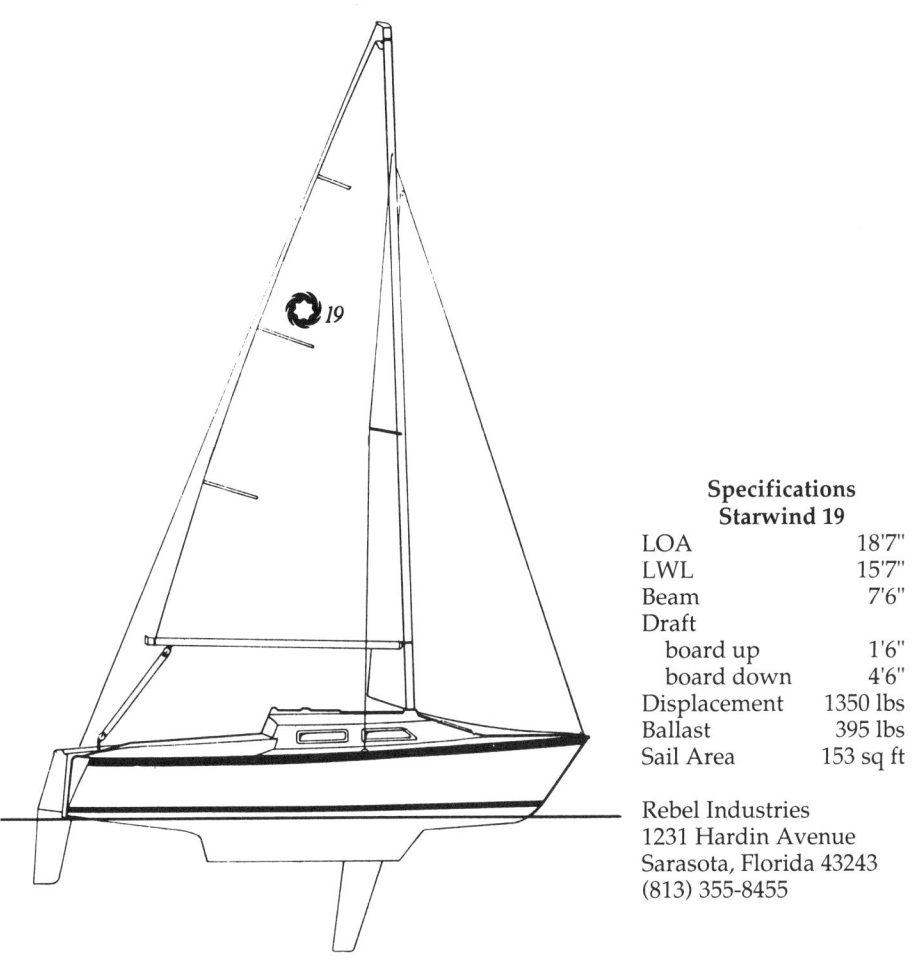

Specifications
Starwind 19

LOA	18'7"
LWL	15'7"
Beam	7'6"
Draft	
board up	1'6"
board down	4'6"
Displacement	1350 lbs
Ballast	395 lbs
Sail Area	153 sq ft

Rebel Industries
1231 Hardin Avenue
Sarasota, Florida 43243
(813) 355-8455

The Starwind 19:
Trailer Sailer of the 1980s

THE BOAT AND THE BUILDER

This is an evaluation that almost "died aborning." The Starwind line of sailboats was sold to a new builder as we were researching this chapter. So, the following analysis is principally an evaluation of the pre-1985 Starwind, not the models built after the transfer of the molds to Rebel Industries.

Nevertheless, the original Starwind 19 deserves review because she is unique. In fact, she deserves an asterisk in the annals of boatbuilding history because she demonstrates that a prosperous powerboat manufacturer—Wellcraft Marine in this case—*can* build a functional sailboat, despite industry prejudice to the contrary. Unfortunately, she further demonstrates that the *economics* of producing a successful sailboat can be poor business for a powerboat builder. Hence, Wellcraft's sale of this product to Rebel Industries.

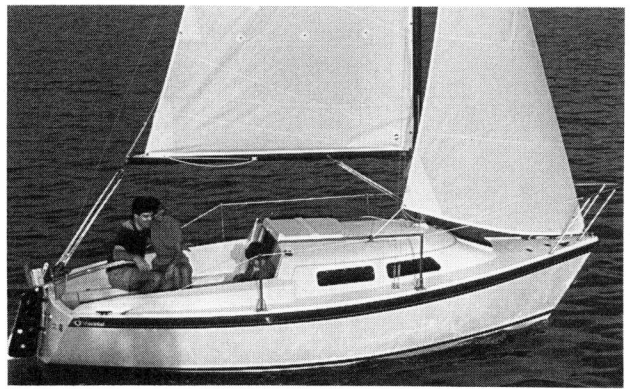

The Starwind 19's conception was a result of the "oil crunch" of the early 1970's. It was then that Wellcraft—the largest boat builder in the U.S. at the time—decided to hedge against an anticipated backlash against "gas-guzzling" powerboats. Sailboats, presumably, would soon rule the waves. Wellcraft began by acquiring Chrysler Marine's sailboat division. Like Bayliner and Glastron—Chrysler's sailboats had suffered from the manufacturer's lack of familiarity with the sailing marketplace. Some boats were poorly designed, others were poorly marketed; none were big sellers.

Wellcraft managed to avoid many of the errors that soured most powerboat builders on the sailboat market. They hired a separate marketing and management staff for Starwind. They set up a separate dealer network. (Only five of the 70 Starwind dealers sold Wellcraft powerboats.) And, the designs chosen were conservative, with a minimum of powerboat glitz, hardware, or high technology.

In the end, however, the primary pitfall wasn't avoided—the basic incompatibility of sailboats and powerboats. Wellcraft was then doing $150 million in business per year. Sprawling facilities were scattered throughout the South and you could literally smell the styrene a mile from their Sarasota, Florida plant. This was the only plant building Starwinds, yet sailboat production was dwarfed by that of powerboats. Only 50 of Wellcraft's 2000-plus employees were assigned to Starwind ... small potatoes, indeed.

Starwind never did turn the corner for Wellcraft. It comprised only two percent of their business. Separate personnel and inventories were both expensive and cumbersome to the primary money maker—powerboats. So, in February of 1985, Wellcraft sold the Starwind operation to a neighbor—Rebel Industries.

Rebel was no newcomer to the boating industry. Under various ownerships, the company had been building small boats since 1947. A move to Florida in 1980, followed by the introduction of a new line of daysailers under the Spindrift logo, had kept the company on solid ground.

The acquisition of Starwind doubled the size of Rebel's production line and gave them access to the trailerboat market, with three Starwind models between 19 and 27 feet. While it tripled the size of their dealer network, the power and sailboat dealers were not mixed, and Wellcraft continued to honor warranties on boats they had delivered.

Spindrift introduced the Starwind 19 with a redesigned cabin house, a few improvements in construction, and a base price of $6995—$500 less than the Wellcraft version of the boat. By the end of 1987 this had risen only to $7995—still a reasonable price for a boat of this type and size. While the builders of most trailerboats were trying to break the $10,000 barrier, here was that rare bird—a boat with overnight accommodations retailing for under $8000. Even fully equipped (trailer, outboard, genoa package, galley package, head, battery, pulpits and lifelines), the Starwind 19 still came in at about $10,500.

For the entry level sailor there were even less expensive (and less comfortable) trailer sailers. Consider the Venture/McGregor 21 at about $7000 fully equipped. Or the Santana 20, with a fixed keel and organized racing, for about $8,500 fully equipped.

For the most part, owners reported being happy with their boats, and their treatment by Wellcraft. Opinions on the dealers were mixed—prospective owners were wise to ensure that the individual dealers knew *something* about sailboats.

CONSTRUCTION

Wellcraft built the Starwind 19 in the only economical way available to them—like a powerboat. We're frankly surprised at how little the boat suffered from such construction. Powerboat techniques just aren't as "high-tech" as those of the typical sailboat. Price sells powerboats, and weight and rigidity are far less critical when you have a hundred or more horses pushing your boat through the water.

Being such a small part of Wellcraft's production, the Starwinds didn't justify their own glass shop. Originally, Starwind designer, Jim Taylor, specified a Klegecell-cored deck, and a layup of 18-ounce fiberglass roving sandwiched between layers of 1.5-ounce mat. But, to fit into Wellcraft's production line, the Starwind 19 was laid up with 24-ounce roving, between layers of mat applied with a chopper gun.

The deck was cored with plywood. Balsa is, of course, the more common core used by manufacturers of sailboats. But balsa is difficult to use in the humid conditions of the South, without air conditioning in the layup shops. (It's cheaper, of course, to use plywood, open the doors, and let nature dispel the fumes.)

There was nothing inherently unseaworthy about Wellcraft's layup methods—it's just harder to control the weight of the finished product. The *designed* weight of the Starwind 19 was 1290 pounds. The substitution of plywood for Klegecell added only a *theoretical* 40 pounds—yet some boats came in at several hundred pounds overweight.

The reasons were probably two-fold. First, precise control of materials is necessary for consistent weights—control rarely found in powerboat construction. Secondly, plywood coring can gain a considerable amount of water weight as a boat ages. Wellcraft cut its plywood into small squares to conform to mold curves. They claimed that this encapsulated each square in resin, and thus avoided water migration.

This would certainly help slow migration, but is it a complete cure? Also, on one deck we viewed on the production line, the wood was unsealed in spots. (The core was not vacuum-bagged, a process which results in more uniform saturation.) The problem of inconsistent weights

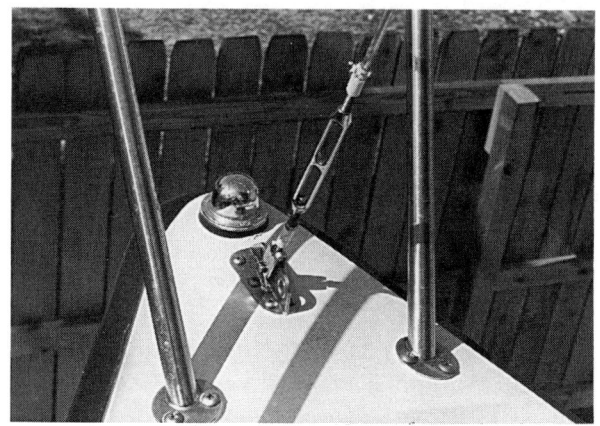

The Wellcraft stem arrangement. Rebel chose pulpit-mounted running lights and a conventional "over the bow" stem fitting.

should not affect the daysailing capability of the Starwind 19, but those wishing to race might be well advised to weigh a proposed boat before purchase.

Rebel chose to follow the designer's layup specifications more closely, but again without vacuum-bagging. Plywood was inserted into the Klegecell deck only as a backup for hardware. Rebel also opted to core the hull, cockpit floor, seats, and some vertical surfaces, with Coremat—a newer core material made up of a relatively thin layer of polyester fibers and microspheres. Coremat is a quick means of adding stiffness to flat panels. It is laid into a mold like any layer of fiberglass. We feel it might prove more brittle than a foam core, so special care should be exercised to avoid "point loading" (poorly placed trailer supports, for example).

It is perhaps amusing that Wellcraft described the Starwind 19 in one of their brochures as having a "high-tech, cored deck." They also said she had a "high impact rubrail." We wouldn't want to hit anything hard with a Starwind 19 however, as she has an outward-turned hull to deck joint, protected from impact only by a snap-on plastic rubrail. Aside from hard knocks, though, this joint should prove more than adequate as it is fastened with #10 bolts at four-inch intervals, and glued with 3M 5200, a semi-rigid adhesive. Rebel chose a similar assembly but substituted stainless steel rivets for threaded fasteners.

Wellcraft used 3M 5200 for bedding all deck hardware and through-hull fittings. While this should effectively prevent leaks, it will also serve to make it almost impossible to remove such hardware without tearing the adjoining deck or hull. A polysulphide or silicone acrylic sealant would have been a wiser choice.

The liner on the Wellcraft model is attached to the hull with extensive fiberglass tabbing, most of it accessible if repair is needed—a good system. Rebel tabbed the liner in a similar manner, in addition to gluing it with a polyester slurry.

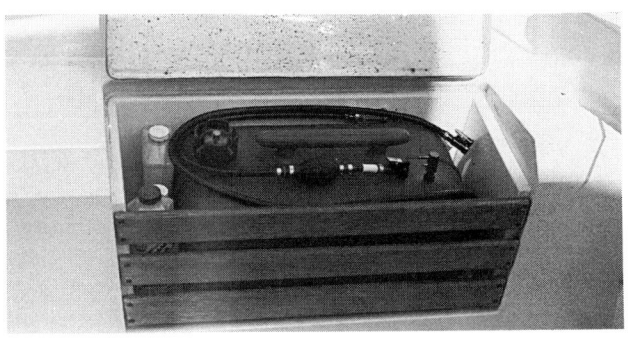

The cockpit locker is safely sealed from the rest of the boat, and well ventilated with teak slats. It will accommodate a fuel tank, but not an outboard.

Wellcraft supported the Starwind 19's deck-stepped mast with an ample compression post, run from the undersurface of the deck, down to the V-berth. The vertical face of the V-berth was then cored with several layers of plywood, and the liner below the V-berth glassed to the hull. Several layers of 24-ounce roving were then added—a solid, in-line assembly. The chainplates are fastened to a plywood partial bulkhead, which is screwed to the liner. This is then tabbed to the hull. As in most boats, the tabbing is the weak link, but on the Wellcraft boats we inspected, the tabbing seemed both adequate and accessible.

The centerboard and rudder were two items that Wellcraft couldn't fit into their powerboat production facilities, so these were contracted out. These Wellcraft "blades" were molded of fiberglass with a poured-in core of high density urethane foam. The mold flanges begged to be sanded off (for better performance) but this would leave the joint between the halves dangerously thin. Wellcraft said the foam was strong enough to stand alone without the fiberglass, but we seriously question this. We would also worry about the instability of urethane foam—which has been known to expand with age, or exposure to heat. Rebel chose to build blades "in-house" with a Klegecell core.

The Starwind has a kick-up rudder for easier trailering. The rudder head is long, which *would* give the rudder blade good support, *if* the blade were butted up beneath the tiller. Unfortunately, the blade doesn't even extend above the lower gudgeon. On one boat we inspected, the rudder head welds had cracked from strain. Mounting the lower pintle closer to the waterline would help, but access to this would involve cutting an inspection port in the cockpit floor. Also, the pintles could be somewhat beefier and some owners complain of a sloppy fit.

While there are generally few complaints about construction among the owners we interviewed, several agreed on a problem with gelcoat cracking and chipping. This is most common along a sharp radius like the turn of the hull flange.

PERFORMANCE

Handling Under Sail
To be truly trailerable, the Starwind 19 had to compromise her performance with shoal draft. This meant a long stub keel housing a centerboard. To im-

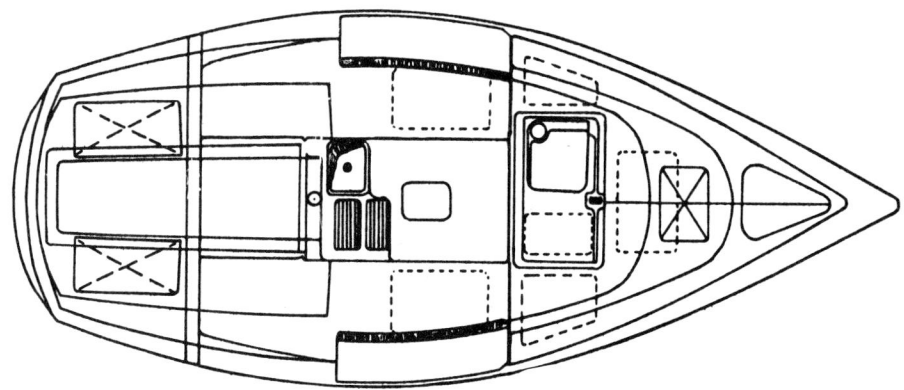

prove performance and safety, she includes several unique features in her keel/centerboard design. The centerboard is ballasted with 35 pounds of lead—just enough to hold the board down when sailing. The board is hoisted with a rope pennant; no mechanical advantage is necessary. The boat's real ballast—395 pounds of lead—is glassed into the forward quarter of the keel stub. This keeps the weight centralized to reduce pitching, and makes the boat safer in the event of a capsize. In such a circumstance, the centerboard can fall back into its trunk with little damage—or effect on righting moment.

To accommodate a centerboard as well as ballast, the keel stub is thick. To minimize drag, this stub is lengthened fore and aft of the centerboard slot, in an effective airfoil shape. The centerboard is also a respectable airfoil. However, the centerboard slot is longer than necessary and is not covered by a gasket. Gaskets are admittedly hard to maintain, but important in reducing drag.

The open centerboard slot is probably one reason that PHRF ratings imply mediocre performance for the Starwind 19. Data on the boat is scant, but the ratings average about 285 seconds/mile, or nearly the same as an O'Day 20. This is slower than a Catalina 22, and significantly slower (by 30 seconds/mile) than an Ensign or Venture/MacGregor 21. For less money, you could buy a Santana 20 and go 60 seconds per mile faster. For real performance, consider that the Holder 20's rating is 180 seconds/mile.

Starwind 19 owners report that performance is above average, compared to similar boats. She is stronger upwind, in part due to her inboard shrouds and working jib leads. Downwind, she is underpowered and a spinnaker is not an option. A genoa package is an option, however, and strongly recommended by owners. Without a spinnaker, an oversized whisker pole is a valuable addition. A boom vang is recommended too, as it will prevent the boom from snagging the backstay during a jibe.

As on most entry-level trailer sailers, working sails were provided as part of the base price. "But," said one owner, "don't expect them to be the equal of a name-brand sail."

Another owner complained that the offset backstay makes the rig difficult to tune because it pulls the mast off center. An adjustable, split backstay would serve better. Fortunately, the untapered mast section seems more than stiff enough to maintain rig tension.

Owners commend the balance of her helm and say she is of average stability. Several report sailing in four-foot seas and 20-knot breezes with no handling problems. They do recommend the pulpit, stern rail and lifeline option however, as handholds are few and far between when going forward.

Handling Under Power/Trailerability

The Starwind 19 comes with a spring-loaded outboard bracket as standard equipment. Several owners complained that the bracket was mounted too high on the transom.

Owners report that the Starwind 19 is easily launched and retrieved with her 18-inch draft. She is also easily rigged because of her deck-stepped mast and swept-back shrouds. Only the headstay has to be backed off to drop the rig.

A trailer wasn't a factory option but individual dealers offered a wide choice of makes and models. When buying a used rig with trailer, look for those with the extendable tongue.

LIVABILITY

Deck Layout

One of the factors that makes a small boat of the 80s stand out from those of the 70s is cockpit design. A modern trailer-sailer is likely to be more comfortable, and the Starwind 19 is a thoroughly modern design. The cockpit coaming is just wide enough, and inclined enough, for practical sitting when heeled. The cockpit seats have angled backrests. The inboard corner of the seat is beveled, so you can kneel against the leeward side when trimming the genoa, or use it as a footrest.

The six-foot cockpit will comfortably seat three or four and the tiller is long enough for easy steering. The solid bar traveler over the tiller keeps the cockpit clear of the mainsheet, but does prevent the tiller from being raised when at anchor.

Aside from minor "annoyances," most of the hardware is of reasonable quality. The jib cleats on a marginally sized swivel cam, but the genoa package includes a Barlow single-speed winch, and there is a Harken mainsheet winch with ratchet.

The mast is a Johnson extrusion with much of the rigging done by the builder. All halyards are rope, and cleat on the mast, with only the main halyard internal. The shrouds are of adequate size and swaged to open-bodied, well toggled turnbuckles. Too many bottom-dollar trailer-sailers skimp on the standard rigging. The Starwind doesn't.

The only parts of the Starwind 19's rig that we didn't like were the undersized spreader brackets and the stainless steel pop rivets used to fasten the shroud tangs to the mast. Stainless rivets are strong, but they corrode the holes in which they're seated. To minimize this problem, Rebel said they would bed the rivets with Lonocote.

An anchor well is molded into the foredeck. While small, it should hold enough ground tackle to allow anchoring in shallow water.

Belowdecks

The Starwind 19 has full sitting headroom on two six-foot-plus settee/quarter berths. The V-berth is also six feet long, but very narrow at the foot. The head of the berth spans a space than can be used for either a portable head or an icebox. Seating in the head is athwartships, behind a privacy curtain. When sleeping, this space is covered by a plywood-backed cushion, which can be flipped and used as a table.

The optional "galley" (a sink with a hand pump) is installed underfoot, below the companionway. We can't see any use for this on so small a boat. Cooking will be done on a camp stove in the cockpit, and dishes can be washed overboard. (Why risk a twisted ankle every time you step below?)

The companionway hatch is large, providing some standing headroom, but it runs on somewhat flimsy teak slides. The companionway is not rain-proof, as the after surface of the cabin house is angled forward. The forward hatch is made of Lexan by Gray. It has sloppy hinges but can be positioned for good ventilation and has an efficient gasketing system.

The Starwind 19's interior has little woodwork, but what it has is clean and attractive. For example, the wiring of the mast light is recessed in a groove in the forward side of the mast compression post, and nicely covered with teak. Wellcraft boasts that it stocks over forty kinds of Formica. Thankfully, they refrained from squandering this on their sailboats.

Wellcraft's first 150 boats had a "speckled" gelcoat overhead. This was subsequently covered with a polypropylene "carpet," glued in place with contact cement. Polypropylene doesn't absorb water and dries quickly. The hull to deck joint is exposed for easy repair, as are most deck fittings.

There are five small sealed bins under the berths, all removable for access to the hull. We would prefer to see larger ones, or as a trade-off for the lost stowage space, the space between them filled with air bags to increase positive flotation. The space under the cockpit seats is also under-utilized, but again, plenty of room for flotation. There is also storage space under the cockpit sole for duffel bags, an outboard, or other bulky items.

CONCLUSIONS

The Starwind 19 should stand as proof that a powerboat builder can build a decent sailboat. But Wellcraft's abandonment of the Starwind line would seem to confirm, alas, that such boats can't be built profitably. The Starwind 19 was built with minimal technology, inexpensive labor, and existing plant capacity. Wellcraft's size and general efficiency should have provided great economy. Their cushion shop alone occupies more floor space than the entire plants of most small sailboat builders. Still, they couldn't make money on her.

Perhaps it was because Wellcraft dedicated a separate staff for the Starwind line, hired competent designers, and farmed out production of components they knew they couldn't make well. But the fact that Wellcraft couldn't make it work would cause us to be skeptical of any sailboat coming from a powerboat builder.

The post-1985 Starwind 19's came from Rebel Industries—a sailboat builder. Unfortunately, Rebel ceased production of the Starwind 19 (and all their boats) in June of 1987, just one more victim of the great middle '80s sailboat shakeout. In all, about 1000 Starwind 19s were produced.

A novice sailor, eager to learn so he can move up to bigger and better things, has several choices. If he or she is young and athletic enough, a good first boat might be such a high-performance dinghy as the Laser.

However, sailors with young families will likely opt for a small trailer-sailer. For them, the cheapest alternative is a used trailer-sailer of early 1970's vintage—like the Venture 21 or the Catalina 22. Such boats can be found, without undue searching, for under four or five thousand dollars. If they can afford it, though, they will be more satisfied with a trailer-sailer of the 80s—like the Starwind 19. Such a boat will have better hardware, handle easier, and be more comfortable—both above and belowdecks.

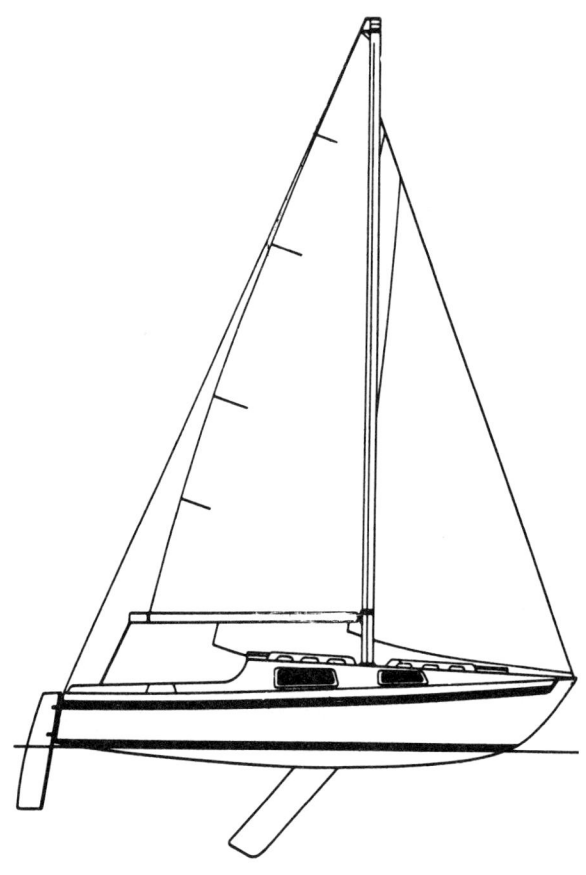

The San Juan 21:
A Trailerboat More Typical Than Not

THE BOAT AND THE BUILDER

The age of the inexpensive "trailer-sailer" began with the design of the Venture 21 in 1965. The San Juan 21 is one of the first in a wave of Venture imitators. Around the time of the Venture's introduction, Bob and Carol Clark began building such one-design sailboats as Lightnings and Thistles in their shop in Washington. Their business relationship with boats was a natural one, because the Clarks were accomplished racers. In fact, success on the race course had been as much a family business as boatbuilding. The Clark's son, Dennis, who managed Clark Boat Company, compiled a record that included national championships in four major one-design classes.

Despite the Clarks' abilities as racers, it wasn't the production of "hot" one-designs that made Clark Boat Company what it was to become. It was a line of

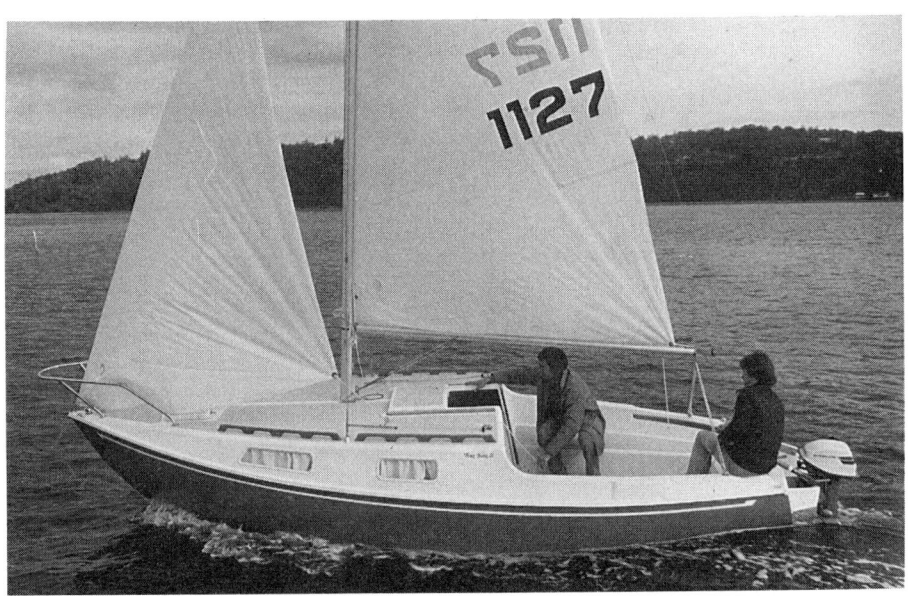

boats that began with the San Juan 21 in 1969. This was the same year that a host of other West Coast builders tried to capitalize on the Venture 21's success. For example, the Catalina 22, Cal 21, and Santana 21 were all designed in 1969.

The inexpensive trailer-sailer has always been intended for the first-time boatowner—the sailor with a young family, a small purse, and limited expectations of both himself and his boat. At first glance, there doesn't seem to be anything that would distinguish the San Juan 21 from its trailerable sisters of this era. With more research, however, it became apparent that many San Juan 21 owners weren't young, and had no intention of "moving up" to a bigger boat. These owners spent a great deal of time racing their boats as one-designs.

The San Juan 21 wasn't intended as a one-design—it was designed to a price that would make it competitive with other trailer sailers. However, the Clarks gave her certain features that are more common on one-design racers than on trailer sailers—most notably a fully retractable centerboard in a gasketed trunk, and an airfoil shape on both the centerboard and rudder.

The Clarks then provided the impetus that got the San Juan 21 one-design class on its feet, organizing the first national championship in 1971. From that point on however, it was the hard work of a few dedicated boatowners that made the class association prosper.

This association operated independently from Clark Boat Company, an unusual but basically healthy situation when a boat is produced by a single manufacturer. The advantage of the association's independence is that the builder can't change the construction of the boat without the association's approval. However, there were three major changes in the San Juan 21's construction, represented by the MKI, II and III versions. And, with each proposed

The San Juan 21

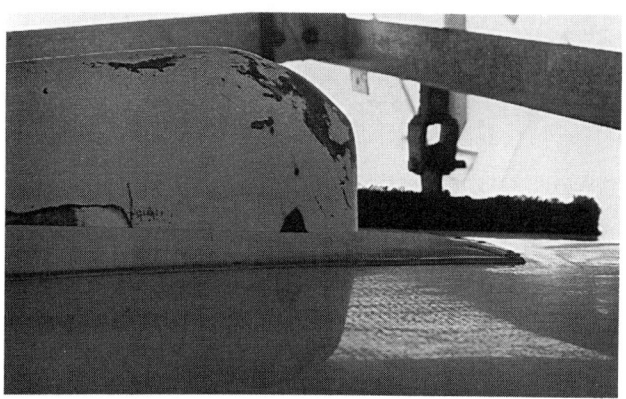

The centerboard retracts into a trunk which is sealed with cloth gaskets.

change, the association took the builder's word that the "one-designness" of the boat was not affected.

Part of this trust may stem from the Clarks' service to their customers. Almost every owner we talked to praised the service they received from the builder. Comments from San Juan 21 owners ran as follows: "Dennis Clark returned a phone call within 12 hours, on a question about balancing the boat." And, "I wrote for information when I bought my boat used and they responded quickly with a personal letter, an owner's manual, and a hand-drawn picture of the genoa track location."

The base price of the San Juan 21, as of March 1984, was $8,495. This included a main and working jib, made by Clark, and an outboard bracket. The list of options was long. For example, a fixed keel option was $400, a self-contained head (Porta-Potti type) was $85, a kick-up rudder $165, a bow pulpit $150, and a trailer $1095. If you added the cost of a genoa and its associated gear ($645), and a spinnaker with its gear ($655), the cost quickly topped $11,000. Freight to the East Coast pushed the price $1000 higher.

This put the San Juan 21 out of the price range of such comparable trailer-sailers as the Catalina 22, and up in the range of the more expensive, higher quality trailer-sailers that have been designed in this decade. Her popularity as a one-design, and Clark's monopoly on her production, may have inflated her price. Perhaps as a result of this, Clark's production of the boat dropped from a high of 400 boats in the mid-1970's to only 25 boats in 1983. Production ended with the 1985 model year.

CONSTRUCTION

Hull/Deck

Don Clark designed the San Juan 21 to be a better boat than the Venture 21—and he succeeded. He also managed to produce an above-average trailerboat, compared to its competition at the time. The consumer must remember, though, that the San Juan 21 was built with 15-year-old trailerboat technology, and that like all trailerboats, she was built with price foremost in mind. There are more modern, trailerable boats now available, that we would consider better built—for the same price.

The original published weight of the boat was 1150 pounds. Later, Clark claimed the boats weighed 1250 pounds. "Not so," said San Juan owners. Two fleets weighed their boats and of the 28 boats tested, the range was from 1500 to 1750 pounds—without sailing gear aboard. Both the deviation from the published weight and the range from lightest to heaviest boat are important. For a tow vehicle of marginal power, the 500-pound deviation could be critical. For the one-design racer the extra 250 pounds on the heaviest boat could be a serious handicap.

The three versions of the San Juan 21 (MKI, II, and III) have changes in the deck molding and the interior. Clark said the changes did not affect the distribution of weight in the boat. The hull molds remained unchanged, but because they are of solid, uncored fiberglass, the hulls themselves change shape easily when stored on a trailer. Dimples, where the hulls sit on trailer supports, are fairly common and can be pronounced. "Print-through" (of the first layer of roving in the laminate) was also common on the older boats we examined.

The deck of the San Juan 2 is cored with balsa. The cabin house and cockpit coaming span the full width of the hull, giving the boat a boxy appearance that can be made more pleasing with contrasting deck and hull colors.

The hull's single-skin construction gives it a certain amount of flexibility. The sides of the cabin house lie in roughly the same plane as the topsides of the hull. When the hull flexes, the cabin house flexes—and gelcoat crazing is the result.

The deck overlaps the hull vertically. This joint is covered by a pop-riveted rubrail which protrudes laterally. The joint is not bedded or mechanically fastened, but is covered with fiberglass inside the hull. The rubrail and the inherent flexibility of the construction protects the boat from damage in small bumps, where a more rigid, fully-cored boat might suffer slight damage.

Rudder/Centerboard
As is common on trailerboats, the San Juan 21 has a weighted centerboard, also called a swing keel. Less common is the ability of her 400-pound centerboard to fully retract into the trunk in the cabin, which makes the boat float off its trailer in shallow water for easy launching. Almost unheard of in trailer-sailers is her

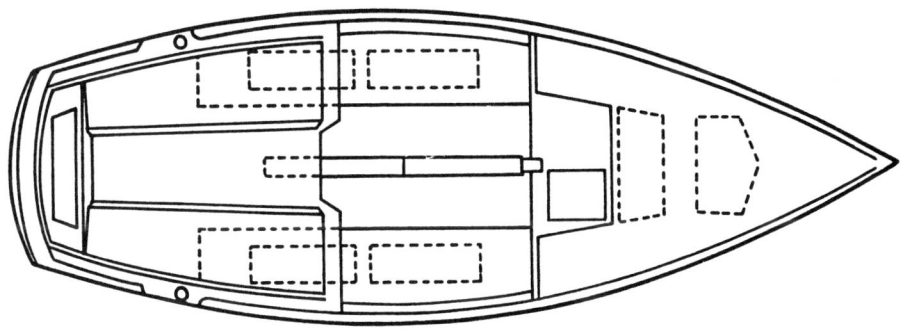

The San Juan 21

use of gaskets in the trunk to reduce the turbulence and drag of an open slot in the bottom of the boat.

This gasket, provided by the builder (and required by the class association) is made of sailcloth, which quickly loses the "spring" it needs to close the slot efficiently. A better system would be to wrap a piece of Mylar with sailcloth, as on most one-design dinghies. Unfortunately, Mylar gaskets are not allowed under class rules. According to owners, the stock gaskets should be replaced every two years for the casual racer, every year for the more serious racer, and *every regatta if you really want to win!*

The centerboard is molded to an airfoil shape. Fiberglass skins are laid into a mold, a piece of lead is inserted, and urethane foam poured in to fill the voids. These centerboards are less than fair and (according to owners) sometimes require up to a quarter of an inch of putty to fill the hollows.

Another performance-oriented feature is the enclosure of the wire centerboard pennant inside the trunk. As the pennant is anchored on the head of the centerboard, the lever arm (raising 400 pounds of board) puts it under great stress. One owner reported that the pennant tore the head from his centerboard, yet said the cable was easily replaced by removing the centerboard trunk cap. The board itself is difficult to remove, both because of its weight, and because its pivot pin is fiberglassed in place to prevent leaks.

The wire pennant exits through a hole at the front of the trunk and leads to a reel winch mounted on the mast compression post. We've heard no complaints about the winch, except that on older models it lacks an automatic ratchet lock. The lack of a ratchet could result in a broken hand if the winch handle ran away.

The San Juan 21's rudder is an airfoil too, and also requires sanding and puttying to make it fair. Older boats were made with laminated wooden rudders, but in the mid '70s, Clark began molding them of fiberglass. A kick-up rudder is an option recommended for trailering and sailing in shallow water. The portion of the rudder blade which "kicks up" is held down by an elastic shock cord, so the rudder lifts automatically upon grounding. Owners say the shock cord holds the rudder down well, even when sailing in heavy air.

The rudder head (on kick-up models) appears strongly built, as do the pintles, which are fabricated specifically for the San Juan 21. However, we have numerous reports of failure of the lower rudder gudgeon. (Failures occur more quickly on boats sailed in salt water.) To prevent the rudder from falling off the pintles (in the event of a grounding or a capsize) it should be tied to the gudgeons.

Spars/Rigging
The rig of the San Juan 21 is not her strong point. The mast is deck-stepped and hinges on a stainless steel tabernacle. Owners report that it is easy for one person to step or unstep the mast. However, the tabernacle can assume a permanent bend in a strong breeze, causing a loss of rig tension.

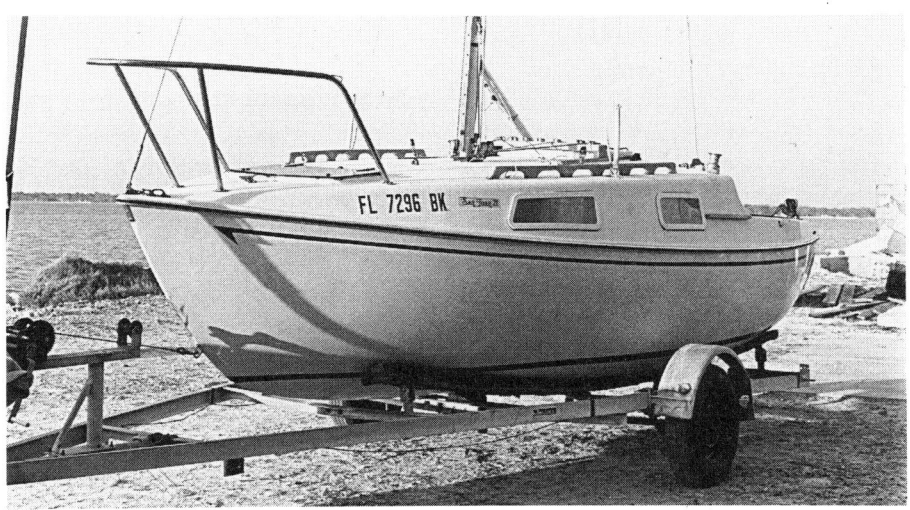

A trailerable boat must have a good trailer, preferably galvanized, with full-length supports for the hull to minimize dimpling. The San Juan 21's trailer filled the bill, although galvanizing was optional.

The mast step position is fixed by class rules, but Clark Boat Company appeared to be careless about placement of the shroud chainplates. On six sample boats, the chainplate position varied as much as three inches.

The shroud chainplates are located as far outboard as possible, which restricts the headsail sheeting angle. Unlike some of the cheaper trailerboats (which use U-bolts through the deck in place of chainplates), the San Juan 21's chainplates extend down through the deck and are securely bolted to small partial bulkheads. The bulkheads are not fastened to the hull, only to the liner, but the liner is fiberglassed to the hull. We have no reports of chainplates or bulkheads coming unglued under adverse conditions. A cap is placed over the chainplate and riveted to the deck to restrict leaks.

On a few boats we inspected, there was gelcoat crazing on the deck under the mast step, but only one boat showed any depression of the deck. Clark changed from plywood coring under the step to solid fiberglass, which should have alleviated this problem on newer boats.

Under the deck, the mast is supported by a compression post, which sits on the hull liner and is supported by its proximity to the edge of the V-berth. There is no support directly under the V-berth for the compression post. In time, the V-berth can deflect from the weight of rig tension and break the glue bond between the liner and the centerboard trunk. We have heard of no complete failures of the compression post, however.

The mast is anodized, untapered, and fractionally rigged. All halyards are led externally for easy maintenance, but at the expense of additional windage. The shrouds are swaged, not Nico-pressed, as on some of the cheaper trailer boats. Until recently, turnbuckles had closed bodies and were fixed with nuts.

Subsequently, the more traditional (and more reliable) open-bodied turnbuckles with cotter pins were used.

The spreader system is antiquated but relatively strong. The spreaders (aluminum tubes) fit over an aluminum stud which prevents them from swinging. Clark provided a list of "tuning tips" which explained that, in very heavy air with the spinnaker up, the mast could invert and bend backwards. He suggested that modifying the spreader brackets (to angle the spreaders aft) would help the problem. But, when we called Clark, he couldn't explain how to modify them. Neither could Yacht Riggers, the company in Seattle that rigged San Juan's spars since 1974. Before then, the spars were rigged by Kenyon.

The upper shroud tangs are securely attached to the mast with a 3/8" bolt, but the headstay tang is attached with a row of pop rivets. While Clark said only stainless steel or Monel pop rivets were used, they are not bedded (nor are any of the other mast fittings). The rivets may be strong enough, but the holes into which they are fastened will corrode without bedding. Despite this dubious design, only one owner reported even *hearing* of a San Juan losing its rig.

The gooseneck is a proven weak point. It is undersized, built with tack welds, and slides up and down the sail track. We've heard several reports of gooseneck failures at the welds. Some owners have had their goosenecks re-welded to prevent problems.

PERFORMANCE

Handling Under Sail

One-design racing in San Juan 21s is done in two divisions: "working sails," and "all sails." In the working sails division, one can only use a mainsail and a working jib. The all sails division allows the addition of a 130% genoa and a spinnaker to the inventory.

The San Juan 21 has a relatively narrow, seven-foot beam and lacks the ability to carry much sail upwind. Most sailors change down from the 130 to the working jib at only 15 knots. Above that velocity, it pays to put a flattening reef in the main (but not a slab reef). Most small, fractionally rigged boats develop lee helm with a slab-reefed mainsail because such a large portion of the boat's sail area is in the mainsail. Lee helm can make it difficult to feather the boat upwind in heavy air.

Despite its light weight, the San Juan 21 is underpowered in light air with its 130% class genoa. This accentuates her tendency toward lee helm. Raking the mast aft (as far as the headstay turnbuckle will allow) helps the situation. So does the use of a 155% genoa, which is only legal for handicap racing. However, the real problem is that the centerboard has a stop which fixes the board at an angle of about 60 degrees to the perpendicular in the "full down" position. Class rules prohibit the modification of this stop to let the board drop farther.

Owners who race under PHRF (Portsmouth Handicap Racing Formula) say the boat is most competitive in light air, assuming you have the 155 genoa and raise the centerboard downwind. If you modify the centerboard stop, the boat can be very fast in light air. With a class inventory limited to a 130 genoa, the boat has trouble sailing to its rating in winds under 10 knots, unless the center-board is raised to allow her to plane downwind. That leaves a boat, with a class inventory, competitive only in a medium breeze.

The San Juan 21's PHRF rating averages 252 seconds/mile. For comparison, the Venture 21 is also 252, and the Catalina 22 is 270. The Merit 22, a modern trailer-sailer, has a rating of 213—significantly faster. The J/22 (semi-trailerable with its fixed keel) is only 185.

There are several other techniques that make a San Juan 21 perform better. Shortening the spreaders to the class minimum of 25 inches allows the genoa to be sheeted tighter. Adjusting the backstay turnbuckle bends the mast (the range in bend should be three to five inches). However, the backstay's effect on headstay tension is limited by the position of the lower shrouds, which are anchored only a few inches aft of the mast.

The boat has no traveler, nor is one allowed by class rules. This makes the boom vang all-important in setting leech tension so the main can be played freely upwind.

Most participants in the working sails division utilize two crew. In the racing sail division, three crew is the norm. Because of the boat's light displacement, extra crew weight can have a dampening effect on light air and downwind speed. Because she is so narrow, extra bodies provide little leverage upwind. The boat does not have lifelines and no hiking aids are allowed. As a result, the crew is hard pressed to utilize its weight outboard. Usually, the forward crew sits on the cabin and hangs onto the shrouds and the cabin's handrail, with the middle crew either on the cabin, or in the cockpit.

Handling Under Power/Launching

A stern-hung, fold-up outboard bracket is standard equipment on the San Juan 21. A long-shaft outboard is recommended. Its primary use is to move the boat when there is no wind. For that purpose, four horsepower should be more than sufficient. Motoring with an outboard in heavy air is often frustrating because the propeller comes out of the water as the boat hobby-horses through seas.

Getting in and out of a dock can often be done without the help of an outboard because the San Juan 21 is so light and maneuverable (thanks, in part, to her stern-hung rudder). Owners report that she is easy to scull with the rudder in light air.

The MK II and III versions have a lazarette in the stern, which is sealed off from the rest of the boat so water can't enter the cabin if the boat is capsized or pooped. This lazarette is a bit small for an outboard so most owners stow their auxiliary on the cabin sole, under the cockpit and between the centerboard trunk and the quarterberth.

A painted steel Calkins trailer was an option, and when requested, these were galvanized to extend the trailer's life. It came with both rollers and bunks. Clark said the boat did not rest on the rollers—a good feature as this would help to minimize dimpling of the hull. The San Juan 21 draws only 12 inches with the board and rudder raised, so trailering is a cinch. At a little over 2000 pounds, including trailer, boat and gear, most mid-sized cars should be able to tow her.

LIVABILITY

Deck Layout
The San Juan 21 was rigged as cheaply as possible, ostensibly to keep the cost of the boat down. Actually, such a practice makes a boat more expensive because you have to re-rig much of it. A significant number of owners complained of Clark's rigging. These comments are typical: "The blocks have parted company under fairly light loads ... the hardware lacks adequate backing plates ... the factory hardware is cheap, undersized, and can't handle racing loads." Most of the gear is Ronstan and some is Nicro Fico. Those planning to race will want to replace such equipment with heavier hardware.

The mainsheet is rigged with a 4:1 purchase, half of which is fixed on each quarter of the transom in a modified "Crosby" rig. The tip of the mainsheet is led from one quarter, down to a swiveled cam cleat on the cockpit sole under the tiller. Owners report that it is very awkward to use. Many have installed a wooden thwart across the after part of the cockpit seats, and mounted the cleat on this. Even so, you have to cross your hands to handle the tiller and mainsheet simultaneously.

If all the mainsheet isn't trimmed in during a jibe, it tends to wrap around the crew, or the tiller. Most experienced sailors prefer to snap the mainsail over without trimming it in all the way. The absence of a traveler, and the manner in which the tail of the mainsheet is led, caused a minor rift within the class association between those supporting change, and those favoring the *status quo*.

On the standard boat, the halyards were cleated on the mast. For $225 extra you got an optional racing package that provided spinnaker gear and brought all the control lines and halyards back to the cockpit. Many owners created their own "racing packages" and brought the running rigging aft to a wooden "control panel" bridging the companionway. This keeps the decks clean and rigging tails out of the cockpit.

The stock boat is rigged only for the working jib. There are no winches, and the jib must be trimmed through a "bull's eye" fairlead to a half cam cleat—which can be difficult in a breeze. Optional genoa gear was available which included tracks and cars and Barient #8 single-speed winches. (On older boats, lower-quality winches are sometimes found.) These winches are mounted on the cabin so they can be used for spinnaker sheets, working jib sheets and halyards. Ratchet blocks on the genoa cars are a worthwhile addition.

In 1975, Clark Boat Company retooled the deck and introduced the MK II version. The MK I cabin house stops at the mast, and the cockpit is longer. The MK II cabin house runs to the bow. This gives the MK II a less traditional appearance (and the MK III has the same deck) but it also gives better footing on the foredeck. The MK I is considered faster than the MK II and III by many

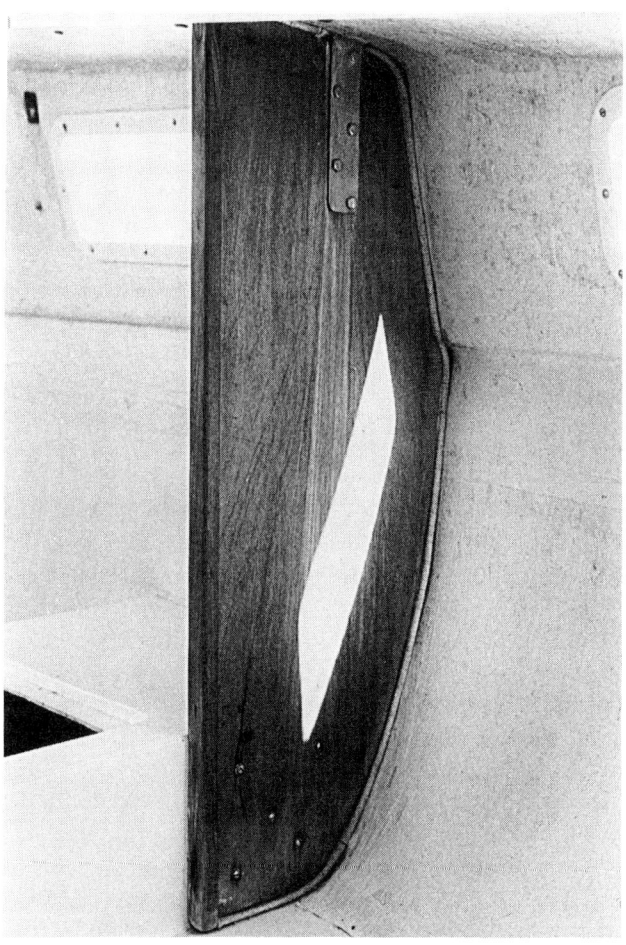

San Juan 21 sailors because its longer cockpit makes it easier for the crew to keep their weight forward, and provides more working room.

Belowdecks

The interior of the San Juan 21 is simple, and like most trailer-boats, unbearable for more than two people for a weekend cruise. She doesn't have the hideaway galleys or flimsy tables of some of her newer, more vivacious trailerable sisters. What she does have, though, is honest sitting headroom for a six-foot person, and a big V-berth with plenty of overhead clearance in the MK II and III models. This gives a couple room to sleep, sit, and dress comfortably.

Chainplates on the San Juan 21 are bolted to semi-bulkheads, which are in turn fastened to the hull liner, which is fiberglassed to the hull. This is far stronger than attaching the shrouds to U-bolts through the gunwale, as is done on cheaper boats.

The quarterberths are long and narrow. Storage space is limited by the flotation tanks. In the MK I and II versions, a small bin is built into the V-berth, and lockers are behind each of the chainplate bulkheads. In the MK III, bins are built into the quarterberths, and the V-berth is raised slightly to make up for the lost flotation.

The centerboard trunk divides the cabin, but since you can't stand and walk around anyway, it's not a big annoyance. The trunk extends under the cockpit, which divides the space normally used to store a cooler. Only very small coolers will fit.

A self-contained head was optional. We feel that *any* boat is too small for a Porta-Potti, particularly a 21-footer. We'd prefer a bucket. The MK I and II models have a platform built into the cabin sole next to the centerboard trunk for the head. In the MK III version, there is a large recess molded into the V-berth, so the person using the head can sit athwartships behind a curtain.

The forward hatch and the cabin windows are a common source of leaks, owners say. On boats built before 1977, the forward hatch was of fiberglass and fit over a raised molded lip in the deck. Owners liked it. Later boats have a flat Lexan hatch that fits on, but not over, the raised lip. Its rubber gasket seal soon wears out, and every wave over the bow sends water into the cabin. "I have to tape it tight every time I go sailing," complained one owner.

CONCLUSIONS

Aside from the complaints about the boat's hardware, San Juan 21 owners have lots of positive comments about their boats. "She accommodates five for family day sailing, and a couple for overnight gunkholing," says one owner.

"Excellent handling, responsive helm, easy to maintain ... a great boat for a novice," says another.

Most say that easy trailering and launching were major reasons for choosing the boat. One owner says he trailers his boat with a 4-cylinder truck, another with a 6-cylinder mid-sized car.

The San Juan is best suited for sailing in protected waters. With the kick-up rudder option, you can sail in shallow water with complete peace of mind. Her high-aspect, airfoil centerboard gives her performance far superior to that of trailerboats with long stub keels. The price you pay is the loss of the interior space taken up the centerboard trunk. We think it's worth the trade-off.

Because the class association tried to keep their boats equal, and perhaps because the builder tried to maintain a profit, the San Juan did not keep up with the times. There are better trailerboats today on the new boat market at realistic prices.

Used San Juan 21s can be bought reasonably, however, with '85s showing up in the BUC lists at from $7750 to $8900, and no doubt selling in some parts of the country for significantly less. If you are interested in getting into competitive sailing, and can't afford a spanking new, cutting-edge-of-technology missile; a used San Juan 21 will provide a platform on which you can be competitive, comfortable, and learn to sail expertly. In fact, the relatively inexpensive Mark I might be even more competitive than the newer MK IIs and IIIs.

That's the end of the saga of the San Juan 21. There were disparate forces within the class association, some seeking modernization of the rules to create a faster and easier to handle boat, while others were dedicated to freezing the boat in time at the moment of its design.

While uncontrolled development can certainly discourage class growth, a boat can become antiquated if all development is stifled. Apparently, this sobering fact finally caught up with the San Juan 21.

Three 22-Footers

The first edition of this book included a comparative look at what in the early 1980s were three of the most popular small "trailerable" boats on the sailboat market, all 22-footers: the Catalina, O'Day and Tanzer 22s. By looking at these three boats "side-by-side," we arrived at not only some conclusions about these particular boats, but about almost all other boats of this size, type, and price.

In updating this book we were tempted to replicate the original comparative evaluation of small boats, replacing the O'Day and Tanzer 22 that are no longer in production with a couple of new versions. The problem we faced was that, given the transitory nature of the market for boats of this size, there would be no guarantee that by the time you read the updated comparison, even the production of the new boats we chose would not already have passed on to that great anchorage in the sky.

As a result, we are reprinting in edited form the original chapter using the same three boats. Two of the three boats are now available only on the used boat market and the third has undergone extensive changes, but the vast majority of their successors are little different in details and essentially identical in concept.

The Impression of Size

The most lingering impression we have of these three boats is that the Tanzer seems to be a small boat enlarged for interior space, whereas the Catalina and O'Day suggest larger boats scaled down. Generally, of course, they are the same—22-foot boats with approximately the same dimensions. The impression is subjective; others looking at the boats might get just the opposite impression.

We also looked at upwards of a dozen other boats of about the same size. We found that they create similar impressions about their size, utilizing a variety of subtle techniques including some that have nothing to do with actual dimensions. Scaling, proportions, and styling all contribute. Buyers should not pick one boat over another just because one looks bigger. Use a tape measure, check by lying on berths, sitting in the cockpit, walking forward on the deck and so forth. In the same way, do not try to judge speed or performance by looks; there are objective criteria (rating handicaps, for instance) that have more validity.

In any boat as small as these, performance may not live up to expectations or hopes. A 22-footer is, after all, a small boat and small boats do not have the capability of sailing as fast as big boats. Moreover, to provide accommodations and safety as well as low price, there have to be compromises on liveliness.

Add to these drawbacks the matter of draft. To be trailered as well as launched and hauled from a ramp, a deep fixed keel (and the better windward performance it gives), must be sacrificed. Instead, the boat must be fitted with some form of retractable keel called a swing or drop keel or with a centerboard in a shallow or stub keel. Increasingly of late the trend has been toward the latter option.

The swing keel is often a complex engineering problem, one reason that in the last few years more and more small boats are being built with other forms of ballast. In the Catalina 22, the keel weighs more than 500 pounds and must be raised and lowered as well as supported during trailering, beaching, and sailing. Add to these drawbacks the reduced stability, lowered performance, more difficult maintenance, and where there is an option, the higher price, of either a swing keel or centerboard. In the end, we think the fixed keel is the answer unless trailerability is a major priority.

Speaking of weight, a word of warning is in order about the weight or displacement figures in builder specifications, in particular where the boat is being marketed for her trailerability. There is no standard for what the term displacement represents. It can mean weight of the basic boat plus some optional equipment or it can even include food, water, and personal belongings of the crew. Of the three boats, only O'Day breaks down the published weights; hull and deck only, minimum trailering weight, and sailing weight with four persons aboard.

Whatever the case, prospective buyers should realize that the published weight is not likely to reflect the actual weight of the boat on a trailer. For such a figure, estimated at best, add about 10 percent to the specified weight. Then add the weight of the trailer itself. This is what the car will actually be pulling.

Cockpits
All three of the boats have a generous beam carried well aft, an important feature. Beam at the cockpit helps stability and, of course, it affords cockpit roominess. Equally important is that the beam gives buoyancy to the after end. The weight of four adults in the cockpit of a boat the size of these could amount to 600 pounds, 25 percent of the displacement. Then there is the weight of an outboard on the transom and a gas tank. Unsupported, this weight would make the stern squat in the water and reduce performance drastically. Beam gives this support. None of these three boats suffers excessively from cockpit loading.

Although cockpit roominess is a virtue, it can also be a fault. Despite the fact that all three cockpits are self-bailing and the boats self-righting from a knockdown, all three would be in real jeopardy if the cockpit filled with water as high as the seats. The three boats all have sills lower than seat level. They will keep incidental cockpit water out of the interior but not major flooding. Moreover, none has a lower hatchboard that can be fixed or locked in place. Owners of boats with low sills and no bridgedeck should make this provision and keep the lower hatchboard in place while sailing in rough conditions.

Worst in this respect is the Catalina. As is typical of most of the boats from Catalina, she has a wide companionway with substantial taper. A hatchboard needs to be raised only a couple of inches before it comes out of the channels on each side.

Accommodations

While our standards call for performance first and comfort second, we did not ignore accommodations. After all, these three boats are cruising boats. In this respect, we think the O'Day 22 is the best. She has the two best berths, usable forward berths (for little folk), and best of all, an enclosed head that incorporates a semblance of privacy not only for the head but also between the two sleeping facilities.

Nevertheless, expectations for overnight comfort for more than two people aboard are unrealistic. A major part of the limitation is the stowage, a vital matter in boats of this size where anything lying about will be in the way. All three boats rely almost entirely on scuttles located under the berths. Not only is this space awkward to get to, but the space may be damp, even wet. The bilges of these boats are shallow. Any water that gets below will tend to slosh under the liner/sole into the spaces below the berths. And even if water does not come in from outside, these are places where condensation will occur, encouraging dampness, mustiness, and mildew.

Although we like the O'Day's berths, the Catalina gets high grades for her decor, which has to be the envy of builders trying to compete with that firm. For sheer space (or at least the illusion of spaciousness) the choice is the Tanzer; there's nothing like carrying the cabin house out to the gunwale to create roominess and the maximum amount of headroom even if it is just sitting headroom.

Auxiliary Power

Most owners of these three boats will, sooner or later, want some form of auxiliary power. All three are designed to take an outboard motor mounted on an optional lift-up bracket on the transom. A long-shaft 4.5-horsepower motor is adequate in a flat calm. However, for powering against any kind of wind or chop, the minimum of a 6- or 7.5-horsepower motor is needed and then don't expect powerboat speed or handling.

Rigs, Sails, and Rudders

In any boat of this size and type, the mast should be capable of being raised and lowered without recourse to a crane. All three of these boats have hinged mast steps on deck for this purpose. Success in hoisting or lowering a mast with these systems depends on smooth water, a gentle breeze, and an experienced crew of at least two. The masts weigh 40 pounds or more and range from 25 feet to 30 feet in length, so getting them up and down requires some care and planning.

All three boats come equipped with a mainsail and working jib (or lapper) as standard. The standard sails are all of routine quality, made to a price commensurate with the price of the boat. Unfortunately it is doubtful if buyers can negotiate enough of a rebate on these sails to justify getting better quality on a custom order with a sailmaker. Again, this is a matter of how high a priority an owner places on performance and how long he expects to keep his boat.

If ramp launching and beaching are high priorities, then so too is a pivoting rudder. A pivoting rudder lets the draft of the rudder match the draft of the boat with the keel or the centerboard retracted. But it may be expensive.

The Bottom Line

Almost all boats of this size and type are built with price foremost in mind. Many are touted merely on the basis of price: "Sail for the low, low price of…"

We wish most buyers had some criteria other than price, even in this rather modest price range. An additional $1,500 or so would make all three of these boats better boats; not necessarily bigger, but better appointed, outfitted and built. But they would not sell as well (if at all). In our opinion, the higher priced Tanzer is a better product than either the O'Day or the Catalina. In our look at a number of other small boats similar to these, the same premise seems to hold true for most of them: the more you pay, the more you get. Or for about the same price a buyer can trade off specific features. For instance, the same $10,000 will buy sparkling performance and a whopping cockpit for daysailing in the 22-foot S2 6.7, but at the expense of accommodations and interior space. The same is true of the snappy 23-foot Sonar for fleet racing.

As initial cost is important, so is resale value. It is especially important because most owners of 22-footers are not likely to keep their boats for more than a few years. Then sale of the 22 is apt to represent a down payment on a larger, more expensive boat, and will usually return much of the dollar value of the original investment.

The value of such a boat for resale is based on many of the same factors that appealed to the owner when the boat was new—price, cosmetics, decor, suitability for the expected use, and so forth. Maintaining the boat, repairing damage, and adding amenities all serve to protect the investment.

In investigating used-boat prices for the earliest boats built, we find the Tanzer 22 has appreciated in value the most; 10-year old boats in good condition are selling for twice what they sold for new, appreciation more than offsetting the inflation rate.

Clearly, the strong owners' associations for the Tanzer and Catalina help in maintaining the resale market. They are strong marketing allies, not only of the builders, but of boat owners. Suggestion: if you buy a boat with such an organization, join it and stay in touch with their activities even if you do not take part in them.

Owners of boats in this range making warranty claims, seeking answers to questions, or asking for special service on orders or service should realize that the relatively low markup on small boats such as these does not make dealers stand at attention. Trial sails, financing, trades up from smaller boats, special options, and so forth are similarly treated. In general, however, the owners of these three boats report satisfactory treatment by dealers and builders.

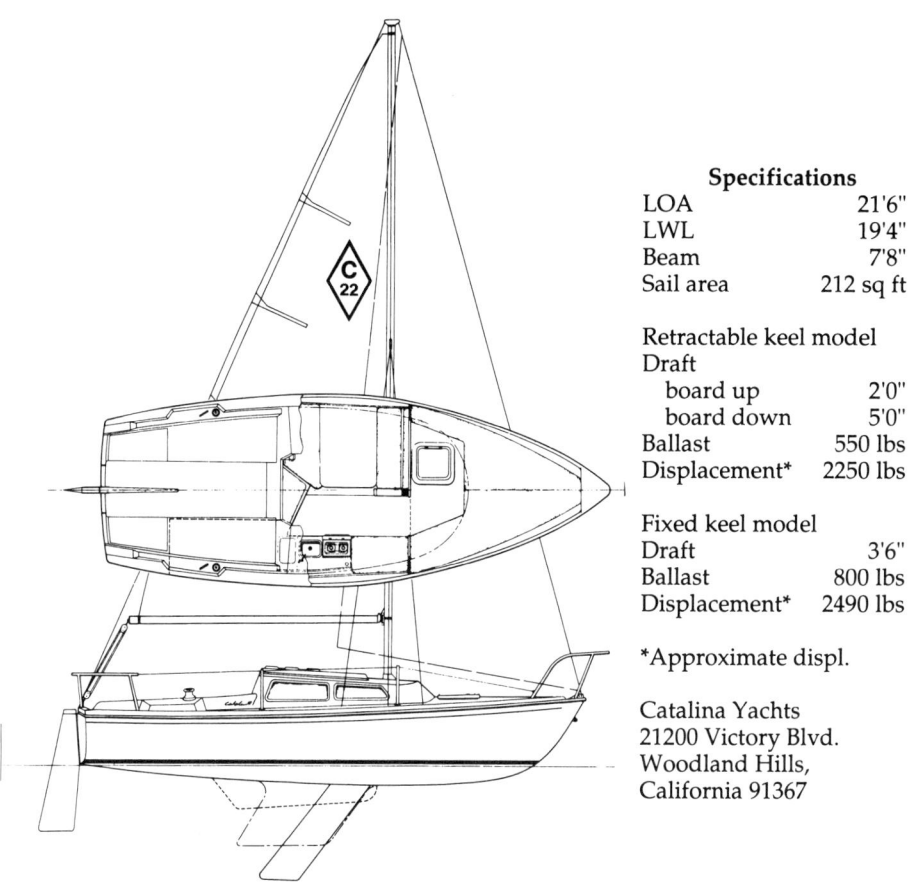

Specifications

LOA	21'6"
LWL	19'4"
Beam	7'8"
Sail area	212 sq ft

Retractable keel model
Draft
board up	2'0"
board down	5'0"
Ballast	550 lbs
Displacement*	2250 lbs

Fixed keel model
Draft	3'6"
Ballast	800 lbs
Displacement*	2490 lbs

*Approximate displ.

Catalina Yachts
21200 Victory Blvd.
Woodland Hills,
California 91367

The Catalina 22

THE BOAT AND THE BUILDER

In its 10th anniversary issue in 1980, *Sail* magazine named the Catalina 22 the boat that had represented the "breakthrough" in "trailer/cruisers" (sic) in those 10 years. We might quibble with its selection over more out and out trailerable boats such as the Ventures, but there is no denying the popularity of the Catalina. More than 10,000 have been built and sales continue to be strong.

For many buyers, the Catalina 22 is their first "big" boat and an introduction to the Catalina line. Many remain with Catalina and buy up within that line.

Catalina is the largest boatbuilder in the world in dollar volume and the firm is one of the lasting success stories in the industry. It foregoes national advertising in favor of local dealer-sponsored ads, and has remained a privately owned (in fact, one man—Frank Butler) company while the trend has been toward conglomerate-owned boatbuilding.

Simply stated, Catalina builds boats to a price—a low price—making the most of volume buying of materials and hardware, long-lived models, a high degree of standardization, and all the cost savings of high volume production. The Catalina 22 was the first boat built by Catalina.

The 22 is a dated boat. A lot has happened in boat design and construction since she was introduced. Not all that has happened has been good, but many of the boats on the market with which the Catalina 22 competes for sales perform better and have accommodations more comfortable than the venerable Catalina. Yet it is to Catalina's credit that the 22 continues to sell and continues to be many sailors' first boat.

CONSTRUCTION

The hull to deck joint of the Catalina 22 is the same joint used on larger boats in the Catalina line. The hull sheer is reinforced with plywood, and the deck molding has a downward turning flange which overlaps the hull and is attached to it with fiberglass slurry and self-tapping screws.

We think it is well suited for use on this smaller boat, although it is not the type of joint we like to see on a larger boat or a boat intended for use in exposed waters.

Catalina Yachts is proud of the contention that the Catalina 22 has remained essentially unchanged for the first dozen years of its production history. Only the pivot for the swing keel version was changed about boat #250 and then, according to a Catalina statement, it was done for production purposes. Later a pop-top option was added and now 90 percent of the boats sold have this feature.

Catalina takes credit for pioneering the one-piece hull liner that has become standard in most high volume small boats. However, it should be noted that the liner is basically a cosmetic component, not a structural member, and the hull must get its strength from the hull laminate and bulkhead reinforcement.

The swing keel, also chosen by 90 percent of the buyers, is cast iron and, in its retracted position, remains substantially exposed (accounting for more than half of the two-foot draft of the shoal draft model). It is a rough, 550-pound iron casting of indifferent hydrodynamic efficiency. Oddly, its configuration in the raised position encourages ropes and weeds hanging up on its forward edge.

The swing keel is hoisted with a simple reel winch located under a small bridgedeck with its handle protruding through a plywood facing. We'd guess that Catalina owners soon become conditioned to its presence, though it can trip those stepping up or down through the companionway.

The drop keel of the Catalina evoked a number of observations from owners. Several note that the keel mounting bolts can loosen and leak in time. Another reports he had to replace his wire pennant twice. Replacing the pennant requires hoisting the boat high enough to have access to the top of the keel.

As with all Catalina-built boats, decor is a major selling point. The line, including the 22, is attractively appointed. They create a highly favorable impression which has to encourage sales, especially for first time boat buyers.

In fact, the Catalina 22 outside and inside is one of the most visually appealing small boats we have seen. She has enough trim and finish to look pretty. Similarly, her hull and rig, although dated, are well proportioned. It is about her performance and livability that we have the most reservations.

PERFORMANCE

By any objective standard, the Catalina 22 is hardly a sprightly performer. There have been too many compromises to performance: trailerability, shoal draft, cockpit space, low cost, and interior accommodations, as well as giving her a placid disposition for novice sailors. The boat needs a genoa jib, a smoother, and more efficient swing- or fin-keel shape and some hardware of the go-fast variety. Even then, the prognosis is that she will remain a relatively slow boat in an age when much of the fun of boats is in their responsiveness, if not speed.

With almost all the Catalinas having been built with the swing keel, the appeal has been her shallow draft for trailering. Yet even with two feet of draft with the keel hoisted, the boat has too much draft for easy beaching. Given the trade-off in performance, the difficulty of maintenance, and reduction in stability, one hopes that indeed buyers of the swing-keel 22 have made good use of it for trailering.

The deck of the Catalina 22 is a decidedly unhandy working platform. The sidedecks are narrow and obstructed by jib sheets and blocks. The three shrouds per side effectively block access to the foredeck, and complicate headsail trim and passage of the jib across in tacking. In fact, so difficult is it to go forward on the 22 we recommend getting rid of the lifelines. They are already too low to offer anything but token protection and they anchor near the base of the bow pulpit where they give no protection. Instead, handrails should be installed on the cabin top.

LIVABILITY

There's a lot of wasted, unused space in the Catalina 22 that could be better utilized. In boats this size, stowage is at a premium. It's surprising to us that there haven't been enough complaints about this wasted space for Catalina to do a minor redesign. The entire area under the cockpit and most of the area under the port cockpit seat (except where the gas tank sits) is all but inaccessible. The loss of this space limits stowage to scuttles under the berth bases.

The convertible dinette, which seats only two with elbow room, is a vestige of the 22's design era and the V-berths forward form that noisome combination of bathroom and bedroom, away from which human beings evolved about the time they moved out of caves.

The result is that the Catalina 22 has but one berth we consider suitable for sleeping, the settee on the starboard side, and even that berth is shared with the optional galley facility that, in use, takes up about half the berth area.

The Catalina 22s now have a pop-top as standard; most of the cabin top lifts

10 inches on four pipe supports. Most owners we have heard from seem to like the system, particularly those in warmer areas. Headroom at anchor is pleasant but we'd rather see room for stowage and sleeping, as well.

One design feature we find unappealing is the stowage for the remote gas tank for a transom-mounted outboard auxiliary. The tank sits on a molded shelf (part of the hull liner) in a seat locker at the after end of the cockpit. This puts the gasoline inside the boat including the cabin. The locker is vented, but it should also be isolated. Spilled fuel can make its way unimpeded to the inaccessible low point under the cockpit. Moreover, there is no way to strap the tank securely nor a way to route the hose without pinching.

It's easy to say that if a feature has existed on a very successful boat for a long period of time, then it must be right. In the case of the fuel stowage arrangements on the Catalina 22, we think they're wrong, no matter how many boats the company has built. In our opinion, a redesign of the fuel stowage compartment would make the boat both more usable and safer.

One of the Catalina's better features is her cockpit. It is long (7') and comfortable, a place where the crew can sit with support for their backs, a place to brace their feet, and with room to avoid the tiller. It is unobstructed by the mainsheet that trims to a rod traveler on the stern.

CONCLUSIONS

Many boat buyers shop for a boat of this type with price foremost in mind. They probably will get no farther than their local Catalina dealer. At $12,000, they can get a boat that is the same size and similarly equipped as boats costing $2000 more. It's apt to be a boat identical to many of those sailing on the same waters. Better still, they are more than likely to have sailing friends who not only have (or had) a Catalina, but belong to one of the most widespread and active owners' class associations in the sport. The whole package has a powerful appeal superbly orchestrated by the Catalina organization.

For performance, accommodations and even construction, they might do better at a higher price, but the prospective buyer of the Catalina is likely to be unsure of what to look for. Understandably they turn to the 22.

At a weight of about 2,500 pounds loaded for the road plus a trailer, the Catalina 22 has marginal trailerability behind the modern small car. For this reason, consider carefully before purchasing a trailer with the boat. Unless and until you are convinced that you will trailer the boat enough to make a trailer's purchase worthwhile, it could be a waste of money.

For the $10,500 "sailaway package" price, the buyer gets some features he might not opt for if he had a choice (e.g. the pop-top, Mercury outboard, and lifelines and stanchions). However, Catalina Yachts, like Hunter Marine, has learned the advantages of packaged boats with bottom-line pricing that is still lower than competitors' so called base boat prices. And boat buyers get what they need (and probably want) without having to know what they need or want.

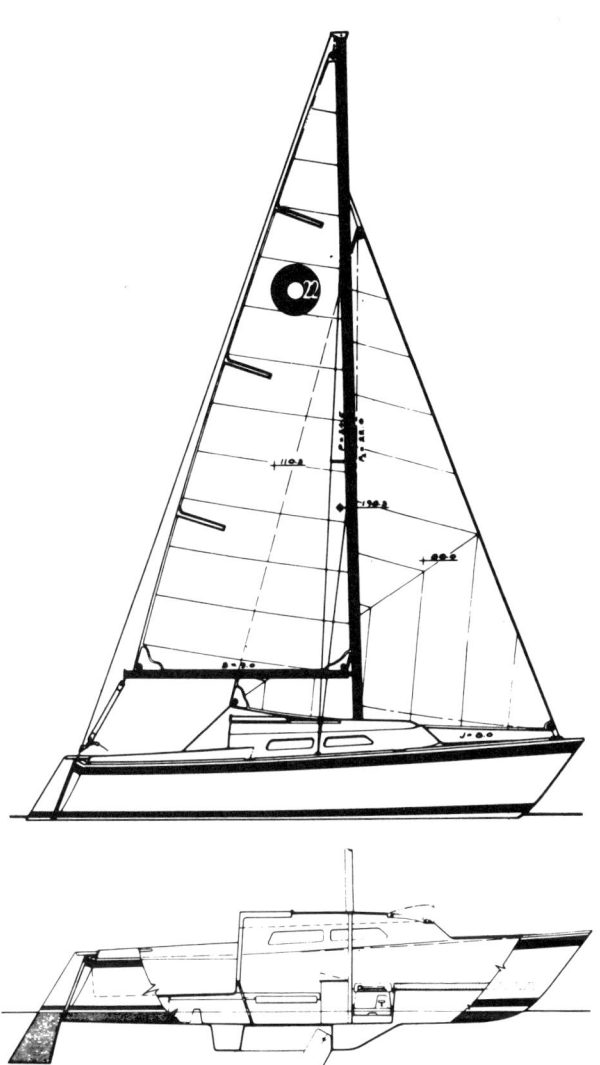

Specifications
O'Day 22

LOA	21'8"
LWL	18'11"
Beam	7'2"
Sail area	198 sq ft
Draft	
board up	1'3"
board down	4'3"
Ballast	800 lbs
Displacement*	2183 lbs

*Approximate displ.

O'Day Yachts
848 Airport Road
Fall River, Mass. 02720
(617) 678-5291

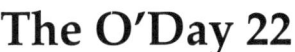

The O'Day 22

THE BOAT AND THE BUILDER

O'Day Boats has been around a long time by fiberglass boatbuilding standards—more than 20 years. Originally the firm was a leader in small boats typified by the Uffa Fox-designed Day Sailer that is still in production.

By the early 70s, O'Day had moved into the trailerable cruising boat market where they have been the leader on the East Coast. In the meantime, the firm was acquired by Bangor Punta along with such other major boat builders as Cal and the now virtually defunct Ranger Yachts. In recent years, with the decline in volume sales of small boats, O'Day has had problems. It was eventually acquired by Lear Siegler and became part of that firm's Starcraft Sailboat Products.

All the cruising-size boats in the O'Day line have been designed by C. Raymond Hunt Associates in one of the most enduring designer-builder relationships in the industry. The result of the relationship is a family resemblance in the O'Day line that is more than superficial. What proves popular in one boat is apt to be adopted in subsequent kin. Therefore, any study of the O'Day offerings over the years reflects a process of evolution.

When she was introduced, the O'Day was touted as a competitive contender on the race course, a contrasting companion to the rather boxy 23-footer which she would soon phase out. The 22 had a masthead rig, a stylish rake to the transom, shallow (23") draft with a short stub keel and no centerboard, light weight (advertised 1,800 pounds) for trailering, and a price under $3,000.

Since then the 22 has acquired a fractional rig, a centerboard, 300 advertised pounds and a price tag almost $7,000 higher.

CONSTRUCTION

O'Day once set a standard for small boat construction and styling. That was before on and off labor problems in its plant, management changes, the decline in sales of boats in its size range, and increasingly fierce competition for buyers who became more cost than quality conscious. The most recent O'Day 22s we looked at have been, frankly, a mixed bag of quality and shabbiness.

The spars, rigging, and hardware are as high quality as we have seen in comparable boats. Our only reservation is with the stamped stainless steel hinged maststep that we know from personal experience requires a steady hand and boat when raising or lowering a mast. We also think that a mainsheet which terminates in a cam action cleat, 16 inches up the single backstay, may be economical and simple, but it is neither efficient nor handy—again a reflection of scrimping to keep price low.

The quality of O'Day fiberglass laminates has always been high, but there have been reader reports of voids in the laminate and there is consistent evidence of print-through (the pattern of woven roving showing through the gelcoat).

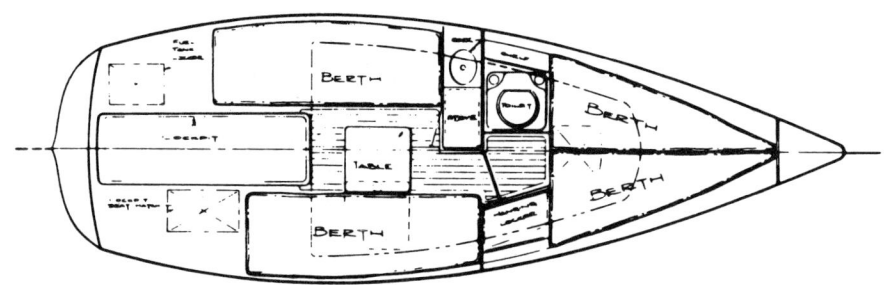

Exterior styling and proportions are superb, an opinion iterated by owners. The O'Day 22, despite her age, is still not outdated.

On a boat of this size and price, a minimum of exterior trim is understandable. What is less understandable is the poor quality of the interior finish and decor. Belowdecks, the O'Day 22 epitomizes the pejorative label, Clorox bottle, often used to describe fiberglass boats. Sloppily fitted bits of teak trim are matched against teak-printed Formica, at best a tacky combination. Cabinetry, such as there is, is flimsy, and in general the whole impression is of lackluster attention to detail.

PERFORMANCE

Without a centerboard, the O'Day 22 simply did not have the performance to go with her racy image. Even with the centerboard she is hardly a ball of fire under sail. She does not point well (tacking through 100 degrees is not uncommon), and she is tender with a disconcerting desire to round up when a puff hits. In light air, with her 3/4 foretriangle and working jib, she is undercanvassed and sluggish. Here, a genoa with substantial overlap is essential.

Since changing jibs is at best a dicey exercise on a 22-footer, the first step in reducing sail is to reef the mainsail. Jiffy reefing is standard and owners of the O'Day should have a system in good working order and know how to use it. Owners of this boat who sail in waters where squalls are a threat, may also want to consider roller furling for the larger jib (trading off the loss of performance and added cost for the convenience and safety).

The O'Day is most hurt in light air downwind and most owners will want either an eight-foot-or-so whisker pole for winging the jib, or a spinnaker. It is a fun boat on which to learn spinnaker handling. With her fractional rig, the spinnaker is relatively small and yet the boat is big enough to provide a foredeck platform for setting the sail.

The trouble is that the O'Day 22 scrimps on the hardware needed for ease of handling with or without a spinnaker. The two #10 Barient sheet winches are, in our opinion, inadequate for anything larger than a working jib and we suggest replacing them with optional #16s. Similarly, the jib sheets lead to fixed blocks, whereas the optional tracks with adjustable blocks are preferable for optimizing sail trim.

The O'Day does not come with halyard winches as standard. It is a large boat for setting and reefing sails with hand tension alone. Most owners will want at least one small winch (#10) on the coachroof, with the jib and main halyards led aft through jam cleats or stoppers to the winch.

The fairing of the O'Day 22 under water is better than average, helped by the fact that the lead ballast is encapsulated in the fiberglass hull molding. The centerboard will, however, be difficult to maintain.

LIVABILITY

Like many other boats of her size, the O'Day 22 is basically a daysailer with incidental overnight accommodations, notwithstanding that her builder (or its ad agency) heralds its comfort, privacy, and space. The cockpit of the O'Day is almost perfect; a spacious 6-1/2 feet long, the seats are spaced to allow the bracing of feet on the one opposite, and the coaming provides a feeling of security and serves as a comfortable arm rest. It is also self-bailing, although the low sill at the companionway means that the lower hatchboard must be in place to prevent water going below in the event of a knockdown.

Seat locker space is excellent for a boat of this size with a quarterberth below, and we like the separate sealed well for the outboard remote gas tank (but not the fact that the hose can be pinched in use).

O'Day's literature boasts berths for two couples in "absolute privacy." Privacy in a 22-footer has to be one of the more relative features. A sliding door encloses the forward cabin and another door, the head.

The layout of the O'Day 22 is a noteworthy example of the trade-off between an enclosed head and berth space. It does indeed have a head area that can be enclosed, a rare feature on a boat of this size. With a conventional marine toilet and through-hull discharge where permitted, this would be a most serviceable facility.

The trade-off is a pair of terrible V-berths forward. Coming to a point at the forward end, there is simply not enough room for two adults on even the most intimate terms. They are thus suitable only for a pair of small children who do not suffer from sibling rivalry.

By contrast the two settee berths in the main cabin are a bit narrow, but are a fit place for two adults to sleep. In contrast to the dinette layout of other boats, we think the more traditional layout of the O'Day would be the choice for most owners, especially those cruising with children. The settees, however, lacking backrests, are not comfortable to sit on. The initial version of the O'Day had the then fashionable dinette arrangement, but was quickly replaced with the present version of a pair of opposing settees. We doubt if many owners would bother setting up the portable cabin table between the berths as it prevents fore and aft passage through the cabin.

The galley with its small sink and space for a two-burner stove is rudimentary but adequate for a boat of this size. Inadequate is the bin/hanging locker opposite the head. Its usefulness escapes us. Enclosed it could have provided more useful stowage space, which the O'Day 22 desperately needs.

CONCLUSIONS

At a minimum trailering weight of 2,200 pounds (more realistically 2,500 plus the trailer), the O'Day 22 is above the maximum for trailering without a heavy car and special gear. If she isn't going to be trailered and launched off a ramp, the two-foot minimum draft is an unwarranted sacrifice of performance and stability. We would look for a fin keel boat unless shoal draft is the highest priority.

On the other hand, with some additional sails and hardware, the O'Day 22 should appeal to the sailor who wants a minimum size (and therefore price) boat primarily for daysailing and occasional weekend cruising (maximum one couple plus two young children).

Clearly the O'Day 22 is a minimum boat built tightly to a price. She is attractively styled. As she is apt to be a first boat, resale is important. O'Day boats have enjoyed good value on the used-boat market; whether the present diminished quality of the 22 will enjoy a similar success in the future remains to be seen.

Yet the price of the O'Day 22 is not all that cheap—about $10,500 (O'Day does not quote prices, leaving that for its dealers). To that base price, add about $1,200 for the extras (genoa and gear, stove, bigger winches, etc.). Thus, for almost $12,000 you get a sleek looking small boat with a good cockpit, a modicum of privacy and two good berths. You also get a schlocky decor and a slow boat.

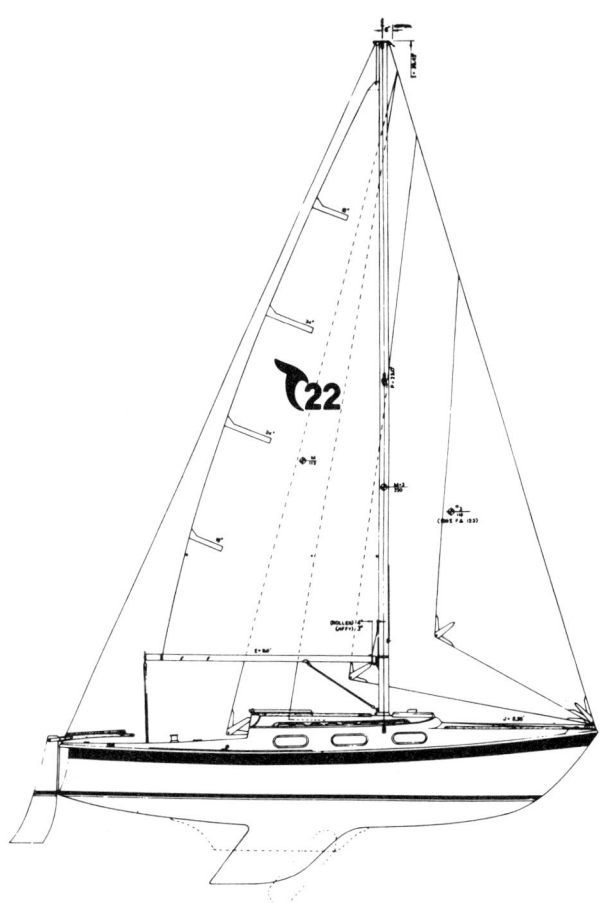

Specifications
Tanzer 22

LOA	22'6"
LWL	19'9"
Beam	7'10"
Sail area	227 sq ft

Keel-centerboard version
Draft	
board up	2'0"
board down	4'0"
Ballast	1500 lbs
Displacement	3100 lbs

Fixed keel version
Draft	3'5"
Ballast	1250 lbs
Displacement	2900 lbs

Tanzer Yachts
Box 67
Dorion, Quebec,
Canada J7V 5V8

The Tanzer 22

THE BOAT AND THE BUILDER

Like the Catalina 22, the Tanzer 22 was a long-time member of her builder's line of boats. Designed by Johann Tanzer, the Tanzer 22 was originally built exclusively in Canada and then had a brief production run in plants Tanzer operated in the U.S. before her builder fell upon hard times in the mid-1980s.

Dating from 1970, about 2,000 Tanzer 22s were built over the next 15 years. Clearly helping that growth has been a strong Tanzer 22 Class Association that boasts 700 members in the U.S. and Canada. This association continues to sponsor both racing and cruising and to promote the Tanzer 22 on the used-boat market. Such an organization, like that of the Catalina 22 association, has much to recommend it, and in areas where the organization is strong, Tanzer 22s have remained a popular boat that has appreciated in value.

One drawback to a boat marketed as a one-design (with the promise that older boats can still be competitive against newer ones) is that the design and construction tend to remain static. Even desirable changes may not be possible. One reason her builder folded was that many of his boats became "old fashioned." The Tanzer 22 was no exception. Her swept-back keel, low aspect rig, and dated profile had been replaced by racier looking, better performing boats in the 1980s. The Tanzer 22 had continued to thrive, outlasting innumerable rivals in the marketplace, but in the end, for all her virtues, she became a victim to changing times and changing tastes.

Still, to look at the Tanzer 22 is to look at a successful small cruiser, one that sails well, was more than adequately built, and continues to give a lot of satisfaction to her owners.

CONSTRUCTION

The Tanzer 22 seems to be basically well built, perhaps better than the average small boat. There is no evidence of flexing or gelcoat crazing, two common symptoms of the under-built or poorly engineered hull and deck structure. The hull to deck joint is now a combination of semi-rigid adhesive and 3/16-inch machine screws on six-inch centers holding together an exterior flange, a construction we approve of in a boat of this size. The resulting flange is one which would be difficult to repair in event of damage. However, it is covered with a vinyl molding that does afford better than average protection.

As is typical of boats of this size, the interior is a molded fiberglass head liner and hull liner. The hull liner incorporates all the basic components of the layout—berths, cabinets, cabin sole, and so forth. In a small boat it is a most practical interior. The disadvantage of such a liner is the difficulty of attaching add-on deck hardware and repairing damage to the hull laminate behind it.

Certain details of the Tanzer 22 are bothersome. For instance, the rudder is a two-part molded piece with a flange around the edge. While strong, it is needlessly crude in this day of well-faired rudders. For another instance, a foredeck well which is standard (and a good feature on a small boat) carries a solid, heavy fiberglass cover, loose and held in place only by flimsy wood toggles. These, however, are correctable details.

PERFORMANCE

The Tanzer 22, particularly the full-keel version, is a peppy little boat, among the best performing boats of her size, weight, price and purpose. She rates and sails with boats two feet longer, years more modern, and touted for their performance. What she might do to windward with an up-to-date keel shape rather than the less efficient swept-back fin makes for interesting conjecture. The same goes for her rudder-blade shape.

Fairing of the cast iron keel is only adequate and of the flanged rudder, poor. If performance in light air is a priority, owners will want to work at getting smoother surfaces.

Performance upwind with the keel-centerboard combination shoal draft version is less snappy, but with the board raised, downwind speed—already the envy of sailors on other boats up to about 26 feet—should be even better. This point may be a moot one, though, as only a small fraction of the Tanzers sold are the shoal draft model. Apparently the Tanzer appeals to more perform-ance-oriented buyers.

As with most boats of her size on the market, the mainsail and working jib are standard. A larger jib is a highly desirable option at a cost from the builder of about $450. With that sail should be included a genoa track and blocks. As sheet winches are all optional, buyers should order the larger two-speed ones when selecting options. Similarly with the spinnaker and gear: opt for pairs of coaming-mounted winches. We also recommend taking the optional cockpit-led halyards. Tanzer 22 owners also mention jiffy reefing, traveler, cunning-ham and vang as highly desirable options, again a reflection of their interest in sail handling and performance.

However, while the Tanzer 22 is a relatively smart performer and with add-on gear can be made more so, do not mistake her potential for that of the hot, light-displacement dinghy types such as the J/24 and its ilk.

LIVABILITY

In keeping with our belief that the cockpit is the most critical area for comfort in a boat of this size, we have reservations about the cockpit of the Tanzer 22. It is large, wider than average, which is a virtue and a fault. On the one hand, there is plenty of space to stretch out; six adults can sit down inside the coamings that offer both protection and support. The distance between the seats allows for bracing with the feet and the short tiller leaves most of the cockpit free of its swing.

On the negative side, though, this width coupled with the 22's low freeboard invites water aboard in the event of a severe knockdown. And it is a big cockpit which can hold much water. Those sitting on the leeward side in a breeze are going to be on intimate terms with the water, although the raised deck does afford protection not found on boats with trunk cabin configurations. There is no bridgedeck, merely a low (too low) sill in the companionway.

Unfortunately the cockpit is complicated by the mainsheet that is fixed to the center of the cockpit floor just forward of the tiller. It is handy to the helmsman and safer than a sheet with traveler mounted on a bridgedeck at the forward end of the cockpit, but it does effectively divide the cockpit and reduce its

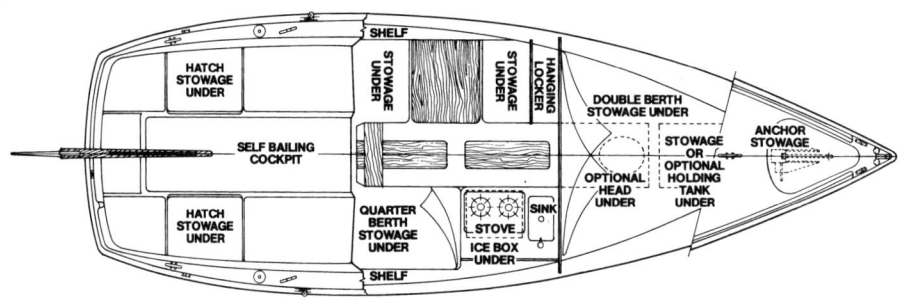

spaciousness. A traveler is optional equipment but does nothing to alleviate the fault with location.

Do not be put off by the fact that the cabinhouse extends to the gunwale, a rather old-fashioned feature. While it does make going forward a bit more awkward, the deck space it provides is welcome. Best of all is the interior space that is obtained in a boat that, with her low sheer, would otherwise be hopelessly cramped below.

The Tanzer 22, like the Catalina 22, is a victim of the time when she was designed. In the late 1960s, the boat-buying public became infatuated with dinettes. Boat builders obliged. The fad expired when owners tried to eat at the table and sleep on the so-called double berth converted from the dinette.

The dinette leaves the Tanzer 22 with but one proper berth, a good quarter-berth, plus a pair of V-berths forward. The V-berths suffer from V-berth syndrome—stacked feet. This coupled with the head (optional Porta Pottie) located under them gives the Tanzer 22 one of the least appealing accommodations we have seen.

As if this were not enough, the icebox (standard) more properly belongs on a powerboat than a sailboat. It is one of those infernal built-in, front-opening types: open the door with the boat heeled on starboard tack and be buried by the contents. Moreover, front-opening boxes such as this lose their cold with every opening (or what is left of the cold; insulation is only 1" of styrofoam).

In an attempt to provide some sunny weather headroom, Tanzer now offers a "convertible hatch" whereby the sliding companionway hatch assembly is hinged and can be raised to boom height. It is a $400 option that can also be retrofitted by owners on older 22s. According to a builder's spokesman, 90 percent of the 22s come fitted with the device. As with the pop-top option on other boats, we'd stay stooped and spend the money on more practical options.

CONCLUSIONS

In sum, the Tanzer 22 is a moderately well-built boat with mediocre accommodations and better than average performance. Buyers in areas with one-design fleets of Tanzer 22s will benefit from an active family racing and cruising program. As with almost all boats of this size, we think the deep keel version is better than the shoal draft version as the boat is apt to be too much for most sailors to trailer.

The deck and the cockpit of the Tanzer should appeal to a family sailor looking for daysailing room. The interior will have much less appeal and we recommend any prospective buyers do some shopping around to see what layouts are most suitable for the type of sailing they plan to do before settling on this boat.

At the bottom line, the Tanzer 22 is a moderately expensive boat with a list base price for the fin keel version at $10,550. Add to that most of the amenities for both comfort and performance and a well-outfitted Tanzer 22 will run at least $12,500. Properly maintained, the Tanzer 22 should at least retain her value for resale, especially in those areas where the boat is well known.

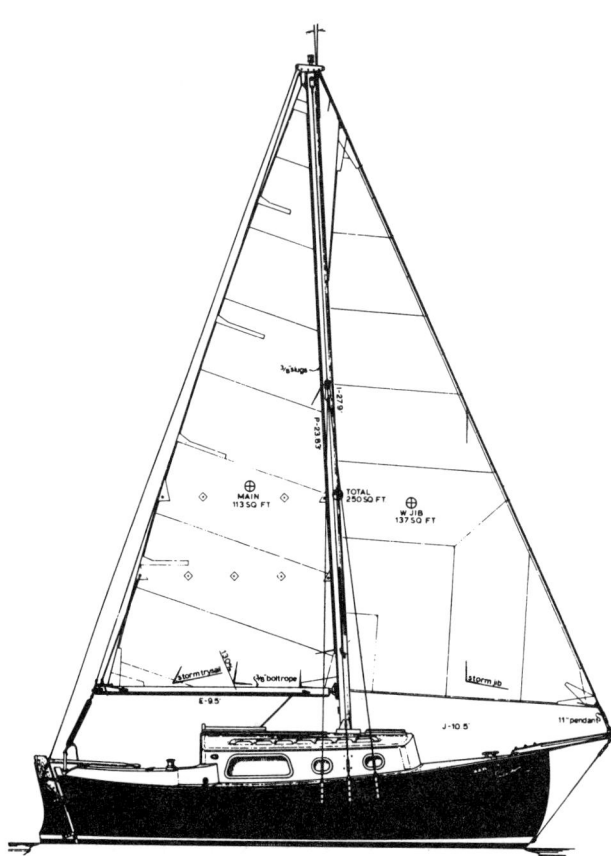

Specifications
Flicka

LOA*	23'7"
LOD	20'0"
LWL	18'2"
Beam	8'0"
Sail area	
Sloop	250 sq ft
Gaff	288 sq ft
Displacement†	5500 lbs
Ballast	1750 lbs

* Includes bowsprit and
  rudder
† Cruising

Pacific Seacraft
3301 S. Susan Street
Santa Ana, Calif. 92704

The Flicka

THE BOAT AND THE BUILDER

The Pacific Seacraft Flicka has perhaps received more "press" in the last few years than any other sailboat, certainly more than any production boat her "size." Publicity does not necessarily make a boat good, but it sure does create interest.

There are few other production boats that offer the Flicka's combination of traditional (or quasi-traditional) styling and heavy displacement in a small cruising yacht.

With the number of Flickas built by Pacific Seacraft at more than 400 plus an indeterminate number built by amateurs early in Flicka history, the boat seems to have become almost a cult object. High priced, distinctive, relatively rare; but with wide geographical distribution, and easily recognized; the Flicka invariably attracts attention and seems to stimulate extraordinary pride of ownership. The owners we talked to in preparing this evaluation all seem to be articulate, savvy, and involved. Moreover, they all show an uncommon fondness for their boats.

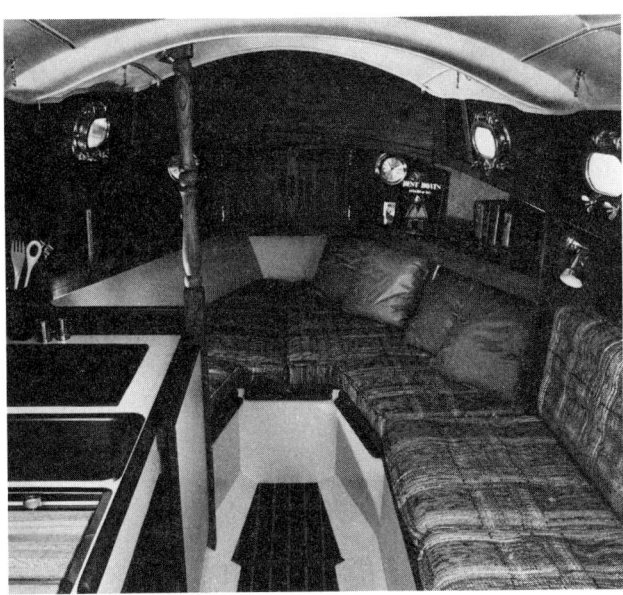

In 1983, a turned post was added to the Flicka's interior to provide a handhold in the otherwise open cabin.

The Flicka was designed by Bruce Bingham, who is best known as an illustrator, especially for his popular Sailor's Sketchbook in *Sail*. Originally Flicka was intended for amateur construction, the plans available from Bingham. She was designed to be a cruising boat within both the means and the level of skill of the builder who would start from scratch. Later the plans were picked up by a builder who produced the boat in kit form, a short lived operation, as was another attempt to produce the boat in ferro-cement.

Pacific Seacraft acquired the molds in 1978 and, with only minor changes, the boat as built by Seacraft remained essentially the same until 1983 when, in response to suggestions from prospective buyers and Seacraft dealers, the interior was redesigned to provide an enclosed head at the expense of one settee berth, and in the cockpit Seacraft incorporated a needed bridgedeck at the companionway and a better engine access hatch in the sole.

Pacific Seacraft is a modest-sized California builder which has specialized in heavier displacement, traditional boats with the construction and engineering that makes its boats among the few on the market that can justifiably be termed as having "offshore" capabilities. The first boat in the Seacraft line was a 25-footer, followed by the 31-foot Mariah, the Flicka, the Orion 27, and more recently the Dana 24, the Crealock 34 and 37, and the Pacific Seacraft 31. William Crealock is designer of the last four additions to the Seacraft line.

Seacraft has dealers nationwide, but has concentrated on the coasts. Apparently the firm was able to survive the hard times that befell some if its competitors, giving credence to the axiom that to succeed a boatbuilder should produce an expensive boat to quality standards that appeals to a limited number of enthusiastic buyers.

The hull of the Flicka is "traditional" with slack bilges, a full keel, a sweeping sheer accented with cove stripe and scrollwork, and bowsprit over a bobbed stem profile. In all, the Flicka is not an actual replica, but she does fulfill most sailors' idea of what a pocket-sized classic boat should look like. The price of the Flicka ranges to $35,000 for a well-appointed standard model that includes inboard engine (9 HP Yanmar), mainsail and jib. This is a high tab for a boat barely 18 feet long on the waterline, 20 feet on deck, and less than 24 feet overall with appendages. With that high-priced package, you get a roomy, heavy and well built boat that appeals to many sailors' dreams if not to their pocketbooks.

CONSTRUCTION

The Flicka looks well built even to an untrained eye. And to the trained eye that impression is not deceiving. This is a boat that should be fully capable of making offshore passages. The basic question any buyer must ask is whether he is willing to pay (in money and performance) for this capability for the far less rigorous cruising on Lake Mead or Chesapeake Bay, to Catalina Island, or up and down the New England Coast.

The hull of the Flicka is a solid fiberglass laminate to a layup schedule adequate for most 30-footers of moderate displacement. The deck has a plywood core rather than the balsa core common in production boats. In a boat of this displacement to length ratio, the heavier plywood reduces stability, but probably only marginally. Its virtue is that installation of add-on deck hardware is easier.

The hull to deck joint is done in a recommended manner: The hull has an inward flange on which the deck molding fits, bonded with a semi-rigid polyurethane adhesive/sealant and through-bolted with stainless steel bolts on four-inch centers. These bolts also secure the standard aluminum rail extrusion. On boats with the optional teak caprail in lieu of the aluminum, the bolts pass through the fiberglass, and the caprail is then fastened with self-tapping screws. As the rail sits atop of half-inch riser, water cannot puddle at the joint. We have heard no reports of any hull to deck joint failure in a production Flicka.

The interior of the boat uses a molded hull liner that is tab-bonded to the hull. Given the ruggedness of the hull laminate, we doubt if this stiffening adds much to the hull itself, but it does make the relatively thin laminate of the liner feel solid under foot.

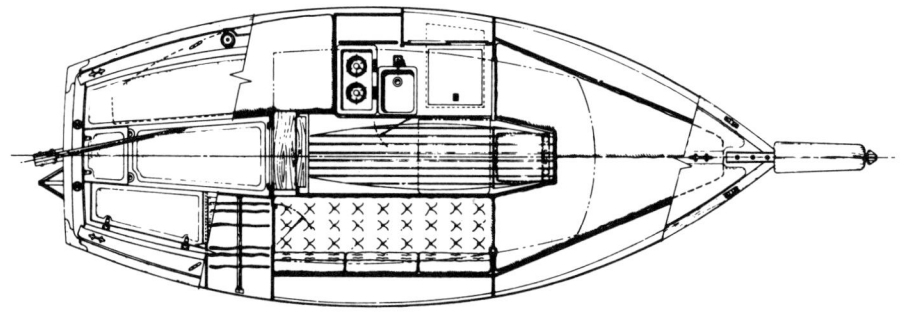

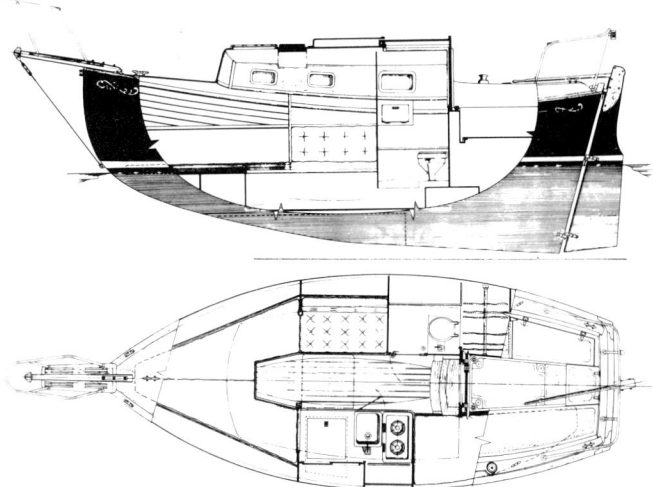

One of the more serious questions we have about the engineering of the Flicka is the under-deck mast support. Reflecting the quest for a completely open interior, the design incorporates a fiberglass/wood composite beam under the coachroof which transfers the mast stresses through the house sides to the underdeck bulk-

Changes in 1983 included a bridgedeck and an enclosed head, which resulted in shortening the settee berth to a mere 4'2".

heads. Apparently these bulkheads are not bonded to the hull, only to the liner.

The builder defends this construction, claiming that it will support over 8000 pounds (more than the Flicka's displacement). In addition, beginning in 1983, a turned oak handhold post was added between the mast support beam and cabin sole, which further increases the strength of the mast-support system.

Cabinetry, detailing, and finish are top quality for a production boat. However, keep in mind that the basic interior component is a fiberglass molding. Functionally the ease of keeping a molded liner clean has much to recommend it; aesthetically the sterility of the gelcoat may offend some tastes.

A few other specific construction details deserve note:

• The hardware on the Flicka is generally excellent, whether it is the standard or the optional cast bronze package, provided your taste allows for a mixture of traditional and modern. Since weight has not been a factor, most of the fittings are rugged, even massive. All through-hull fittings are fitted with seacocks. Particularly impressive is the tabernacle maststep, a contrast with the flimsy sheet-steel versions on cheaper boats. A notable exception to this endorsement are a pair of inadequate forward chocks.

• The scribed "planking seams" in the fiberglass topsides as well as the scrollwork are especially well done. However, any owner of a wood boat who has spent untold hours fairing the topsides to get rid of real seams has to wonder at anyone's purposely delineating phony seams in fiberglass.

• There is a removable section of cockpit sole over the engine compartment that gives superb access for servicing the engine and permits its installation or removal without tearing up the interior. It is a feature many boats with under-cockpit engines should envy given the chronic inaccessibility of such installations. Access to the Flicka's engine from the cabin is no better than that on most boats, even for routinely checking the oil level.

The Flicka

• External chainplates eliminate a common source of through-deck leaks but at the expense of exposing the chainplates to damage.

• There is good access to the underside of the deck and coaming for installation of deck hardware. The headliner in the cabin is zippered vinyl.

• Anyone with a modern boat with its vestigal bilge sump has to appreciate the Flicka's deep sump in the after end of the keel.

• The ballast (1,750 pounds of lead) is encapsulated in the molded hull, risking more structural damage in a hard grounding than exposed ballast, but eliminating possible leaking around keel bolts.

PERFORMANCE

Handling Under Sail

In an era that has brought sailors such hot little boats as the Moore 24, the Santa Cruz 27, and the J-24, any talk about the performance of a boat with three times their displacement to length ratio has to be in purely relative terms. In drifting conditions, the Flicka simply has too much weight and too much wetted surface to accelerate. Add some choppiness to the sea and she seems to take forever to gain way.

When the wind gets up to 10 knots or so, the Flicka begins to perk up, but then only if sea conditions remain moderate. With the wind rising above 10 or 12 knots, the Flicka becomes an increasingly able sailer. However, she is initially a very tender boat and is quick to assume 15 degrees of heel in contrast to lighter, shallower, flatter boats that carry less sail but accelerate out from under a puff before they heel.

In winds over 15 knots the Flicka feels like much more boat than her short length would suggest. As she heels, her stability increases reassuringly. Her movement through the water is firmer and she tracks remarkably well, a long lost virtue in an age of boats with fin keels and spade rudders. Owners unanimously applaud her ability to sail herself for long stretches even when they change her trim by going forward or below.

Those looking at—and reading about—the Flicka should discount tales of fast passages. While it is certainly true that the boat is capable of good speed under optimum conditions, she is not a boat that should generate unduly optimistic expectations. In short, there may be a lot of reasons to own a Flicka but speed is not one of them.

One mitigating factor is that performance consists not only of speed, but also ease of handling, stability, steadiness, and even comfort. In this respect, the Flicka may not go fast, but she should be pleasant enough to sail that getting there fast may not be important.

The Flicka comes with two alternative rigs, the standard masthead marconi sloop and the optional (about $1,500) gaff-rigged cutter. Most of the boats have been sold as sloops. The gaff cutter is a more "shippy" looking rig, but for good reasons, most modern sailors will forego a gaff-mainsail.

If you regularly sail in windy or squally conditions, you might want to consider a staysail for the sloop rig. However, for a 20-foot boat, a sail inventory of a mainsail fitted with slab reefing, a working jib, and a genoa with 130 to 150 percent overlap should be adequate. For added performance the next sail to consider is a spinnaker and, if offshore passages are contemplated, a storm jib.

Handling Under Power

Any observations about handling under power raise the question of inboard versus outboard power. In fact, this may be the most crucial issue a potential Flicka owner faces. In making the decision, start with this observation: At a cruising displacement of over 5,000 pounds, the Flicka is at the upper limit for outboard auxiliary power. Then move to a second observation: Small one-cylinder diesel engines such as the Yanmar fit readily into the Flicka, albeit at the expense of some valuable space under the cockpit sole.

The Flicka is a boat that seems to beg for inboard power; she has the space, and weight is not critical. Moreover, cost should not be critical either. Inboard power adds about 10 percent to the cost of the boat with outboard power, a small percentage of an expensive package. Much of the additional cost is apt to be recoverable at resale, whereas the depreciation on an outboard in five years virtually amounts to its original value.

LIVABILITY

Any discussion of the livability of the Flicka should be prefaced by a reminder that above decks this is a crowded, cluttered 20-footer, and belowdecks this is a boat with the space of a 26-footer. The Flicka is a boat with a enough space below for a couple to live aboard and yet small enough for them to handle easily.

Deck Layout

Nowhere is the small size of the Flicka more apparent than on deck and in her cockpit. The short cockpit (a seat length of barely over five feet, too short to stretch out for a nap), a high cabinhouse, sidedecks too narrow to walk on to windward with the boat heeled and always obstructed by shrouds, the awkwardness of a bowsprit, and lifelines that interfere with jib-sheet winching are all indicative of the crowded deck plan.

The stern pulpit is an attractive option, but it does make manual control of a transom-mounted outboard motor difficult. Originally this pulpit incorporated the mainsheet traveler, but the lead for close sheeting was poor. After the 1983 redesign, the traveler moved to the bridgedeck where it is much more effective and handy, albeit adding more clutter to a relatively cramped cockpit.

For a boat heralded for use "offshore," the lack of a bridgedeck to keep the water in a flooded cockpit from getting below was a notable shortcoming. One of the most common occurrences in heavy seas are waves breaking into the cockpit and some means—a bridgedeck preferably, but at least a stoutly secured lower dropboard—is vital to keeping that water from finding its way below. Thus the 1983 improvement was crucial if the Flicka was to deserve to be called an offshore cruiser.

Belowdecks

In the original design of the Flicka, every effort was made to keep the interior open from the companionway to the chain locker, a noble endeavor that gave the impression of spaciousness that rivaled 30-footers.

Two notable drawbacks of that interior are conspicuous as soon as the impression wears off. The layout, featuring four full-sized berths, leaves no room for an enclosed head compartment and sleeping privacy. How important these factors are is purely a matter of individual taste and priorities, but for a cruising boat of 20 feet long on deck, four berths seems an unconscionable waste of space.

Incidentally, this observation about berths is not meant to imply any special deficiency in the Flicka. It is true of too many boats on the market. They are built for a boat-buying public that seems to think the number of berths in a boat is almost as important as whether the boat will float.

Frankly, the lack of an enclosed head in a boat that otherwise can boast of being a miniature yacht is the most serious drawback to her interior, surplus berths notwithstanding.

That is why in 1983 Pacific Seacraft redid the Flicka's interior, cropping more than two feet from the starboard settee berth, making it a seat, and incorporating the space into an enclosed midship head compartment. The enclosure stole from the openness of the original layout but is a decided improvement in the livability—and civility—of the Flicka.

The other contributors to the sense of openness have been retained. Headroom is almost six feet for the length of the main cabin (find that in another boat-shaped 20-footer!). Better yet, good height extends over the galley counter, the cabin settee, and the after section of the forward berths. Moreover, the Flicka's high topsides permit outboard bookshelves and galley lockers, stowage under the deck over the V-berths and enough air over the head of the quarterberth that it does not seem like a coffin.

CONCLUSIONS

Buyers put off by the price of the Flicka should consider the fact that this is a 20-foot boat with the weight and space of a 26- to 28-footer of more modern proportions. That still may not put her all-up price tag for the "deluxe" model of $35,000 in crystal clear perspective. It shouldn't. The Flicka is still an expensive boat. She still has a waterline length of only 18 feet, true accommodations for two, a too-cozy cockpit, and a lot of sail area and rigging not found on more conventional contemporary boats. Nor does she have the performance to rival more modern designs. (One owner reports a PHRF rating for his Flicka of about 300 seconds per mile, a figure that drops her off the handicap scale of most base-rating lists we have seen.)

Recognizing the limitations of the Flicka for buyers looking for "a bit more" in a small cruising boat, Pacific Seacraft introduced the Crealock-designed Dana 24 in 1984. The 24, retaining the "traditional" look and proportions as the Flicka, but almost four feet longer on deck, gives a crew of two a more practical layout with only two berths, over six feet of headroom, and a larger and more comfortable cockpit. Moreover, the Dana 24 has an inboard diesel engine as standard and better sailing performance than the Flicka, befitting her six-foot longer waterline length.

At the same time the Flicka is a quality package that should take a singlehander or a couple anywhere they might wish to sail her. There are not many production boats anywhere near her size and price that can make that claim.

The faults with the Flicka have to be weighed against her virtues as is the case with choosing any boat. Fortunately, though, her faults are the type that can be readily seen; they are not the invisible ones of structure, handling, or engineering so typical of other production boats. Similarly her virtues are traditional and time tested. She is built by a firm to whom the owners give high marks for interest and cooperation, and the few Flickas that have come on the used-boat market have maintained their value better than the average production boat. At the bottom line is a boat with much to recommend her.

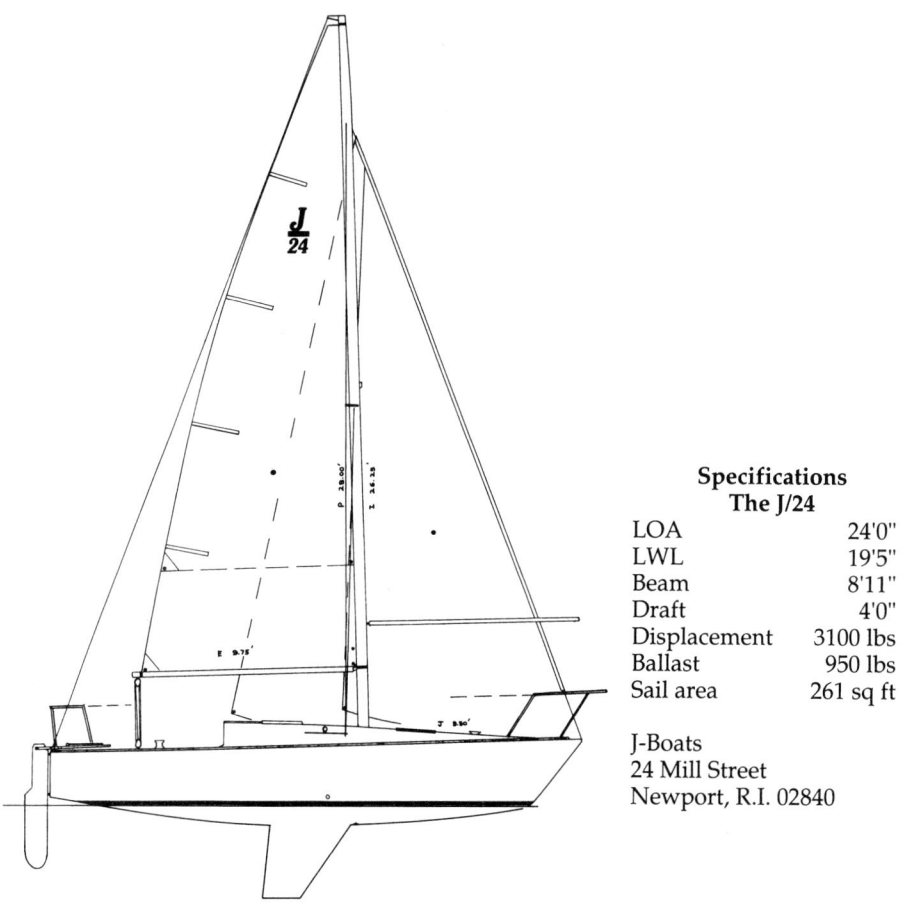

Specifications
The J/24

LOA	24'0"
LWL	19'5"
Beam	8'11"
Draft	4'0"
Displacement	3100 lbs
Ballast	950 lbs
Sail area	261 sq ft

J-Boats
24 Mill Street
Newport, R.I. 02840

The J/24

THE BOAT AND THE BUILDER

The J/24 is one of those boats that happened along at just the right time, with the right marketing to a ready market. Some may wonder whether the tale of her success would make a better textbook or a better storybook. Either way, much of the marine industry has studied her story, and then flattered her with emulation. However, no imitation or variation of the J/24 has yet to achieve her popularity.

Since her humble beginnings in 1976 in the garage of an amateur designer, over 4000 boats have been sold from factories in Rhode Island, California, Australia, Japan, Italy, England, France, Brazil and Argentina. All of the builders are licensed by a company called J-Boats to build the J/24 to strict one-design tolerances.

J-Boats is owned and run by two brothers—Bob and Rod Johnstone (the J in J-Boats). Bob is the marketing whiz and Rod is the designer. Conservative estimates put their total revenue from the J/24, after buying the boats from the builders and selling them to the dealers, at upwards of $4-$5 million. Not bad considering how it all began...

Ragtime was a 24-foot inspiration evolved by Rod Johnstone and his family in their garage as a two-year, weekend project. Rod was a salesman for a marine publication and an avid racer with a successful background in high-performance one-designs. He had undertaken, but never completed, the Westlawn home-study course in naval architecture (although he has since been awarded an honorary degree so the school could use his name in its advertisements). *Ragtime* was launched in 1976, and was an instant winner, taking 17 firsts in 19 starts in eastern Connecticut. People began asking for their own "Ragtimes."

At this time, brother Bob, also a respected racer, was working in the marketing department of AMF Alcort (Sunfish, Paceship, etc.). When Alcort declined to produce the J/24, Bob quit and formed J-Boats. Tillotson-Pearson, builder of the Etchells 22 and the Freedom line of boats, was more receptive and production began in 1977. The first J/24s were as fast as *Ragtime*, and dominated regattas like the 1977 MORC Internationals. Bob made sure that the favorable results were well publicized; more than 200 boats were sold that year, and nearly 1000 the next.

The boat was a big hit for a number of reasons. She moved into a void, appealing to two groups of sailors who were ripe for her type of racing; those who had outgrown athletic small boats, yet still yearned for the competition of one-design racing, and those who wished to compete without the expense, hassles and uncertainties of handicap racing.

The J/24 is a one-design's one-design. Like the Laser, Windsurfer, and Hobie Cat, she is built under the supervision of one company. Unlike most proprietary one-designs, sails are not provided by the J/24's builder. This was a particularly astute move by the Johnstones as it meant that sailmakers could become involved in the class. Sailmakers comprise many of the big names in racing; by getting them into the regattas, the Johnstones added instant credibility to the J/24's budding status as a "hot" class. By the J/24 Midwinter Cham-

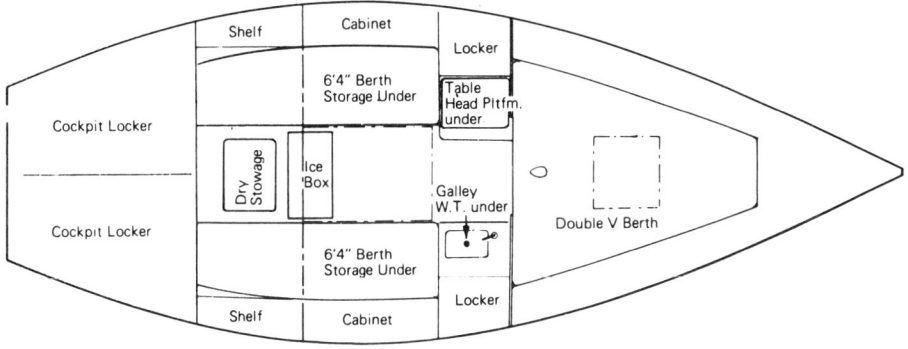

The J/24

pionship in 1979, almost every boat among the top 15 finishers had a sailmaker on board.

The big advantage that proprietary one-designs have over "independent" one-designs (classes with competing builders) is the power of centralized, big-bucks promotion. J-Boats has organized and promoted regattas and had a heavy hand in running the class association. J/24s got a lot of press, thanks to J-Boats. Full color, multi-page advertisements appeared monthly in the slick sailing magazines. Promotion has been primary; money, no object. J/24s have been donated for several high visibility USYRU championships. Big discounts have been given for fleet purchases (sometimes to effectively crush interest in competing one-designs). With the help of British enthusiasts, the Johnstones were able to make the J/24 a class recognized by the International Yacht Racing Union. More international lobbying got the J/24 into the Pan-American Games.

There are some disadvantages to proprietary one-designs. First, the class is in a real bind if the builder goes bankrupt. Likewise, if the builder should ever abuse his power by ignoring the class administration or changing construction of the boat to suit economic demands. Although a proprietary builder faces competition from other types of boats, there is no competition building *his* boat. This can inflate the price, especially when there are three substantial markups in the pricing structure (builder, J-Boats, and the dealer).

The J/24 is not cheap. Base price is $15,900. When you include sails, an outboard, lights, battery, and halyard winches, the price is over $20,000. If you want to go to distant regattas, a trailer runs about $1800. Used boats appear to hold their original value. Even the oldest J/24s, which originally sold for $9800, are now selling for $14,000 or more. In areas where the J/24 has been popular for years, used boats are readily available.

CONSTRUCTION

The J/24 has the distinct advantage of having been produced in great numbers and been subjected to the rigors of hard racing. It's safe to say that nearly everything that could have broken, has broken, and that the J/24 is now almost bulletproof. J-Boats has done a commendable job in correcting nearly all of the "bugs" in the J/24. However, if you are planning to purchase a boat several years old, you should be watchful for some of the older problems.

Boats built during the first two years of production had problems with leaking along the hull to deck joint, delamination of the main bulkhead, and the attachment of the keel to the hull.

The hull to deck leak was due to failure of the silicone sealant in the joint. The inward-turning hull flange is overlapped by the deck, which is bedded in sealant and through-bolted at close intervals through a teak toerail. Now the joint is bedded with 3M 5200, a pliable and strong adhesive, and leaks are infrequent. Fortunately, the internal side of the joint is exposed throughout the J/24's interior, so recaulking is not difficult.

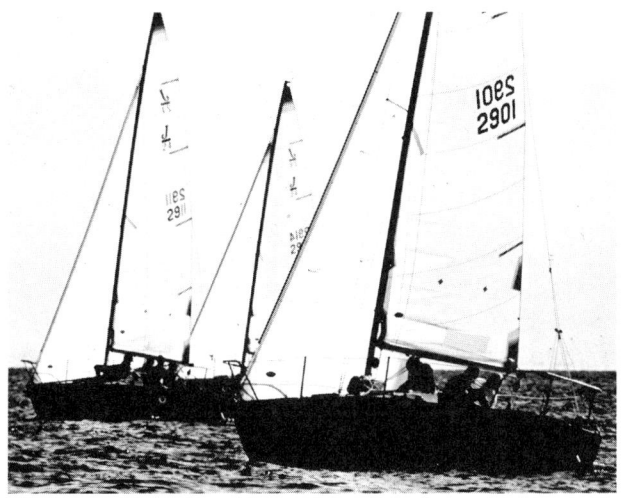

Harder to rectify is the problem of delamination of the main bulkhead. J/24s are raced hard, often with substantial rig tension. The chainplates pierce the deck and are bolted to the main bulkhead. The plywood bulkhead is tabbed with fiberglass to the hull and deck. The mast is stepped through the deck and sits on an aluminum beam, which is also tabbed to the main bulkhead. Rig tension pulls upward on the bulkhead while mast compression pushes downward on the beam, resulting in tremendous shearing forces on the bulkhead and its tabbing.

On some of the older J/24s, the plywood has delaminated, letting the mast "sink" 1/4 inch or more. Owners of these boats have either returned them to the factory for replacement of the bulkhead, or ground off the delamination and reglassed the bulkhead themselves. The builder now uses a better grade of plywood and installs screws to reinforce the bulkhead tabbing. As an added precaution, the boat owner may wish to bolt the mast-bearing beam to the bulkhead with an angle-iron.

The third problem with some of the older J/24s is the keel-to-hull attachment. The builder used to fill the keel sump with a mixture of resin and fiber. The keel bolts were fastened through the mixture which, when saturated with water, is less rigid than solid laminations of fiberglass. After several years of sailing or a hard grounding, the keel bolts would begin to work, and the keel would loosen enough to be able to be wobbled by hand with the boat suspended from a hoist. The first sign of this problem is the appearance of a crack along the keel stub. Tightening of the keel bolts, which are quality stainless steel, is a simple but temporary fix. What is needed is a backing plate for the bolts.

There was a variety of other problems with early J/24s: The mast has three internal halyards; two jib halyards exit below the headstay with the spinnaker halyard above. On the older boats, a large square hole was cut in the mast to accommodate the sheaves, leaving an open, poorly supported space adjacent to the spinnaker sheave. This space is sometimes the source of mast cracks; the fix is to weld a plate over it.

In 1980, the J/24 got much-improved companionway and forward hatches. The hatches on older boats were molded of thin fiberglass and had a tendency to leak and fracture under the weight of heavy crewmembers. The new forward hatches are Lexan, and the companionway hatch is now much heavier with a lower profile.

The J/24's rudder is heavy and strong. The builder claims you can hang a 900-pound keel from the rudder tip without breaking it. Although the J/24's rudder pintles appear more than adequate, after several years of use they have been known to develop corrosion cracks where the pintle is welded to its strap. In 1981, the builder began equipping J/24s with weldless pintles; the builder also offers the new system as a replacement for older boats.

The starboard chainplate bolts through both the bulkhead and the hull liner. The port chainplate bolts through only the bulkhead. After the first two years of production, the port bulkhead was reinforced with fiberglass in the chainplate area. On earlier boats, a backing plate should be added to prevent the chainplate bolts from elongating their holes.

The hull and deck of the J/24 are cored with balsa, which makes them stiff, light, quiet and relatively condensation-free. We have heard of occasional delaminations resulting from trailering with improperly adjusted poppets.

The Kenyon mast section is the same as that used on the Etchells 22, a bigger boat. It is more than adequate for any strength of wind.

The J/24 does not have positive flotation, and she has been known to capsize in severe conditions. This is usually not a problem as she floats on her side with the companionway well out of the water. However, should the leeward cockpit

---

J/24: How Trailerable?

The J/24 is not launchable from a boat ramp, unless the ramp is steep, whether paved or of hard sand, and unless you use a long extender between the tongue of the trailer and your trailer hitch. Her 3100 pounds (fully loaded) require a big, 8-cylinder vehicle to tow her. She is easily launched from a 2-ton hoist which can attach to a strap on her keel bolts. However, the main hatch slides just far enough forward to allow the hoisting cable to clear it, so the hatch tends to get chewed by the cable.

The J/24 was originally designed to sail at a displacement of 2800 pounds. The class minimum was later increased to 3100. The original single-axle trailer provided as a factory option was barely adequate for the intended, 2800 pound boat, and totally inadequate for a fully loaded boat. Tales abound of blown tires and broken trailer welds. The factory now offers both a single and double axle trailer; we recommend the double axle.

If you want to seriously race a J/24, trailering is a necessity. Local fleets grow and shrink each year with the whims of their members, but national and regional regattas continue to attract many participants. Make no mistake, however; trailering is expensive. The original cost and maintenance costs of a big car, the gas and tolls of trailering, and the housing of crew are not cheap.

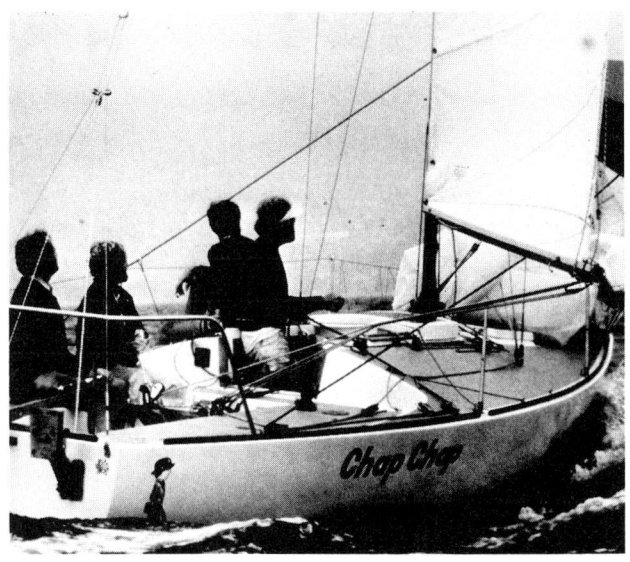

locker fall open, water can rush below, filling the cabin and causing her sink. While fastening the lockers in heavy weather prevents the problem, the manufacturer began to seal off the lockers from the cabin with an additional bulkhead several years ago as an added safety measure.

Of the J/24s sold in the US, more than 2500 of them have been built by Tillotson-Pearson in Rhode Island. The others were built by Performance Sailcraft in San Francisco, which is now defunct. New boats are now shipped cross-country. Top West Coast sailors tell us they favor the East Coast-built boats, claiming the keels and rudders on the West Coast-built boats are too thick to be competitive. The West Coast keels are thick because they are covered with injection-molded gelcoat. Tillotson-Pearson fairs the keels with autobody putty.

PERFORMANCE

Handling Under Sail

The J/24's PHRF rating ranges from 165 to 174, depending on the handicapper. She rates as fast as or faster than a C&C 30, Santana 30, or Pearson 30. One must remember that, because the J/24 has attracted competent owners, her PHRF rating is probably somewhat inflated. While the J/24 is an excellent training boat because she is so responsive, a beginning racer may have an especially hard time making her perform to her PHRF rating.

Aside from her speed, the J/24's greatest asset is her maneuverability. With her stern-hung rudder she can be turned in her own length, sculled out to a mooring in light air, and brought to a screeching halt by jamming the rudder over 90 degrees.

The J/24 has a narrow "groove;" it takes a lot of concentration to keep her going at top speed. She is sensitive to backstay trim, sheet tension, weight placement and lower shroud tension. The lower shrouds act like running backstays because they are anchored aft of the mast. They must be loosened in light air to create some headstay sag, and then tightened in heavy air to straighten the mast, making backstay tension more effective in removing headstay sag.

Sheet tension is also critical. Top crews rarely cleat the genoa sheets, having one crewmember hold the tail while hiking from the rail. Some of the best sailors even lead the jib to the weather winch so the sail can be trimmed without sending crew weight to leeward.

The class rules allow you to race with a mainsail, a 150-percent genoa, a working jib and a single spinnaker. This makes sail selection simple and the inventory affordable (about $2600 total). However, the one genoa must carry the boat all the way from a flat calm up to 20 knots or more. To be competitive in light air, the genoa must be full; yet to hold the boat level with this full genoa in a strong breeze, you need a lot of crew weight. Most of the top crews are now sailing with five people on board for a total crew weight of 800 to 900 pounds. The J/24 is a small boat, and the additional fifth crew really makes the boat cramped. Add to this the increasing trend of some skippers making the crew sit in the cabin on the leeward bunk in light air, and you have a boat on which it can be less than fun to crew.

There are two worthwhile improvements that can help a J/24's performance. To decrease the boat's slight tendency toward a lee helm in light air, the mast should be cut to minimum length allowed in the class rules, and the headstay should be lengthened to the maximum allowed to give the mast more rake. The other improvement is fairing the keel to minimum dimensions. The keel is much thicker than is necessary for optimum performance. It comes relatively fair from the builder, but most owners will want to grind off the builder's filler and sharpen the trailing edge. On some of the older boats, the trailing edge is twice the minimum thickness. Some racers go so far as to spend $500-$1000 to have the keel professionally faired.

The J/24 is best suited for racing; there are many boats in her size range that are far more comfortable and practical for daysailing. However, the J/24 is a joy to sail under mainsail alone. Unlike most boats, she balances and sails upwind at a respectable speed, and her maneuverability gives her tremendous freedom in crowded harbors.

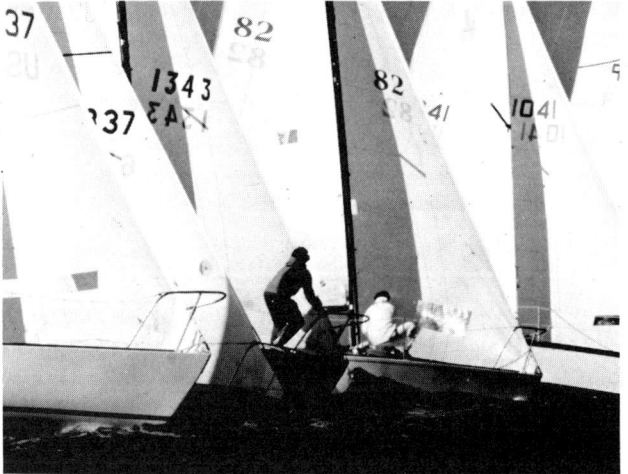

Handling

Under Power

The J/24 is powered by an outboard engine; an inboard is not feasible or available. Class rules require that an outboard with a minimum of 3.5 horsepower be carried while racing. Most owners opt for a 3.5-4 horsepower outboard. It provides adequate power and is as much weight as you want to be hefting over a transom. Although the cockpit locker is plenty big enough, most owners stow the outboard under a berth in the cabin to keep the weight out of the stern. This makes using the outboard inconvenient. The factory-supplied optional outboard bracket has a spring-loaded hinge to lift the engine for easy mounting; we recommend it. Because the outboard is likely to be stored in the cabin, a remote gas tank will keep fuel spillage and odor to a minimum.

LIVABILITY

Above Decks

The J/24 is well laid out, yet she is still not a comfortable or easy boat to crew on. When she was first launched, sailors said her layout could be no better, and she was copied by manufacturers of competing boats. However, after years of racing, sailors have discovered several things that could be improved.

Cockpit winches are located just forward of the mainsheet traveler, which spans the middle of the cockpit. Many sailors have moved the winches forward, so the crewmember tacking the genoa can face forward instead of aft during a tack.

The standard mainsheet cleat is attached to the traveler car so that, when you trim the sheet, you inadvertently pull the car to weather. Many sailors have solved this by mounting a fixed cleat with a swivel base at the center of the traveler.

On older boats, the backstay was single-ended at the transom. Boats now come with a double-ended backstay led forward to the helmsman on each side of the cockpit. Foot blocks need to be mounted on the traveler to keep the helmsman from falling to leeward as the boat heels (you must steer from forward and well outboard of the traveler).

For those who plan to try cross-sheeting to the weather winch, leading the jib sheets through Harken ratchet blocks is advised. Most sailors will also want to mount barber haulers to pull the genoa sheet outboard in strong winds. Cam cleats for the barber haulers should be mounted on the companionway so they "self-cleat" when led to the weather winch.

Cabin-top winches for the halyards and spinnaker guys are optional and essential. Because the J/24 has single spinnaker sheets, most sailors mount "twings," which pull the guy down to the deck outboard of the shrouds when reaching.

In the search for a cleaner deck, it is common to mount the spinnaker halyard cleat on the mast. Most sailors use only one jib halyard. Although a second jib halyard is optional, it is necessary only for long-distance handicap racing. On short one-design courses, it is better to struggle along overpowered than to place crew weight on the bow to change headsails. Instruments are also unnecessary in one-design racing. There are more than enough boats on a one-design race course to judge your speed without the help of a speedometer.

The J/24 comes equipped with a Headfoil II grooved headstay system, which works smoothly. Early boats came with Stern Twinstays, which have occasionally failed when the bearings freeze up with age. Some sailors have exchanged the grooved headstay system for cloth snaps on their headsails (you seldom change sails anyway). We applaud this idea, as it makes the sails all the more manageable in severe weather.

Although the flat decks are well suited for racing, the cockpit is less than comfortable for daysailing. There are no seat backs and the boom is dangerously low. Visibility with the deck-sweeping genoa is terrible and is often the cause of nightmarish collisions on crowded race courses. Lower lifelines are optional and recommended for those who sail with children, but they interfere with fast tacks when racing.

The boom is rigged with a 4:1 vang, which is swiveled to be adjustable from either rail on a windy spinnaker reach. The boom is also rigged with reef lines which exit through stoppers at the gooseneck. Top sailors have discovered that the boat always sails better without a reef, which is a good thing, because the stoppers are both difficult to operate and have a history of slipping.

Belowdecks

The interior is simple and functional. On most boats it is used for little more than sail storage. However, for a couple who enjoys roughing it, it could make for occasional weekend cruising. The first thing you notice when you go below is the lack of headroom. You can sit in comfort, but to move about you must crawl.

The interior is finished in white gelcoat. Early boats had coarse, non-skid gelcoat on the overhead. While this may have been more attractive than smooth gelcoat, it was hard on elbows and bald heads. It also tended to collect dirt and mildew.

A molded hull liner is used to form the two quarterberths, the cabin sole, and two lockers and a galley just aft of the main bulkhead. One locker is deep enough to serve as a wet locker for foul weather gear; the other is best used to store the rudiments of a meal. The galley consists of a sink with a hand pump. A small, two-burner stove could be mounted in the small, removable "table" forward of the port quarterberth. The icebox, a large portable cooler made by Igloo, has a piece of teak glued to it and doubles as a companionway step. After a season or two of jumping on the ice chest, tack after tack, the lid disintegrates.

The forward V-berth, although divided by the mast, is still large and comfortable enough for a couple. The boat does not come equipped with a head. To avoid the extra drag of a through-hull fitting, portable toilets are often used. We would rather use a cedar bucket—there simply isn't enough space in the cabin of a J/24 to cohabitate with a portable head. If you plan to seriously race, you won't want to load the boat's lockers with cruising equipment. If you do cruise, it will probably be out of a duffel bag.

CONCLUSIONS

The appeal of the J/24 is as a racer. If you plan to do anything else, she is not for you. Although the J/24 is relatively easy to sail, she is very difficult to sail well. To many people, she represents a chance to compete in the big leagues; by traveling to major regattas you can sail against some of the best sailors in the country. However, the big leagues are tough—if you like to race with a pick-up crew and a hangover, you'd also better be satisfied with finishing at the back of the pack.

One appeal of the J/24 is that, unlike many big league boats, you can always sail in your home waters because the boat has so big a following. There are enough boats to race one-design almost anywhere; and in a pinch, there is always handicap racing. As long as you don't want to travel, the boat is inexpensive to maintain.

Despite our effort to highlight every flaw that has appeared throughout the J/24's evolution, we'd like to emphasize that she is more hardy than most boats of her type. Few boats can take the punishment that a J/24 gets during a season of hard racing and come through with so few scars. No racing boat is ever a good investment—that is, she won't appreciate; but the J/24 has shown that she can at least keep her value.

The dream boat with the fairy-tale success story has turned out, after all, to be a rugged winner in the real world.

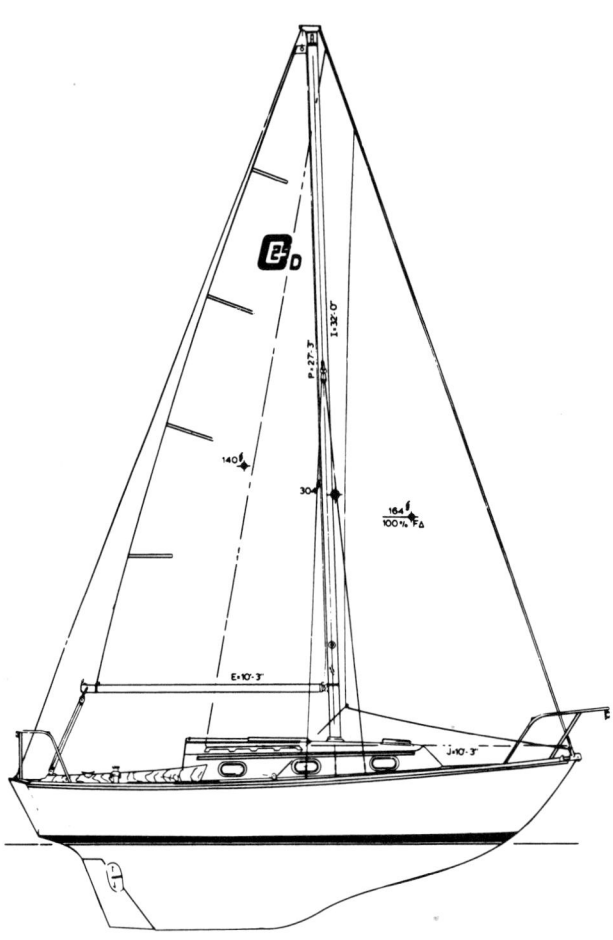

Specifications
Cape Dory 25D

LOA	25'0"
DWL	19'0"
Beam	8'0"
Draft	3'6"
Displacement	5120 lbs
Ballast	2050 lbs
Sail area	304 sq ft

Cape Dory Yachts Inc.
160 Middleboro Avenue
East Taunton,
Massachusetts 02708
(617) 823-6776

The Cape Dory 25 and 25D:
Sisters, But Not Twins

THE BOATS AND THE BUILDER

Cape Dory Yachts is one of the more conservative firms in the boatbuilding industry. With the exception of a brief fling with modern cruiser-racers (the Intrepid series), the company's stock in trade since the late 1960's has been traditional, full keel auxiliaries and sailboats.

Most of the Cape Dorys have been from the board of the late Carl Alberg, long the dean of traditionalist American designers. It is ironic that a man, who began his career drawing schooners and Universal Rule racing sloops in the office of John Alden, should find his greatest popularity designing production fiberglass boats some 60 years later. The Cape Dory line has included more than a dozen boats from 18 feet to 45 feet, each a larger or smaller development of her sisters. Since he picked up the tooling for the well known 18-1/2 foot

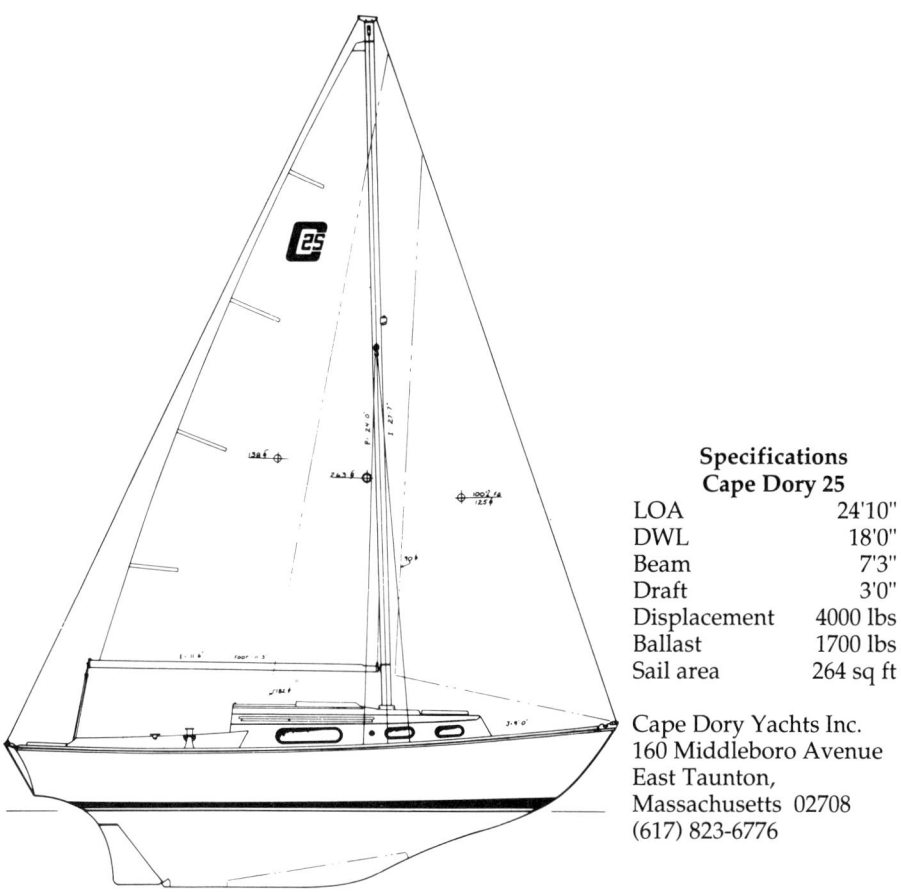

Specifications
Cape Dory 25

LOA	24'10"
DWL	18'0"
Beam	7'3"
Draft	3'0"
Displacement	4000 lbs
Ballast	1700 lbs
Sail area	264 sq ft

Cape Dory Yachts Inc.
160 Middleboro Avenue
East Taunton,
Massachusetts 02708
(617) 823-6776

Typhoon in 1969, Cape Dory owner Andrew Vavolotis showed an almost unswerving loyalty to the long keel with attached rudder, and to designs by Alberg. Only two non-Alberg designs have been part of the Cape Dory line of larger boats: the Ted Hood-designed Cape 30 (the company's first big boat, and totally different from the current 30), and the Cape Dory 25.

Credit for the basic design of the Cape Dory goes to George Stadel. The boat was originally built by Allied as the Greenwich 24. Vavolotis purchased the tooling during one of Allied's frequent business disasters, redesigned the boat to suit his own ideas, and put the Cape Dory 25 into production in 1973. In the next nine years, almost 850 25s were built, and the boat has rightly been termed a modern classic.

In November of 1982, the last 25 went down the line, and March of 1985 saw the 25D take the same trip, marking the 189th 25D produced. But, fortunately, they did not sink into oblivion. Cape Dory 26s and 26Ds took their place, and are selling well today. Current price of the 26 (the outboard version), is $29,750, while the 25D (as in diesel), runs $36,990.

It was the fall of 1981 when the 25D was introduced, but there's much more than power plant that differentiates the two boats. The only thing the 25 and the 25D have in common is overall length. The 25D is an entirely different boat; wider, heavier, deeper, with inboard engine, a dramatically different interior, and a price tag 50% higher than that of the 25.

In a time when retrenchment was the watchword in the boatbuilding industry, Vavolotis had the grin of a Cheshire cat on his face when he said, "We've found our niche in the industry."

For a number of years, that niche was narrow indeed. While racer-cruisers proliferated in the 1970's, while the fat fin-keeler with the high aspect ratio rig became the industry vogue, Cape Dory continued to espouse long keels with attached rudders, relatively narrow beam, attractive sheerlines, moderate freeboard, and substantial overhangs — "old fashioned" boats.

While there are a number of companies that offer a few traditional, heavy displacement boats, no other builder can claim a full line of ultraconservative designs. It might seem that Cape Dory has created so many models that their prime competition is between boats in their own line, but apparently there is enough product differentiation to support five different models between 25 and 30 feet.

Cape Dory customer loyalty is tremendous. Probably more owners trade up through the line than change builders when the time comes to upgrade. The cynic might say that it's because no other builder caters exclusively to buyers of "traditional" boats. In fact, a large percentage of the product loyalty is generated by consistently good quality, high resale value, and excellent builder support on warranty work.

While Cape Dory offers the fairly standard one-year warranty, owners report that the company has consistently made good on problems well after any legal liability to do so. We think this policy is a key to customer satisfaction and long term loyalty, and one that other builders should emulate.

Cape Dory boats are not for everyone. By any standard, the 25 and the 25D are heavy displacement boats. Interior volume of both boats is substantially less than that of "modern" 25-footers due to their relatively narrow beam and short waterline. (By way of comparison, the Ericson 25 is almost three feet longer on the waterline and over a foot wider than the Cape Dory 25D, with almost identical displacement, ballast, sail area, and price.)

The Cape Dory 25 is really a daysailing and weekending boat. Although the boat has berths for 4, accommodations are cramped and creature comforts minimal. The 25D is a very different concept. She is a miniature cruising yacht. Inevitably she will be compared to that star of an earlier generation of pocket cruisers, the Laurent Giles-designed Vertue.

CONSTRUCTION

Construction of all boats in the Cape Dory line is similar. Hulls are moderately heavy solid glass layups of mat and woven roving. Ballast in all cases is a lead casting. The casting is carried in a hollow keel molding, with voids between the casting and the molded shell filled with polyester slurry. The casting is heavily glassed over on the inside of the hull. While the workmanship and materials used in these ballast installations are excellent, we prefer an external, bolted-on lead casting for its shock absorbing qualities.

Decks and cabin tops are cored with end-grain balsa. This results in a firm, stiff surface with good sound-absorbing and insulation properties. Gelcoat quality of the 25 and 25D is excellent. Light roving print-through is evident, but there are neither external hard spots nor evidence of distortion of the hull from the attachment of the deck.

Cape Dory uses a wide internal flange for attachment of the deck molding. The deck is joined to the hull using a semi-rigid polyester compound. This joint is also reinforced by the screws which attach the toe rail, by the through-bolts of the pulpits and lifeline stanchions, by the chainplate bolts, and by deck hardware bolts. Our belt and suspenders approach to construction would prefer through-bolting of the joint at close intervals in addition to the chemical bond and random fastening.

Cape Dory's chainplate installations merit special comment. On the 25D, shrouds are attached to cast bronze lugs which rest on the deck, over the hull/deck flange. Each of these lugs is bolted through the flange with two 3/8" diameter stainless steel machine screws. On the underside of the hull flange, a heavy aluminum plate is glassed into place, using unidirectional roving which also extends down the inside of the hull.

This is an immensely strong installation for a boat of 5,000 pounds displacement. The chainplates are less prone to leakage than conventional flat bar plates bolted to bulkheads. The only disadvantage of this system is that it locates the chainplates at the outboard edge of the deck. This gives the shrouds a wide base for supporting the mast, but interferes with close sheeting of overlapping headsails.

All Cape Dory rudders are hung from the back of the keel. The primary advantages of this type of rudder is strength and relative invulnerability to damage. The only real drawback to Cape Dory's rudder installation is that dropping the rudder for repair is fairly complex. The cast bronze heel fitting must be removed by grinding off the heads of its fastenings at the base of the keel. Then the rudder and stock are pulled out from below, necessitating either a deep hole under the boat, or lifting the boat with a Travelift while the rudder is being removed. Fortunately, repairs should be infrequent, and most can be made without removing the rudder.

All deck hardware is through-bolted using stainless steel bolts and aluminum backing plates. The forestay fittings on both the 25 and 25D are heavy bronze castings, as are cleats, winch islands, and portlights.

We have one reservation about Cape Dory's hardware installations. The mixture of bronze castings, stainless bolts, and aluminum backing plates strikes us as less than ideal. While the deck hardware is not immersed in an electrolyte, there is a difference in voltage potential between the aluminum backing plate and the manganese bronze casting. The type 304 stainless fastenings are relatively inert, but they do join very dissimilar metals. Below the waterline, Cape Dory uses silicon bronze fastenings in their bronze castings.

The Cape Dory 25
61

Seacocks are used on all through-hull fittings below the waterline on the 25D, including head intake and discharge, cockpit scuppers, engine cooling water intake, and galley sink drain. Engine exhaust and bilge pump discharge exit through the transom, and have no provision for shut-off. On the 25, bronze ball valves are used in place of seacocks.

The 25D uses a full molded hull liner which incorporates all the major furniture components. Interior trim and systems are installed in the liner before it is fiberglassed into the hull. The liner itself is a heavy solid layup almost as thick as the hull. The only disadvantage to the full hull liner is limited access to the inner surface of the hull in the event of damage. Bilge access in the 25D, for example, is only through a small trap in the main cabin sole. Repairs requiring access to the inside of the hull skin will require major surgery.

The general standard of workmanship in Cape Dory boats is very good, and both the 25 and 25D display this standard. The 25D, with its emphasis on serious cruising, is a far more complex boat than the 25 in both systems and construction. The 25D is probably one of the strongest boats of her size on the market.

PERFORMANCE

Handling Under Sail
While both the 25 and 25D are cruising boats, neither is a dog under sail. Owners of the 25 report average speed compared to boats of similar size.

Thanks to a ballast/displacement ratio of almost 43 percent, the 25 is a reasonably stiff boat, despite her narrow beam and slack bilges. Stability is enhanced by a short, low aspect-ratio rig. Owners report that a 150% genoa is a must to keep the 25 moving in light air.

The 25D may actually have better performance potential than the 25. The 25D's rig is substantially more modern in design, with a mast 4-1/2 feet taller than that of the 25, a J-measurement over a foot longer, and a higher aspect mainsail. The extra six inches of draft, nine inches of beam, hard bilges, and 350 extra pounds of ballast should make her quite stiff.

The 25D comes with a recessed inboard jib track, as well as the rail-mounted genoa track common to both boats. Both also have full width mainsheet travelers mounted at the aft end of the cockpit.

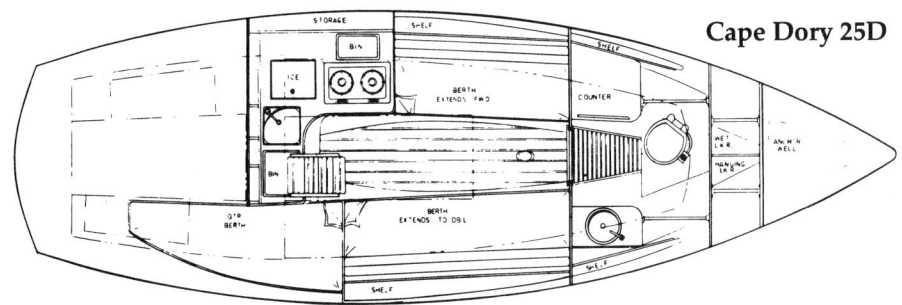

Cape Dory 25D

Cape Dory boats of 30 feet and under come with factory supplied sails built by several different lofts. Though the stock sails may be adequate while you're learning to sail the boat, they may not be when you become interested enough in good performance to appreciate the difference between a mediocre suit of sails and a really good suit. With either the 25 or 25D, the first sail you'll want to add to the boat is a 150 percent genoa, no matter where you sail. A lot of sail area can compensate for a lot of wetted surface when sailing in light air.

Both the 25 and 25D have deck-stepped masts. In the 25, most of the mast compression is carried by the main cabin bulkhead. In the 25D, an aluminum compression column directly under the mast transfers the rig compression to the keel. Cape Dory's support systems for deck-stepped masts are among the best we've seen.

The mast on the 25D was originally designed to step through to the keel. The sales department feared that a large mast tube in the main cabin might turn off potential buyers, so the mast tubes were shortened, and a complex deck stepping arrangement was incorporated.

The main boom of the 25 is equipped with roller reefing, a method of sail reduction that has, thankfully, just about vanished. Jiffy reefing, which is standard on the 25D, is preferable to roller reefing in almost every way.

In performance, neither the 25 nor the 25D will be mistaken for a racer-cruiser. Nevertheless, the owner concerned about improving performance can make real improvements by fairing in through-hull fittings, wet sanding the factory-applied KL-990 bottom paint, and adding higher-performance sails.

Handling Under Power
A major difference between the 25 and 25D is their mechanical propulsion systems. The Cape Dory 25 has an outboard well at the aft end of the cockpit, while the 25D has inboard diesel power.

The outboard engine installation of the 25 is less than 100% successful, according to owners responding to a *Practical Sailor* reader survey. The cover to the engine compartment must be kept open to provide adequate air for the outboard engine when running under power. The engine well resonates loudly, making the 25 noisy under power.

The 25 will accommodate engines up to 15 horsepower, but the most commonly used engines are the Johnson and Evinrude 9.9 horsepower units, which

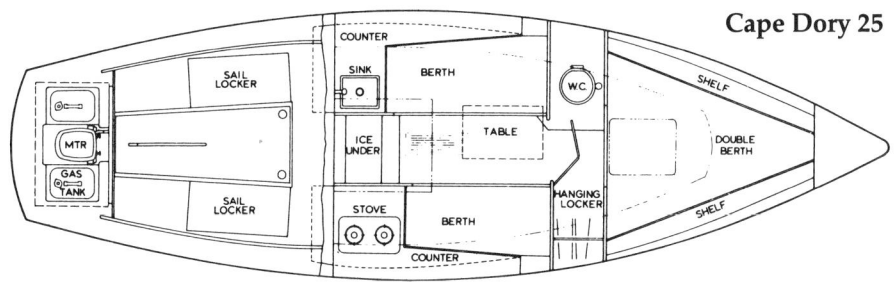

Cape Dory 25

The Cape Dory 25

provide more than adequate power for the boat. The engine's location aft of the rudder means that there is no prop wash against the rudder to multiply rudder effect at slow speed. Coupled with the 25's long keel, this means that the boat will be slower to respond under power than a modern fin keeler of similar displacement. Handling the 25 in reverse is a problem, according to owners. A large percentage reported in our survey that the boat "doesn't maneuver in reverse worth a damn."

The 25D has a conventional inboard engine installation, using a raw-water-cooled Yanmar 1QM 7-1/2 horsepower diesel. At 154 pounds, this is one of the lightest small diesels available. The 13-gallon fuel tank, mounted under the cockpit, should give the 25D over 50 hours of operating time under power, or a range of about 250 miles.

A two-bladed solid bronze prop is standard, tucked in an aperture at the aft end of the keel. The aperture extends into the rudder, which will cause some cross ventilation and a slight loss of rudder efficiency under sail. The 2.62:1 reduction gear should allow the little engine to achieve full power in driving the 25D.

The engine installation is excellent, and meets ABYC standards for the installation of gasoline engines, as well as the far simpler standards for diesels. A lift-out plastic storage bin in the top of the engine box is removable for routine service of belts and filters, as well as for checking the oil level. More complete access to the engine can be gained by removing the companionway ladder and the plywood front panel of the engine box. The compartment is not sound-proofed.

LIVABILITY

Deck Layout
The 25 and 25D share a simple, uncluttered deck layout, although the 25D has some features lacking in the 25. The 25D has a large foredeck anchor well capable of holding the normal working ground tackle for the boat. The 25D's stemhead casting incorporates an anchor roller. We would add a large eyebolt to the anchor well to secure the bitter end of the anchor rode.

While the 25 has a single centerline foredeck cleat, the 25D has twin cleats outboard of the well. Bow lines should be secured to the cleat on the opposite side from the bow chock to avoid blocking access to the well.

You can have any hull and deck color from Cape Dory as long as it's Cape Dory off-white and tan. The white of the cabin house is a warm brownish white, and will not unduly reflect light on bright days. Tan non-skid areas avoid the desolate appearance of white on white found on some boats.

The 25 and 25D both have teak toerails and rubbing strake, teak cabintop handrails, and teak cockpit coamings. We strongly recommend that these be kept in good shape by the application of a teak dressing. Despite the fact that teak is reasonably forgiving of neglect, it does require some maintenance to avoid warping and checking.

Bow pulpit, stern rail, and single lifelines are standard on the 25D. A bow pulpit is standard on the 25, but lifelines and stern rail are optional. The 25D incorporates Aqua Signal international-style running lights in the pulpits.

Cockpits of both boats are large and reasonably comfortable, although the coaming sides are vertical rather than being slanted at an angle more conducive to comfortable seating. Older models of the 25 had a low cockpit sill, with the lowest companionway drop board six inches above the cockpit sole. Newer models have a substantial bridgedeck.

Both the 25 and 25D have large cockpit scuppers leading to through-hull fittings with shut-off valves. The scuppers are properly located at the forward end of the cockpit, which prevents flooding by the quarter wave.

There are large lockers under both cockpit seats on the 25. The 25D has a shallow locker to starboard over the quarterberth and a deep locker to port. Access to the stuffing box on the 25D is through the port locker.

The tiller on both boats takes up a lot of the cockpit whether sailing or at anchor. A few 25Ds have been delivered with pedestal steering, which seems a little presumptuous on a boat this size, but does free up the cockpit for seating.

With a good solid bridgedeck, big scuppers, and a companionway that is almost parallel sided, the 25D has a cockpit suited for offshore use, although its volume is at the upper limit for a small boat. The use of plywood drop boards is rather disappointing on a boat of this quality. A properly made solid board is as warp-free as plywood, and certainly looks better.

Belowdecks

The most obvious difference in the two boats is down below. The 25 is a minimal short-term cruiser for two adults and two children, while the 25D has a genuine cruising interior for a couple.

The 25 has what could best be described as "stooping headroom." The forward cabin has a sharply tapered V-berth that is too small for two normal sized adults. Immediately aft is a cramped toilet compartment, divided from the V-berths by a curtain and from the main cabin by folding doors.

The main cabin settees doubles as berths. Actually, they are berths doubling as settees, as there are no backrests for comfortable sitting. Because the galley sink hangs over the foot of the port settee, owners report that as a berth it is only comfortable for a fairly short person.

The galley consists of platforms port and starboard at the foot of the settees. The starboard platform can hold a two burner stove, which is optional, or can be used for navigating. The port counter contains the aforementioned sink. There is a small icebox under the companionway step.

Stepping from the 25 to the 25D is a confusing experience. On a marginally larger hull, Cape Dory has produced a boat with an interior that a couple could find comfortable for fairly extended cruising. Without substantially raising either freeboard or cabin trunk, the 25D has headroom of about five feet eleven inches. One way this has been accomplished has been by dropping the cabin sole well into the bilge, gaining headroom at the cost of cabin sole area. In this case, it's a fair trade-off. The only real impingement into the headroom is the teak finishing piece for the overhead companionway hatch, which extends down a full two inches. Many people will find this a real headcracker.

The interior of the 25D is unusual in that a forward cabin has been eliminated, and a huge head, which can be fitted with a shower, installed in the space that would otherwise contain a cramped berth. The head compartment has headroom of 5'9", two hanging lockers, a small sink, and two solid towel rack/grab rails. Anyone who has spent any time in the head in rough weather will appreciate the grab rails. Although there is little storage space in the head for sheets, towels, medicine, or other small items, there are two large blank bulkheads crying out for the handy boatowner to install cabinets or shelves. The shower, if installed, drains directly into the bilge, an arrangement that leaves something to be desired. A Bomar hatch over the head provides good ventilation, as do the two opening ports in the head compartment.

Attractive is an overused word, but it is truly descriptive of the main cabin. The hull outboard of the settees is lined with an ash ceiling, a welcome change from the teak used by most builders. The main cabin settees extend through the head bulkhead into alcoves that form the dresser surfaces in the head. These alcoves are handy for storing bedding or other loose items under sail.

Cape Dory gets an A-plus for comfortable settees in the 25D. The settee backs are nicely padded, properly angled, and the settee tops have been reduced to the proper width for comfortable seating. For sleeping, the backs fold up on hinges and latch out of the way.

The starboard settee extends, with minimal maneuvering, to form a double, giving the 25D *nominal* accommodations for four adults. A 20-gallon polyethylene water tank is mounted under the starboard quarter berth — undeniably the best berth in the boat — but one that is likely to be used more for storage than sleeping when the boat is cruised by a couple. Ironically, this water capacity is four gallons less than that of the Cape Dory 25, which would presumably be used more as a daysailer.

With a little imagination, the galley of the 25D could probably be made far more serviceable for the serious cruiser. There is little storage space for any quantity of food, although there is enough room under the bridgedeck and outboard of the stove to create much more. The sink is tucked away under the bridgedeck, and is almost impossible to use. The fresh water pump is all but unreachable. The galley stove is a two-burner, recessed Kenyon alcohol model with integral tank, a type of stove about which we have grave reservations.

Cross ventilation of the main cabin is excellent, with four bronze opening ports. Cowl vents in dorade boxes should be fitted at the aft end of the main cabin for foul weather and offshore ventilation.

With the exception of the galley, the interior of the Cape Dory 25D is one of the most functional we have seen for a small cruising boat. Putting the head in the forepeak and eliminating the cramped V-berth are excellent ideas in a boat of this size. The lack of privacy in the head, a major complaint in small cruising boats, is a problem Cape Dory has solved in one bold stroke.

CONCLUSIONS

For two boats of similar size and type, the Cape Dory 25 and 25D are radically different. The 25 is a daysailer and weekender, with cramped accommodations. The 25D has the potential to be a comfortable long-term cruiser for a couple, with a roomy interior whose only real flaw is a mediocre galley arrangement.

Construction of both boats is solid, and they are well finished, although not perfectly so. Finish detail is substantially better than on Cape Dorys of five years previous. The 25D is tough enough to be a serious cruising boat.

Cape Dory boats are for traditionalists. In a time when traditionalism and conservatism seem to be growing in popularity, the popularity of boats such as those produced by Cape Dory is bound to grow. Yes, Cape Dory has found its niche in the market, and that niche isn't nearly as small as it was just a dozen years ago.

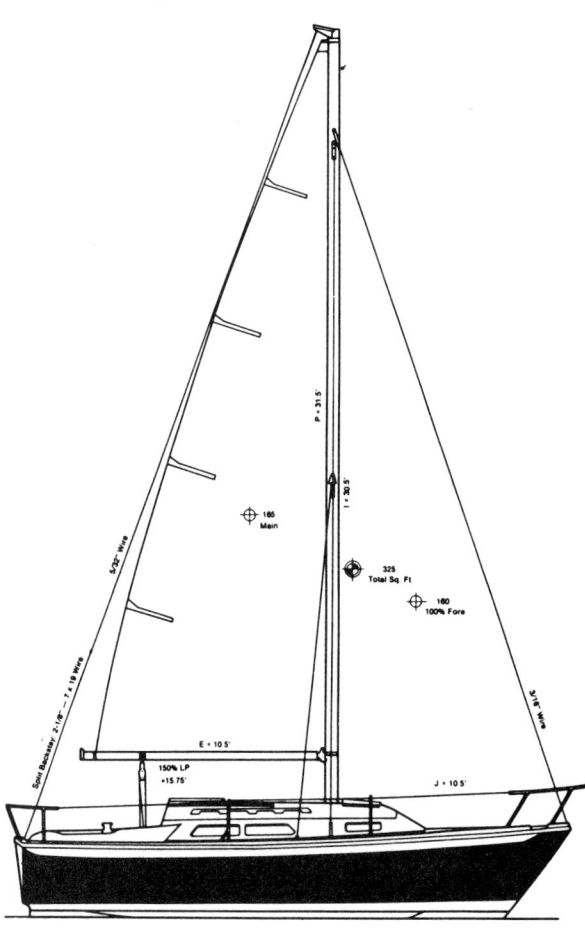

Specifications
Ericson 25

LOA	25'5"
DWL	21'10"
Beam	9'3"
Draft	
standard	4'11"
shoal	3'11"
Displacement	5000 lbs
Ballast	2000 lbs

Ericson Yachts
1931 Deere Avenue
Irvine, California 92717
(714) 250-7000

The Ericson 25:
Big Cruiser for the Small Family

THE BOAT AND THE BUILDER

Not too many years ago, the prospective buyer of a 25-foot sailboat knew that serious compromises awaited him. His 25-footer would probably have little more than sitting headroom, might have four rudimentary shelves masquerading as "berths," and have a head stowed under the V-berth. The galley? With luck, a two-burner alcohol stove, perhaps a sink, and a water tank holding ten gallons. Auxiliary power usually meant a six horsepower outboard hanging from a bracket on the stern, or in a well in the lazarette.

This wasn't anyone's vision of cruising heaven, of course, but the late '70s and early '80s saw economic developments that caused a rethinking among many who had been fantasizing about boats in the low to middle 30-foot range. Suddenly, as petroleum-inflated prices and astronomical interest rates became reality, economic necessity made the mid-twenty-footer a desirable target for many (opposed to no boat at all).

Enter the new generation of small cruising auxiliaries. Today the state of the art in modern 25-foot "family" sailboats has a six-foot headroom, berths for five (if privacy isn't a high priority), an enclosed head, and perhaps a diesel inboard — a veritable miniature yacht.

The Ericson 25+ is a good example of this current trend toward "more boat in less length." Proof of the popularity of this concept lies in her numbers. Over 660 units were built in the first three years after the Ericson 25+ was introduced in late 1978.

Designer Bruce King has enjoyed a long and successful relationship with Ericson Yachts, starting with the Ericson 23, 30, 32, and 41 of the late 1960s, and going on from there. He has not been Ericson's only designer, but the vast majority of Ericson's boats have come from his board. King and Ericson have found a formula not unlike that of Bill Shaw and Pearson: build a wide range of boats of similar type in two to three foot increments, develop customer loyalty, and watch the customers move up through the ranks. Keep the really popular models, such as the Pearson 35 or the Ericson 35, and bring out other models every few years to catch the latest trend. That formula works whether you're on the East Coast or the West, and like Pearson, Ericson has the formula down pat.

With the exception of a few forays into the cruising market with the clipper-bowed Cruising 31 and the Cruising 36 (later to be called Independence), the Ericson formula has been to produce a well-finished cruiser-racer with good sailing characteristics. The Ericson 25+ is the continuation of this successful formula.

CONSTRUCTION

The hull of the Ericson 25+ is a solid hand layup. A molded fiberglass body pan is glassed to the inside of the hull, functioning as the base for much of the interior furniture and adding to the rigidity to the hull. The deck, cockpit, and cabin trunk molding are balsa cored, with plywood replacing the balsa in high stress areas such as under the deck-stepped mast and where deck hardware is mounted. Exterior glasswork is of good quality, with little roving print-through. Gelcoat work is also good.

The hull to deck joint depends on a secondary chemical bond. Both the hull and deck have an external molded flange. Glass-reinforced polyester resin is used as a bedding compound between these flanges. The inside of this joint is then lapped with four layers of fiberglass mat and cloth. This joint is covered on the outside by a plastic extrusion with a soft plastic insert which functions as a rubrail.

The deck of the 25+ has a remarkably solid feel, thanks to its cored construction. Neither the deck, cockpit, nor coachroof has any of the sponginess frequently associated with small boats.

Deck hardware on the 25+ is well mounted. Stanchions, pulpits, cleats, and winches have adequate aluminum backing plates. The tiller head is a substantial chrome-plated bronze casting. The transom is cored with plywood, greatly adding to its rigidity.

The mast of the 25+ is a black, deck-stepped extrusion. The stainless steel mast step looks surprisingly fragile. Because the mast is designed to be owner-stepped if desired, the forward lower half of the base of the mast is cut away to allow the mast to pivot forward for lowering. The design of the mast step greatly reduces the bearing surface of the heel of the mast. We doubt, in any event, that there are many owners who will want to step their own masts.

In contrast to the mast step, the chainplates are of surprisingly heavy construction. The 25+ utilizes Navtec chainplates, shroud terminals, and turnbuckles. The chainplates are strongly tied to the hull.

All through-hull fittings below the waterline have Zytel valves, made of a reinforced plastic. Although modern plastics are strong, we suggest that you carefully inventory through hull fittings, as they are a major culprit in many sinkings of otherwise undamaged boats. Plastic valves may be immune to electrolysis, but they cannot be forgotten any more than bronze seacocks can be ignored.

PERFORMANCE

Handling Under Sail

Despite the chubbiness of the 25+, owners report that she is a fast boat under sail. There are a number of features that contribute to this speed. She has minimum wetted surface, despite a displacement that is average for her overall length (though fairly light for a waterline length of almost 22 feet).

The Ericson 25+, 28+, and 30+ all feature Bruce King's trademark, the "delta" fin keel. King states that this keel form has very low induced drag, and the 25's performance reinforces this belief. The optional shoal draft keel reduces draft a foot, reduces lateral plane, and no doubt reduces windward ability. Unless one is determined to have a boat drawing under four feet, the deeper draft version seems to be the better alternative.

The rig of the 25+ is a high aspect ratio 7/8 sloop rig. The mainsail hoist of 31.5 feet is unusual for a 25 foot boat. In light air, tall rigs are usually faster, and we would expect the boat's best point of sail to be upwind in light air. Since a great deal of sailing seems to be upwind in light air, this approach to the rig is a rational one.

With the addition of a backstay adjuster (a simple modification because of the split backstay) it is possible to induce a reasonable amount of mast bend to control sail shape. A full-width mainsheet traveler mounted on the cockpit bridgedeck greatly enhances mainsail control.

The chainplates are set well inboard, allowing narrow headsail sheeting angles. The genoa track is also located inboard, almost against the cabin side.

There is no main boom topping lift. We think this is pretty indefensible on a cruising boat, and despite the additional windage, a topping lift is greatly to be

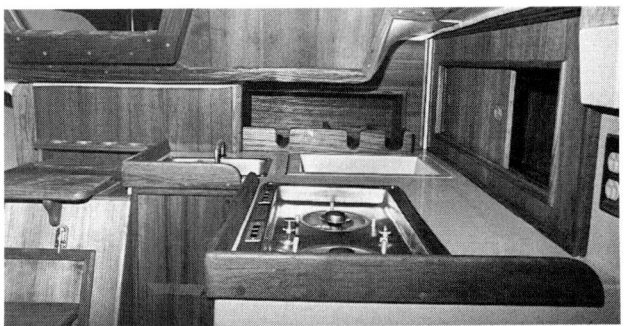
The galley is suprisingly complete for a 25-footer.

desired on a racing boat. Without a topping lift, reefing becomes a real exercise in agility. Dropping the mainsail is greatly complicated, especially when cruising short-handed. Should the main halyard break when sailing close hauled, the main boom could injure anyone sitting on the leeward side of the cockpit.

Two-speed Barient headsail sheet winches are now standard. There is room on the cockpit coamings both for the addition of secondary winches for spinnaker handling and the replacement of the standard winches with larger ones. A single halyard winch is mounted on the mast. There is no main halyard winch.

The 25+ should sail with almost any other production cruiser-racer of her size. Her wide beam and deep draft should offset the additional heeling moment of the tall rig. Like all wide modern boats, she should be sailed on her feet. Get the crew weight out on the weather rail in a breeze, and she should carry sail well.

Handling Under Power
There were probably more power options for the 25+ than any similar-sized boat on the market. They included: outboard power, OMC gas saildrive, Volvo diesel saildrive, and Yanmar diesel inboard.

The 25+ is small enough to be driven fairly well by a 10 horsepower outboard. There is about a $3500 difference in equipping the boat with an outboard engine versus the diesel inboard. The choice depends largely on how the boat is to be used. Few boats of this size are used for long-distance cruising. For daysailing and racing, an outboard engine is more than adequate.

If extended coastal cruising is to be the boat's primary activity, then one of the inboard options should be considered. Frankly, we have little love for saildrive installations. If you really want an inboard engine, the new Yanmar single-cylinder inboard diesel is the real choice. At resale time, the Ericson 25+ with diesel inboard in good condition is likely to be worth about $2000 more than the same boat with an outboard. As a pure investment, choosing the diesel would appear to be an irrational decision. At the same time, the boat equipped with an inboard diesel is a very desirable package, one that will definitely be more salable in the future.

No matter which engine is ordered, the boat is equipped with a 20-gallon aluminum fuel tank. With a one-cylinder diesel engine, given a four-knot cruising speed and fuel consumption of about 1/4 gallon per hour, the range under power is almost 350 miles — a truly astounding range for a 25 foot boat. That's probably more range under power than the average boat is likely to need for an entire season.

LIVABILITY

Deck Layout

With shroud chainplates set well inboard, and a reasonably narrow cabin trunk, working on the deck of the 25+ is fairly easy. There is adequate room between the shrouds and the lifelines to walk outboard of the shrouds with ease.

There is a small foredeck anchor well, adequate for the stowage of a single Danforth and rode. There are no bow chocks, but there are two cleats located forward at the outboard edge of the deck.

Molded-in nonskid of color contrasting to the primary deck color is standard. This relieves eyestrain in bright sunlight and reduces the basically austere external appearance of the boat.

The cockpit of the 25+ is comfortable. Coamings are angled outward rather than being vertical, allowing a more natural sitting posture. As in most tiller-steered boats, the sweep of the tiller occupies a large percentage of the cockpit volume. In port, the tiller swings up and out of the way, providing uncrowded seating for up to six adults.

A single cockpit scupper, 1-1/2 inches in diameter, is recessed in a well at the back of the cockpit. The well allows water to drain on either tack. A stainless steel strainer over the scupper reduces its effective area by over 50 percent. A single 1-1/2 inch diameter scupper has more cross sectional area than two one inch drains, and is less likely to clog. We would, however, be inclined to remove the strainer for sailing.

There are two cockpit lockers. The starboard cockpit locker is a shallow pan, suitable for storing small items such as winch handles and sail ties. At its after corner in a deeper bin which makes a handy icebox for cold drinks. The port locker is a large, deep affair which suffers from the common failing of not being adequately separated from the underside of the cockpit area. A snap-in Dacron bag would convert this locker to reasonable sail stowage.

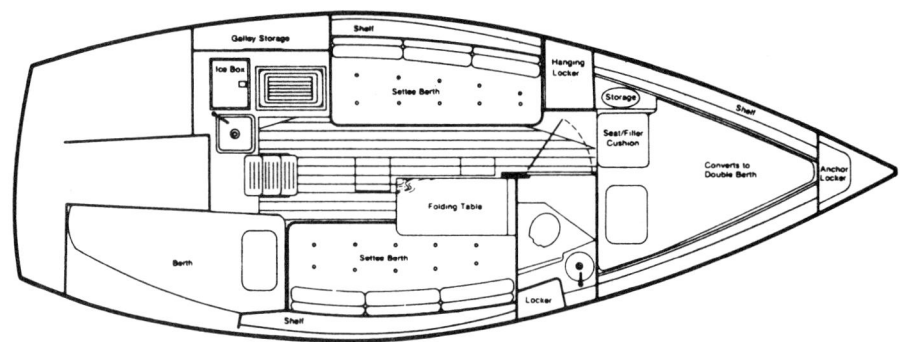

The companionway uses thick, solid teak dropboards with proper step joints to prevent water from working below. Unfortunately, the very strong taper to the companionway slides allows them to be removed by lifting less than an inch. For sailing in rough water, a positive means of securing these slides — a sliding bolt, for example, should be installed.

It is gratifying to see a real bridgedeck in a boat this size. Except for the strong taper to the companionway sides, this is one of the best designed cockpits we have seen in a small boat.

Belowdecks

The amount of interior volume in the 25+ is truly remarkable. The boat easily has the headroom and elbow room of most 30-footers of ten or fifteen years ago.

The forepeak contains the usual V-berth with filler to form a nominal double. We truly mean nominal — two normal-sized people do not fit in the forward berth of the Ericson. Consider it a large single, or a double for two children. Water and holding tanks occupy the space under the berth.

The 25+ has a genuine enclosed, stand-up head, an almost unheard of luxury in a boat this size. The head has an opening port for ventilation. There are two small lockers in the head, but both are largely occupied by plumbing hoses. Opposite the head is a small hanging locker. This locker is fully lined with teak plywood, a nice finishing touch.

It is in the main cabin that the 25+ really shines. Headroom is an honest six feet. Two comfortable settee berths seat six in comfort. A fold-down drop-leaf table is big enough to serve four, and is one of the sturdier tables of this type that we have seen.

The main cabin is well finished with a combination of off-white fiberglass and teak. This is a very successful decorating job, with just enough teak to give a well finished appearance, but not so much as to create a dark, cave-like interior. Hull ceiling of teak strips is now standard, and the cabin trunk sides are veneered in teak. A teak and holly cabin sole is standard, with two access hatches to the bilge.

There is a real bilge, unusual in a boat of this size. The strum box (strainer) for the cockpit-mounted Whale Gusher pump is accessible through one of the cabin sole hatches.

Under the settee on each side of the cabin there are storage bins. These utilize molded polyethylene drop-in liners, a most practical solution which recognizes the reality that under-seat storage is rarely completely dry. An optional extension to the starboard settee converts it to a double berth, but at the expense of easy access to the storage bins underneath.

The galley is surprisingly complete for a 25-foot boat. There is a well-insulated icebox of five cubic foot capacity. The insulation is exposed in the port cockpit locker, and will be vulnerable to damage from items stowed there. It could easily be sealed off with either plywood or fiberglass to protect it. The icebox lid is an uninsulated molding advertised as a "removable serving tray."

The Ericson 25

If it is used as a serving tray, then the icebox is uncovered, of course, allowing the ice to melt.

There are storage lockers both above and below the galley counter. The stove is a recessed Kenyon two-burner alcohol unit with a cutting board cover. These stoves have the fuel fill located between the two burners, and we feel they are a poor choice for use aboard a boat. The burners must be absolutely cool before the fuel tank is filled to eliminate the possibility of explosion or fire.

A human-sized quarterberth is a welcome feature. With adequate headroom over, it eliminates the coffin-like aura of so many small-boat quarterberths, and is without a doubt the roomiest, most comfortable berth on the boat. With an outboard engine, the room under the cockpit that would normally house an inboard is given over to storage. The tiny one-cylinder Yanmar diesel would easily shoehorn into the same space.

Without a doubt, the interior of the Ericson 25+ is a real accomplishment. It is well finished, generally well designed, and remarkably roomy for a boat of this overall length. There is some miniaturization of components, such as the galley sink, head sink, and hanging locker. Nonetheless, she's a big little boat, and would be truly comfortable for extended coastal cruising for a couple. That's something that can rarely be said for a 25-foot boat.

CONCLUSIONS

Ericson has come very close to achieving their goals in the 25+. She is about as much boat as can be crammed into this overall length.

An interesting option is an E-Z loader trailer. With a beam of over 9' and a weight of 5,000 pounds, the 25+ is no trailer-sailer. It takes a large, powerful car or truck to tow a boat of this size, and the beam could present legal problems in some states. The trailer would be most useful for taking the boat home for winter storage, rather than frequent over-the-road transport.

Workmanship and finish detail are generally of good stock boat quality. Exposed joinerwork is good. Fillet bonding varies from good to only fair, with the glasswork generally good.

The Ericson 25+ is probably a good example of something to be seen more and more often as slip prices, fuel prices, and boatyard prices increase. She is a good small cruiser for a young family, and offers enough sailing performance to be a reasonable choice for club racing.

Unlike many small cruiser-racers which concentrate on interior volume and forsake sailing ability, the 25+ really will sail. This means that the new sailor will not quickly outgrow her as he learns to make the boat go fast.

With good hardware, such as Barient and Navtec, and a fairly high degree of finish detail, it is easy to see why this boat sold at nearly $30,000 sailaway with outboard power, and considerably higher with inboard. For those used to the less costly 25-footers, this price was sometimes a shock. At maximum price for her length, she was never intended as an example of "more for less." But, as Ericson has pointed out, there are no free lunches in the world of sailing.

Production of the Ericson 25+ ended in 1984 when the Ericson 26 was intro-

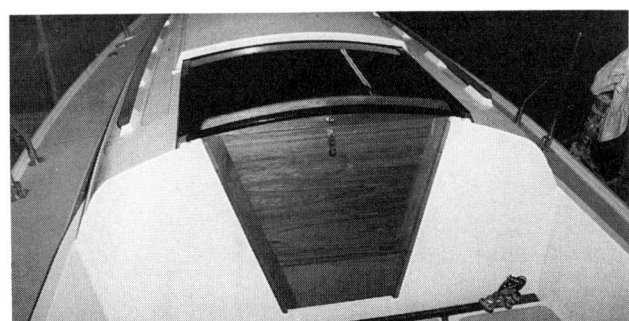

The sharp companion-
way taper mars an
otherwise fine cockpit.

duced. The Ericson 26 uses the 25+ hull, but incorporates a number of deck and interior refinements. Base price of the Ericson 26, depending on freight, will run about $27,000.

With an inboard diesel, a good light air rig, and lots of interior volume, she's a good little cruising boat for a couple. A maximum boat in minimum length, she represents a good solution to the high cost of sailing.

The Ericson 25

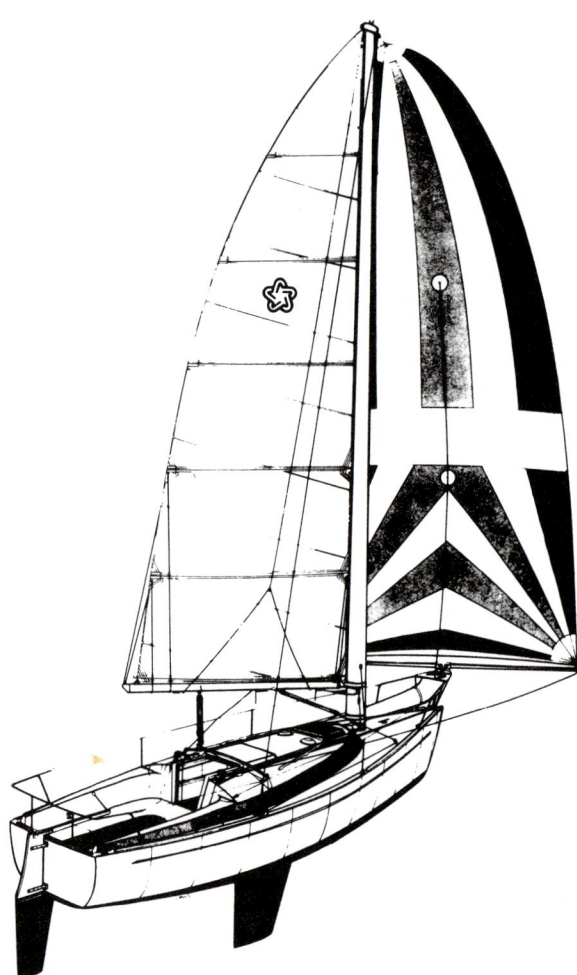

Specifications
Freedom 25

LOA	25'8"
DWL	20'0"
Beam	8'6"
Draft	4'5"
Displacement	2500 lbs
Ballast	1025 lbs
Sail area	260 sq ft

Freedom Yachts
Bend Boat Basin
Newport, R.I. 02840
(401) 683-3500

The Freedom 25:
Wave of the Future

THE BOAT AND THE BUILDER

"Why evaluate the Freedom 25," you might well ask. There are many more popular 25-footers around, but none of them scream for attention like the Freedom 25. She was truly a radical departure from the run-of-the-mill cruising daysailer. Her unstayed mast is still the trademark of the Freedom line, and has spawned several less sophisticated imitators. The Freedom 25 takes this trademark a step further—such a giant step in fact—that we suspect it will take some copycat rigs years to catch up. Because some of her innovations will be showing up on more conventional sailboats in the future, we think she deserves documentation as a legend—or at least a technical breakthrough—in her own time.

Garry Hoyt was the moving force behind Freedom yachts, which are built by Tillotson-Pearson. (See the subsequent Freedom 33 evaluation for more on Hoyt and Tillotson-Pearson.) Hoyt's unusual career began when he retired from his advertising executive position (and championship one-design sailing exploits) to look for a cruising boat that performed well and handled easily. He couldn't find one that suited him. The typical racer-cruiser didn't satisfy him because racing rules dictate stayed masts and multiple headsail—which are difficult for a shorthanded cruising crew to handle. "Uncompromised" cruising boats err in the other direction, he felt, tending to be undercanvassed and overweight, which make them slow and sluggish, especially upwind.

Hoyt's solution was the unstayed mast with wrap-around sails and wishbone booms. The unstayed mast offers strength and simplicity—no maintenance, no worry about losing the rig to a cracked turnbuckle, an so forth. "Airplanes did away with stayed wings 40 years ago," argued Hoyt. The wraparound sails helped overcome the aerodynamic drag of the larger section of the unstayed mast (albeit at doubling the cost of a sail and causing chafe problems.)

A line of Freedoms, beginning with the Freedom 40, were designed by Hoyt (with help by professional naval architects like Halsey Herreshoff) with his unstayed, wrap-around rig. Except for the Freedom 44, none had fin keels; hence, upwind performance, especially in light air, was less than sparkling. They did perform well off the wind however, and true to Hoyt's predictions, were easier to handle than boats with conventional sloop rigs.

When Hoyt got the high-performance bug, his ever creative mind wandered off in a different direction. After years of co-designing Freedoms, he drew the lines for a 25-footer by himself. In the time since the first Freedom 25 was built, the boat has undergone a radical metamorphosis. She started with a foot less freeboard, a ketch rig with wrap-around sails set on two stubby unstayed masts, a bulb-ballasted daggerboard, hiking wings hinged outboard of the gunwale, and the earliest version of the Gun Mount spinnaker pole system. Hoyt managed to get a MORC rating and entered his creation in the 1980 Block Island Race Week. However, upon planing into the harbor on a reach, Hoyt aroused enough consternation among his competitors to get his rating revoked (hiking wings and wrap-around sails did not fit "the rule").

Hoyt also learned at Block Island that, although his 25 was a flyer on a windy reach, she was just as lacking as the larger Freedoms upwind. So the ketch rig was discarded, in favor of a single, wing-shaped, rotating mast, made of wood by the Gougeon Brothers. This wooden mast was so heavy that it nearly capsized the little 25-footer. It was removed from the boat and used as a plug to mold a lighter spar out of carbon fiber. These spars were too light; Hoyt broke the first seven prototypes before finding the optimum section.

Somewhere during the lengthy story, Hoyt decided that his racy 25-footer would never collect in the number required for one-design racing, nor would

The Freedom 25
77

the evil arbiters of "the rule" ever allow her to compete in handicap races. So he raised the freeboard, added a keel and an interior, and made her the little cruising boat with the funny rig that she is today.

Hoyt made a wise choice in Tillotson-Pearson as the builder of the Freedom line. Not only is Tillotson-Pearson a leader in the development of balsa-core sandwich construction (they build J/Boats as well as Freedoms), but they also have extensive experience with carbon fiber, having made tennis rackets and oars of that material. This experience enabled Hoyt to replace the aluminum masts standard on the early Freedoms with a lighter and stiffer spar of carbon fiber.

Coincidental with the development of the Freedom 25, Tillotson-Pearson was also tooling up for the production of large fiberglass windmill blades. This defrayed the research and development costs needed to fabricate the Freedom 25's wing mast. There are very few, if any, production boat builders who have the technology to laminate unstayed masts of carbon fiber. Tillotson-Pearson and Hoyt appear to have cornered the market.

CONSTRUCTION

Construction of the Freedom 25 is comparable to that described later in this volume in the evaluation of the Freedom 33. Tillotson-Pearson's construction is among the best in the production boatbuilding industry. The boat's hull and deck are cored with balsa, which offers the advantages of a lighter, more rigid hull that is less prone to condensation and deadens sound better than an uncored hull. The hull to deck joint is the standard Tillotson-Pearson inward turned flange, sealed with semi-rigid 3M 5200 adhesive and bolted through the teak toerail — a strong, seaworthy system.

The external, 1025-pound fin keel is bolted into a small but adequately deep sump. In their years of building J/24s and J/30s, Tillotson-Pearson has learned to build rudders and rudder fittings strong enough to withstand heavy air. The Freedom 25's outboard rudder has gudgeons and pintles beefy enough for a 30-footer.

Tillotson-Pearson does not part easily with details of the construction of their carbon fiber spars. From what we understand, the spars, which are hollow, are not molded in two separate halves and joined together because the resulting

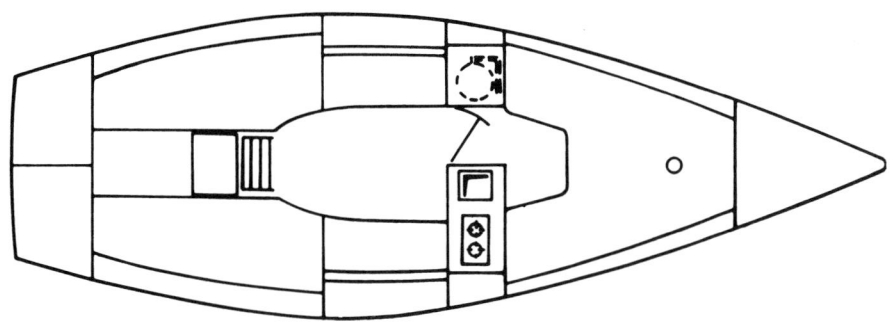

seam would be a weak point. Unidirectional carbon fiber is laid onto an inflatable bladder, and then a mold is clamped around it. When the bladder is inflated, it "vacuum bags" the mast into the shape of a wing. The mast is sanded smooth before being painted with polyurethane. A plastic sail track is then riveted to the trailing edge of the wing.

While the idea of a mast without stays might be unsettling to some sailors, there is no need to worry as long as the mast step, partner, and section are properly engineered. This engineering is relatively simple with a round, non-rotating wing mast. The 25's wing section begins above deck; below deck it is round, to enable it to bear evenly on the step and partner. A wing section is inherently strong in the fore and aft plane, but it is susceptible to side bend because it is so thin in the athwartships plane. There are two ways to break an unstayed wing mast; either sail upwind in a strong breeze with an unreefed main and the mast rotated in the wrong direction (right angles to the boom), or set a large staysail from the masthead without the support of running backstays. Both of these mistakes put extreme side loads on the mast. Running backstays were part of the optional spinnaker package. The builder said the 135-pound mast had a safety margin which allowed it to withstand an accidental casting off of a backstay in winds up to 25 knots.

To allow free rotation and prevent excessive wear and tear on the step and partner, the Freedom 25's mast is stepped in a stainless steel bearing race and sleeved at the deck with Delrin. Maintaining those two pressure points should be infinitely easier than the upkeep on all the standard rigging of a conventional spar. The mast fittings are fastened with aluminum rivets, and bedded with 3M 5200 adhesive sealant. Bedding is essential, as Tillotson-Pearson claims that corrosion of aluminum in contact with carbon fiber is even more severe than aluminum in contact with stainless steel. The gooseneck lever controlling rotation was bolted to early masts, creating a weak point that caused several to fail. This lever was glued on in later models.

PERFORMANCE

Upwind

We doubt that there is any cruising boat with a more efficient rig than the Freedom 25. Wing masts have been used for years on catamarans and iceboats because the drag of a wing is so much less than a conventionally shaped mast. A typical cruising boat mast usually creates enough turbulence to render the forward quarter of the mainsail useless, reducing effective sail area. A round unstayed mast, as is used on the larger Freedoms, is larger in diameter than a stayed mast, so drag can be even worse.

A wing mast, however, causes little turbulence because it is so thin in the athwartship dimension. When a wing is rotated so it is aligned in the plane of the leading edge of the mainsail, it acts as an extension of the sail and effectively increases sail area. This is how the Freedom 25 can be efficiently powered by a 260 square foot mainsail alone, while comparably sized, conventionally rigged boats usually have more sail area in their combined main and working jib.

A wing spar must be able to rotate independently of the boom. To align with the mainsail's leading edge it must be rotated about 20 degrees beyond the boom's angle off centerline. Sail trim fanatics might want to adjust the rotation slightly as they adjust the draft of the mainsail, or to affect the side bend of the mast. The Freedom 25's rotational control line has no purchase, so it is difficult to adjust.

The independent rotation of the Freedom 25's wing mast, although necessary for good performance, does create some minor problems. While sailing, mainsheet tension keeps the mast in place. However, when the mainsheet is lightly trimmed in light air the mast has a tendency to swing as a powerboat wake or big sea passes under the boat. Whenever the boat is not sailing, the mast must be lashed to keep it from rotating back and forth.

When tacking in a strong breeze, the mainsheet must be eased to allow the mast to rotate. If it doesn't rotate, the leech puts extreme side load, instead of fore-and-aft load, on the tip of the mast if the mainsail is not reefed. This shouldn't be a problem with the Freedom 25 as she begs for a reef in winds over 15 knots.

As is common on boats with wing spars, the Freedom 25 has a fully battened main. Full-length battens make the mainsail an almost rigid airfoil — the sail never luffs. Luffing is quickly destructive to a sail. Because the Freedom's sail won't luff, it should last two to three times as long as a conventional sail (and all this at nearly half the price of a wrap-around sail.) This sail is also easier to furl. As Hoyt says, it folds like a venetian blind, between the lazy jacks rigged at either side of the boom.

The problem with full-length battens is that, because the main won't luff, the boat doesn't slow easily when docking, mooring, or anchoring under sail. Owners tell us that they have to drop the main before they make a landing, and sail the rest of the way on the power of the wing spar. (Owners also tell us that the wing spar makes the boat sail back and forth on the mooring.) This difficulty in landing is offset by the Freedom 25's maneuverability. (Like a J/24, she turns in her length.) However, most sailors will take the security of the optional inboard engine.

Mainsail trimming on the Freedom 25 is different from that of a conventionally rigged sloop. If you center the boom, trim the mainsheet hard, and pinch her (like a jib-headed boat) you will go nowhere. Like any catboat, you have to let the boom out over the quarter, twist the leech, and foot the boat. Since the full-length battens don't allow the sail to luff as you feather into the wind, you have to sail by telltales placed on both sides of the sail, a few inches back from the luff — just as you would with telltales on the jib of a sloop-rigged boat.

When Hoyt designed the Freedom 25's rig, he envisioned a boat that would go to windward like a J/24, yet handle with the ease of a catboat. Despite the efficiency of her wing spar, the Freedom 25 still lacks the windward ability of racing sloops in her size range. This is most noticeable in light air. However, she is the equal of any cruising boat and she does handle with virtually no effort. (We have heard that Hoyt is experimenting with "spoiler" foils attached to the wing to accelerate the wind flow on the leeward side of the mainsail, as would a jib.)

The Freedom 25's reefing system, although not a new idea, is nonetheless ingenious. We wish all boats had it. Instead of using a hook or a separate line for securing the tack, there is one continuous line to secure both the tack and the clew. It runs from the clew, through the boom, then out a

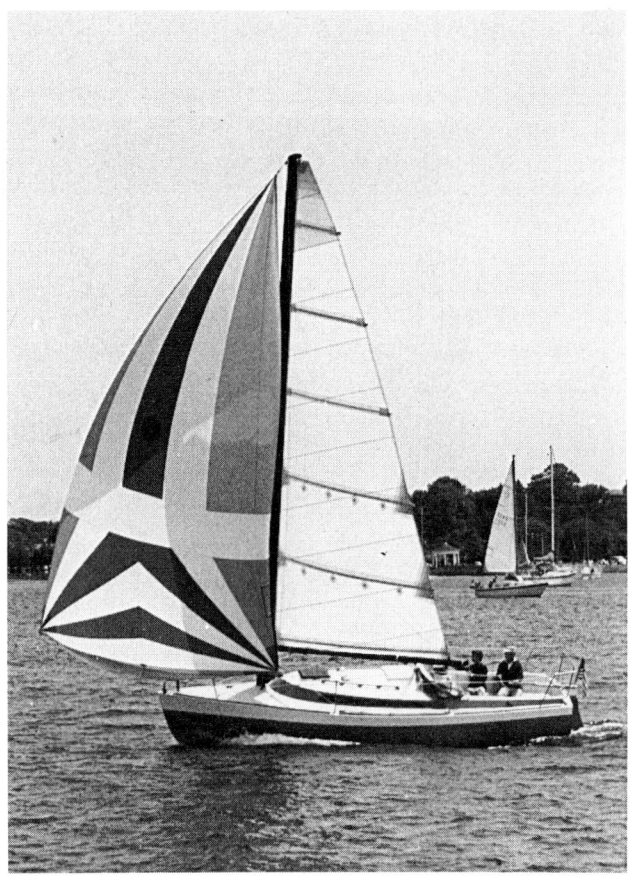

sheave at the gooseneck, up through the luff grommet, then back to the base of the mast and aft to a stopper. Ease the halyard and pull this one line and the sail is reefed in seconds—without sending a crewmember out of the cockpit.

Offwind

On a broad reach the Freedom 25 is at least the equal of most racing boats in her size range, and she blows the cruisers out of the water. Her speed can be attributed to her relatively light, 3500-pound displacement, and the positioning of most of her sail area well forward in the boat. The patented Gun Mount puts most of the spinnaker forward of the bow. The result is a boat that has virtually no tendency to round up on a heavy air reach. Even in a strong puff the rudder does not load up as it would on a sloop-rigged boat with a normal length pole. With the Freedom's unstayed mast, you also don't have to worry about wrapping the spinnaker around the headstay.

We were skeptical of the Gun Mount at first. It's hard to believe that anything that looks so awkward and complicated can possibly live up to its billing. The Gun Mount, which consists of an oversize spinnaker pole run through a sleeve on the bow pulpit, rests on the lifelines when not in use. You can't store it on deck, so visibility is always obstructed. The spinnaker is hoisted out of, and retrieved into, a long sock tied to the deck. The spinnaker feeds into the sock via a wide-mouth plastic scoop hung on the bow pulpit. This adds to the visibility obstruction, but the scoop and sock can be removed for storage below deck.

There are 16 lines leading back to the Freedom 25's cockpit—nearly twice as many as you might find on another 25-foot daysailer (the builder specifies over 500 feet of line for the Freedom 25). Ten of those lines are needed for the optional Gun Mount package. However, if you can overlook the cluttered bow, and keep the rat's nest of lines coiled, the Gun Mount works like a charm.

To set, jibe and douse the spinnaker, you never have to leave the cockpit. You adjust two lines to center the pole in the Gun Mount, then pull two more lines to haul the clews of the spinnaker to the ends of the pole, and then set one of the running backstays if it is windy. To ease the task of hoisting, it helps to put the boat on a reach so the spinnaker will luff. Once up, the spinnaker is fixed to both ends of the pole. You adjust the pole with two "reins." Because the pole is balanced, there is absolutely no pressure on either rein, and there is no need for winches to trim the sail. You can jibe at will, and adjust the pole at your leisure as there is no tendency to round up.

We took the Freedom 25 for a long sail on a tight reach in a shifty breeze. When the wind shifted aft we hoisted the chute. When it shifted forward, we took it down. We must have done this every five minutes for nearly an hour — and all without leaving the cocking or raising a sweat.

There are a few drawbacks to the Gun Mount. Aside from its windage and obstruction of visibility, the Gun Mount works poorly on a beam reach, because as one end of the pole is let forward for tight reaching, the other end of the pole pulls the clew almost into the mainsail. This so closes the slot that the sail tends to stall. If you sail without the spinnaker, the boat is just as slow. A separate staysail is needed for tight reaching.

The other problem with the Gun Mount is that *it makes flying the spinnaker too easy*. Sailors without much heavy air downwind experience are tempted to set the spinnaker in winds of 20 to 30 knots, because the boat is so easy to control. However, if you should accidentally jibe and slam the boom against the running backstays, or accidentally let off one of the backstays, you stand a fair chance of breaking the mast. If the spinnaker hoists were 3/4 of the way up the rig, instead of at the masthead, or if there were diamond shrouds to control side bend, the mast would be far less likely to fail. (In fact, on a Freedom 21 currently under development, there were plans to use a wing mast with a 3/4 spinnaker hoist.)

If you are thinking that you might want a Gun Mount on your current boat, you might as well forget it. Hoyt is not selling Gun Mount kits, although he is planning to license certain builders to offer the Gun Mount as an option on their own boats. The Gun Mount wouldn't work well on sloop-rigged boats, because the headstay would interfere with the launching sock. Hoyt admits that the Gun Mount was an "afterthought" on the Freedom 25, and says he might recess the sock and funnel into the hull on future models. If this were done, we don't see why he couldn't also remove the lifelines forward (you never leave the cockpit anyway), and lower the pole and Gun Mount to deck level to improve visibility.

Handling Under Power

Inboard power was a $4600 option. The Freedom 25 is probably as large a boat as can be powered with an outboard engine. We don't think anyone—especially if there is a tendency toward back problems—should try to lift a large outboard over the transom. This effectively limits the potential outboard to 4.5 horsepower, not really enough for a boat of this size. We therefore favor the inboard option. The Yanmar 7-1/2 horsepower auxiliary offered with the Freedom 25 has a Martec folding propeller, weighs only 154 pounds, and pushes the boat at more than six knots.

The inboard is mounted under the companionway, the top step of which lifts for supposed access to the oil dipstick. However, try as we did, we could not reinsert the dipstick without removing the whole engine box. This difficulty will tempt owners not to check the oil as frequently as they should. The engine box removes easily, but is heavy and awkward to reset on its mounts. Access to the engine is relatively good, however, with the box removed.

Even though the propeller shaft is mounted slightly off center to compensate for the pull of its rotation, the boat still pulls hard to one side when the engine is opened up. You can't let your eyes off the compass for a second without wandering off course. If you release the tiller, even momentarily, the boat will fall off into a screaming 360-degree spin. In short, it's a lot more work to power a Freedom 25 than it is to sail one. Like most single-cylinder diesels, engine vibration is excessive at low RPM. Fuel capacity is 10 gallons for a range of about 100 miles.

LIVABILITY

Deck Layout

The center of all activity on the Freedom 25 is the cockpit. Those 16 lines that constitute the running rigging lead into the cockpit through Easylock stoppers to Barient #10 winches mounted on either side of the companionway. The Easylock stopper has a clutch action that enables you to cast off a line without taking up the tension on a winch, a feature that helps the Gun Mount work so handily. We recommend installing several cloth bags on both sides of the companionway to separate and store all of the control lines.

It's a good thing that you never have to leave the cockpit to sail the Freedom 25; with the mast stepped on the foredeck, the Gun Mount and spinnaker sock occupy the little remaining space. There is no anchor well, although there is plenty of space to set one into the huge forward locker. However, unless the funnel for the spinnaker sock is unhooked from the bow, access to an anchor well would be difficult. You cannot store the anchor on a bow roller either, for the exposed prongs of the anchor could tear the spinnaker. Luckily, the ground tackle needed for a 25-footer is light enough to be easily carried from a cockpit locker to the bow.

The cockpit of the Freedom 25 has deep seats, with a substantial coaming for dryness and security, and angled seat backs for comfort. There is backstay to obstruct the cockpit. The cabin table is portable and can be used in the cockpit, fitting easily and securely onto brackets attached to the transom. The tiller lifts out of the way to let 4 to 6 people eat in comfort.

The mainsheet traveler is mounted over the companionway hatch. To minimize visibility obstruction, the builder used a low-profile traveler by Harken. Although the traveler is bent to match the camber of the deck, it is not radiused to follow the swing of the boom. If it were radiused, the mainsheet might not have to be eased during a tack to allow the mast to rotate. The traveler is easily adjusted by the helmsman, but the mainsheet is just out of reach. We would recommend that owners install a boom knocker cam cleat on the end of the boom, and lead the dead-ended part of the mainsheet to it.

The running backstays were led to cam cleats in the cockpit in early Freedom 25s, but after losing several masts, the builder later installed Barient #8 winches for extra safety. There are two low-profile Beckson ventilators mounted on the coachroof, and a Lexan hatch made by Gray.

Belowdecks

The Freedom 25 has what we feel is an attractive and sensible interior. She does not have standing headroom. To have standing headroom, a 25-footer must have either a high cabin house, which can be ugly, produce excessive windage, and limit visibility from the cockpit; or it must have deep bilges, which often means poorer performance. A six-foot person can move freely about the cabin of the Freedom 25 in relative comfort, though stooping is required.

There is has an enclosed head, which we feel is almost essential for comfortable cruising. Instead of the portable toilet common on most small cruisers, the Freedom 25 has a Groco head, which is equipped with a Y-valve for overboard or holding tank discharge.

The interior is trimmed in blond-colored ash, which lends a more open appearance than teak. The cabin sole is teak and holly, and the companionway steps are also teak. There is ash veneer on the settee berth risers, so they are easily blackened with scuff marks from shoes, and any salt water that may penetrate the finish will discolor the wood.

The settees in the main cabin have straight seat backs, which make for comfortable seating, but less comfortable lounging. The portable cabin table is fastened to the companionway steps with Faspins. When the table is set up, you have to climb over it to leave the cabin. Stepping on it is no worry, though, as it is one of the sturdiest tables we've seen on a sailboat of this size.

The settees extend aft under the cockpit, and widen into quarter berths that *could* be used as double berths in a pinch. The forward cabin is enclosed by the door to the head and contains a V-berth divided in half by the mast. There is a bulkhead separating the head and main cabin from the V-berth. To make it easier to climb through the opening in this bulkhead, the front of the V-berth is cut back. This not only completes the separation of the V-berth's occupants, it also makes the halves of the berth uncomfortably narrow. One owner we interviewed has added a filler cushion across the front of the berth so he could sleep with his mate.

The galley consists of a small sink with a hand pump and a two-burner, pressurized alcohol stove by Seaward. It can be a chore to use a galley in a boat without standing headroom. To solve this problem, the Freedom 25's galley is laid across the main bulkhead, so you can work at the galley while sitting on the settee. There is space under the sink for a medium-sized cooler. Storage space is ample, but the absence of a good clothes locker means you will be living out of a duffel bag. If you forego the inboard option, you gain storage space under the companionway.

There is no headliner on the Freedom 25. The overhead is sanded and finished with white gelcoat. All the deck fastenings are exposed for easy service. Bolts are capped with barrel nuts. On the boat we sailed, the finish was smooth in the main cabin, but unusually sloppy for Tillotson-Pearson around the companionway and cockpit.

CONCLUSIONS

We think the Freedom 25 is a pretty neat little boat. She's well built. Her interior is pleasing to the eye and comfortable for weekend cruising. The interior joinerwork is well above average. She provides reasonable performance upwind, and a real thrill downwind—and all for much less crew effort than is required by a conventionally rigged boat. While she is a great coastal cruiser and singlehanded daysailer, the Freedom 25 is not a trailer sailer. With her fin keel and heavy, keel-stepped mast, she is not easily launched from a trailer without a crane. There are also few cars on the road today that can easily handle her 3500 pounds.

The Freedom 25 was not cheap, but she was less expensive than many contemporary 25- and 26-foot pocket cruisers. The base price was $21,900; the inboard a $4600 option; and the Gun Mount a $1200 option. Sails ran about $1400 for the main, $750 for the spinnaker, and $100 for the spinnaker sock. This meant that the sailaway price was still under $30,000.

The Freedom 25's rotating unstayed wing mast, fully-battened mainsail and Gun Mount spinnaker may be a bit too radical for the boat to be widely accepted in this decade. After all, it took Garry Hoyt nearly ten years to convince the public of the merit of the simple unstayed mast and wrap-around sail found on the older Freedom models.

While production of the Freedom 25 ceased in 1985, the rationality of her founding principles are validated by the fact that Tillotson-Pearson stands today as one of the rare success stories among sailboat builders during the mid-1980s. Today they're building (and selling) Freedom 28s, 30s, 36s, and 42s—all of which contain many of the ideas pioneered by the Freedom 25.

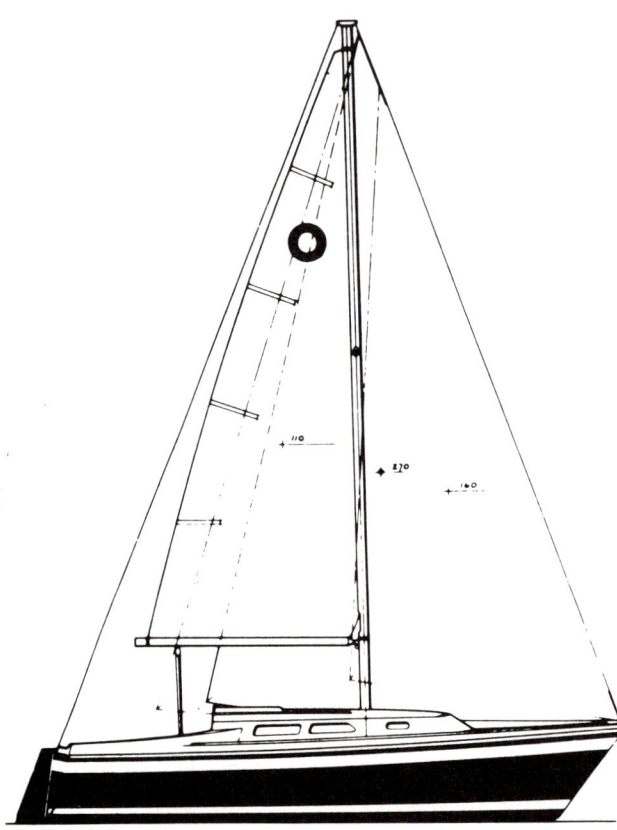

Specifications
O'Day 25

LOA	24'10"
LWL	21'0"
Beam	8'0"
Draft	
centerboard	2'3"
keel	4'6"
Displacement	
centerboard	4007 lbs
keel	3962 lbs
Ballast	
centerboard	1825 lbs
keel	1775 lbs
Sail area	
centerboard	270 sq ft
(100% foretriangle)	
keel	290 sq ft
(100% foretriangle)	

O'Day Yachts
848 Airport Road
Fall River, Mass. 02720
(617) 678-5291

The O'Day 25 and The Montego 25: A Tale of Two Cruisers

THE BOATS AND THE BUILDERS

The O'Day 25 was one of the most successful of all 25-footers. Almost 3000 were built during the first eight years of its production. The O'Day 25 tried to be all things for all people; the all-purpose 25-footer with short or tall rig, deep or shallow draft, and with inboard or outboard power.

In trying to be the 25-footer for everyone, the O'Day 25 made a number of compromises:

• Beam was limited to 8 feet for uncomplicated trailering.

• The shoal draft version lacked the stability to carry the tall rig the boat needs for really good performance.

• The boat was heavy enough to require a large, awkward-to-handle outboard engine.

At the same time, the sheer volume of production of the O'Day 25 meant it was a boat whose costs were kept to a minimum, a boat with an established market value and good resale potential, and a thoroughly debugged boat.

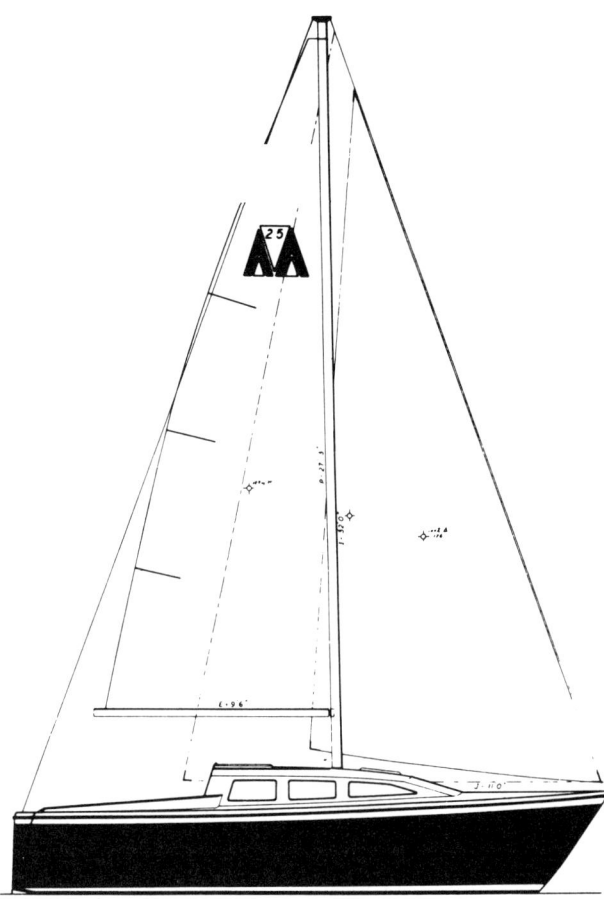

Specifications
Montego 25

LOA	25'3"
LWL	20'6"
Beam	9'1"
Draft	
standard	3'6"
deep	4'6"
Displacement	4550 lbs
Ballast	1800 lbs
Sail area	306 sq ft
(100% foretriangle)	

Offshore Technology
7921 Bradenton Road
Sarasota, Florida 34243
(813) 351-7747

These were all important considerations for the prospective buyer of a 25-footer, who might also be looking forward to owning a 27- or 28-footer a few years down the line.

In addition, the keel-centerboard version of the O'Day 25 provided a maximum-sized trailerable cruiser with adequate accommodations for normal vacation-length coastal cruising. This assumed, of course, that you had a vehicle capable of towing over 4000 pounds, in addition to a heavy trailer. Owners suggested a trailer rated for 6000 pounds—which added up to a big package for trailering.

By all indications it's a popular package. Almost 90% of the O'Day 25's sold have been the trailerable keel-centerboard version.

Surprisingly, fewer than half of the owners we spoke to considered shoal draft or trailerability of primary importance in their decision to buy an O'Day 25. This may be a reflection of a common phenomenon: Owners of maximum sized trailerables often find the hassle of trailering, launching, and rigging more than they care to go through for a day or weekend of sailing. After a year or two of this, the boat ends up in a slip or on a mooring.

With the Montego 25, the decision has already been made to move from a trailerable to a non-trailerable boat. Despite such characteristics as a shoal draft option and outboard power, the Montego 25 buyer makes a conscious commitment to move into a boat whose home for the sailing season will be a marina, rather than the driveway at home. The choice of shoal draft and outboard power for the Montego 25 are determined by the waters sailed and the depth of the buyer's pocket, rather than the need to keep weight and draft to a minimum for trailering.

CONSTRUCTION

The O'Day 25 and Montego 25 are generally similar in construction. Both are uncored hull layups with wood-cored deck moldings. The Montego 25 has plywood coring. The O'Day is cored with end-grain balsa.

Both boats use what we consider to be "small boat" hull to deck joints. The O'Day 25 uses a simple coffee can or shoebox joint, fastened with self-tappers and adhesive compound. The Montego 25 uses an outward-turning flange which is riveted and glassed over on the inside. Vinyl rubrails cover the hull-to-deck joints on both boats.

This is the maximum size boat suitable for external hull to deck joining. External joints are subject to damage in collisions or even in hard docking. Covering the external joint with a rubrail may give the impression that it's okay to use the joint as a bumper. It isn't.

Neither boat uses faired-in through-hulls. A handy owner can resolve this lack in a couple of hours using epoxy and microballoons and a little elbow grease. Gelcoat quality of both boats is good.

Although both the Montego 25 and O'Day 25 come in shoal and deep draft versions, their approaches to the problem are quite different. Both the shoal and deep draft versions of the Montego 25 use external cast iron keels, bolted to a shallow keel stub. On the deep draft boat we examined, the keel had been faired to the stub using fiberglass cloth, which had begun to separate from the iron keel in several places after a season of use.

Any dings in an iron keel, such as that of the Montego 25, should be ground to bright metal and coated with coal tar epoxy before applying bottom paint. Direct application of copper or tin bottom paint to an iron keel will create severe surface erosion if the boat is used in salt water.

The shoal and deep draft versions of the O'Day 25 are very different in character. To make the boat trailerable, the shoal draft O'Day uses a long, shallow keel stub with inside lead ballast. A centerboard gives additional lateral plane for going to windward, but adds little to stability. Over the years, O'Day has gradually added several hundred pounds of inside ballast to the shoal draft 25 in order to improve stability, which has, of course, increased the weight for trailering.

In the deep draft O'Day 25, a deep glass stub keel replaces the long, shoal keel box of the centerboard boat. A high-aspect-ratio fin keel is bolted to this stub keel, giving a substantial draft of 4'6". The external keel casting is lead, but

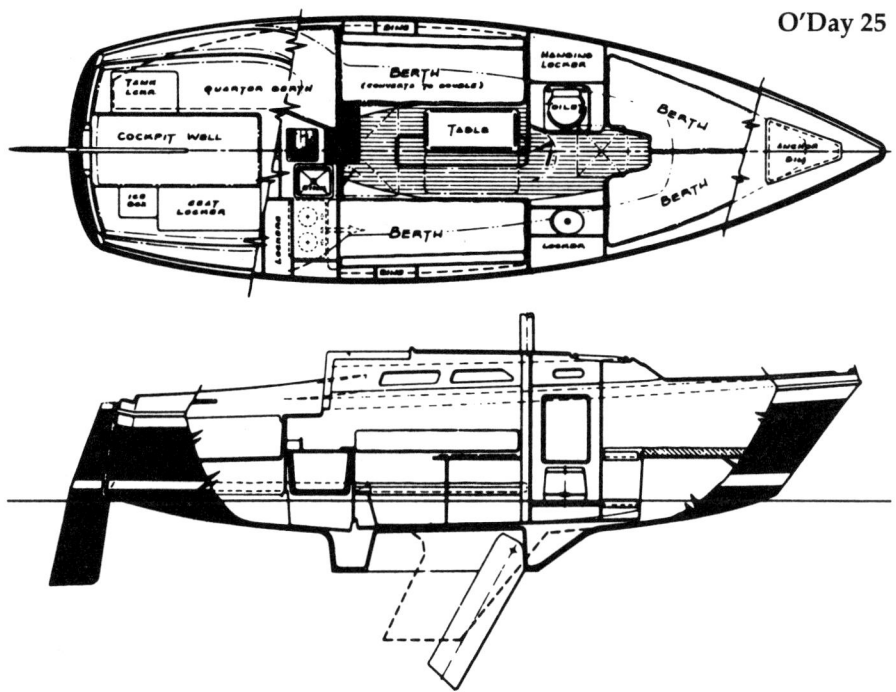

it took a little work to figure that out. Some at O'Day said the keel was iron, others insisted it was lead. The argument was settled by drilling into the keel casting. It is, we can report with confidence, lead.

It's a good thing that the keel is lead, because it needs a bit of fairing to improve efficiency. The trailing edge is blunt, and the keel casting is poorly faired to the fiberglass stub keel. Lead planes almost as easily as hardwood, so refairing the keel of the deep draft O'Day 25 is a simple task. Of the dozen or so deep draft O'Day 25's we looked at, about half the owners had taken the time to fair the keels. It should be worth the effort in improved performance.

Some owners report trouble with the rudder of their O'Day 25s. In the centerboard version, the rudder is five inches deeper than the keel stub. This means that the first part of the boat to contact the bottom when you run around could be the rudder. If you're moving along at a fair clip, a grounding can tear the rudder off the stern of the boat.

Construction of both boats is perfectly adequate for usage up to and including coastal cruising. We would not particularly want to take any boat of this size offshore, independent of the quality of construction.

PERFORMANCE

Handling Under Sail
The fin keel, tall rig O'Day 25 and the deep draft Montego 25 have identical PHRF ratings of 219. The rating of the O'Day 25 changes significantly with

different rig, keel, and engine combinations. The outboard-powered keel-centerboarder, for example, has a rating of 234, 15 seconds per mile slower than the deep keel, tall rig boat. This difference reflects the vastly different character of the two versions of the same boat. The deep keel boat has a more efficient lateral plane and a lower center of gravity, giving much better performance than the keel-centerboard model. Owners report the keel-centerboard boat to be tippy, and the fin keel boat to be stiff.

In addition, the tall rig of the deep keel boat gives slightly greater sail area—enough to make the boat a competitive family racer. Unless very shoal draft and trailerability are essential, the deep keel, tall rig version of the O'Day 25 is the obvious choice. The extra stability, extra sail area, and underbody efficiency add up to a boat that behaves more like a big boat than a small boat.

Both the deep keel and shallow keel versions of the Montego 25 are good performers. If the depth of your sailing waters allows, we would choose the deep keel version for the greater stability and extra lateral plane.

The rigs of the O'Day 25 and the Montego 25 are almost identical Kenyon rigs, but halyards of the Montego 25 lead aft to winches, while O'Day's winches are mast mounted.

These are big boat rigs, with substantial mast sections, airfoil spreaders, and good-sized standing rigging. Booms are set up for jiffy reefing. Mast fittings, tangs, and chainplates are substantially heavier than would be found on boats only marginally smaller.

In other words, these boats have transcended the "toy boat" syndrome so often seen on boats in the 20' to 25' range, and have rigs strong enough for more than fair-weather sailing.

Handling Under Power
The 4000-pound O'Day and 4,500-pound Montego 25 are at the outside limits for using outboard power. With high freeboard and no remote controls, starting and throttle operation are a bit of a nuisance, since the outboard must be mounted far down the transom to keep the prop in the water. Remote outboard controls are a must.

Most owners will use a 10-horsepower outboard on either boat. In a flat calm, it should easily be able to push the boat. However, once there is any wind or sea, the weight and windage of these boats mean that a 10-horsepower outboard is marginal. Unfortunately, a larger outboard is heavier, more expensive, and stretches the capacity of most outboard brackets.

The O'Day 25 has a molded-in outboard fuel tank holder in the port side of the cockpit. The Montego 25 has none, so right away you must figure out where you'll keep the gas tank.

There is a growing tendency to put small diesels in boats of this size. Both the Montego and the O'Day were offered with the Yanmar 1GM as optional auxiliary power. O'Day charged $3900 for this option, Montego $4500.

Inboard power adds over 100 pounds to the weight of the O'Day 25, compared to the outboard version. For a boat that's already pushing the upper

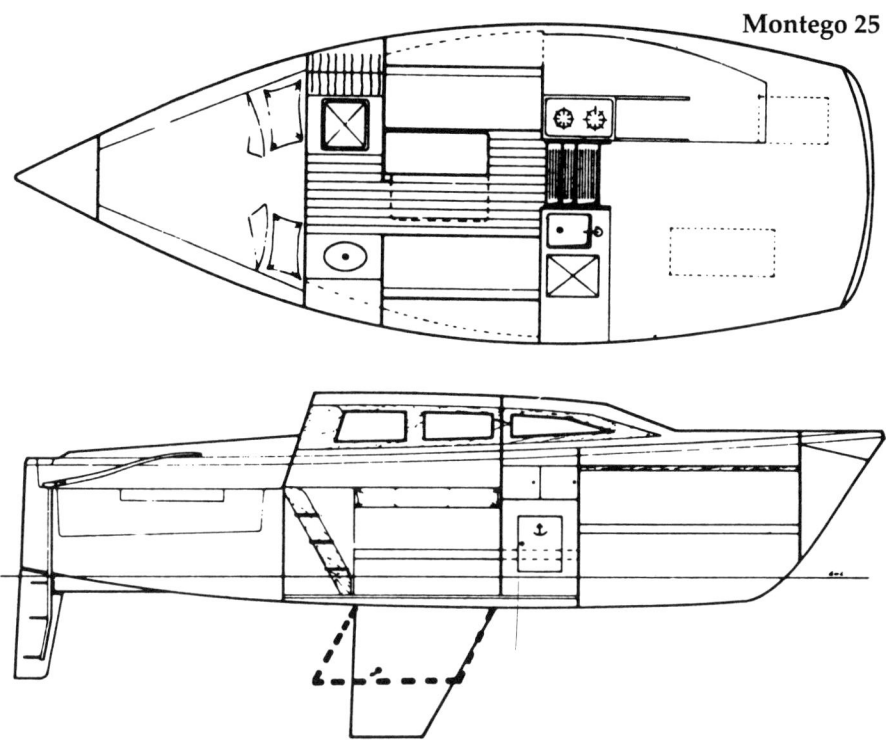

limit of easily trailerable weight, every pound hurts. However, inboard power greatly adds to either boat's function as a cruiser. If all your sailing is done on a lake where strong winds and seas are not likely to be a problem, inboard power is probably an unnecessary expense. On the other hand, if you plan to do a considerable amount of cruising along the seacoast or in the Great Lakes, the convenience, range, and power of an inboard engine begins to make sense.

If we trailer-sailed on Lake Lanier, Georgia, for example, we might choose the centerboard O'Day 25 with outboard power. If we kept our O'Day 25 on a mooring in Newport, Rhode Island, and cruised to Block Island, Nantucket, and the Elizabeth Islands, we'd be more likely to choose the tall rig, deep keel O'Day 25 or the deep keel Montego 25 with inboard power.

These boats are really at the break-even point for the inboard power option. Most of the cost of the inboard installation will come back at resale time, unless you sail in a small inland lake. A five-year-old outboard, on the other hand, adds little or nothing to the value of the boat.

LIVABILITY

Deck Layout
Neither boat has a particularly complicated deck layout. Both have an anchor-well forward, single lifelines, and a fairly large cockpit. Because its shrouds are

set well inboard, it's far easier to get to the foredeck of the Montego 25. The inboard shrouds should also produce narrower sheeting angles and give better upwind performance.

Both boats have cockpit seats long enough to double as fair-weather berths. Both boats also have substantial bridgedecks, fitted with a mainsheet traveler. The mainsheet traveler on the O'Day 25, however, is merely a flat piece of track with a slider. Several O'Day 25 owners said they'd prefer a ball bearing traveler, such as that on the Montego 25. We would, too.

The tiller on both boats takes up a lot of the cockpit. In addition, the tiller fitting of the Montego 25 we examined had a fair amount of play in it. O'Day 25 owners report the same problem. This can frequently be remedied by the owner.

Belowdecks
The trade-off between a trailerable 25-footer and one not constrained in beam by the highway laws is immediately apparent when comparing accommodations of the Montego 25 and the O'Day 25. The extra foot of beam of the Montego 25 gives the boat much greater interior volume than the O'Day 25. Much of the $4000 difference in price can also be explained by the interiors of the boats.

O'Day has mass production boatbuilding down to a fine art. Nowhere is this better demonstrated than in the interior of the O'Day 25. Much of the interior furniture is incorporated in the body pan. A fiberglass headliner finishes off the overhead. This saves a lot of time in building the boat, and therefore results in cost savings.

On the other hand, the Montego 25 also used a molded body pan, but not a deckliner. Instead, the inside of the cabin trunk was faced with teak veneer, and the overhead finished with a vinyl liner. The cabin sole of the Montego 25 is teak ply, and the boat has a solid teak companionway ladder and solid teak dropboards.

By contrast, the O'Day 25 has a fiberglass cabin sole, and uses a molded box step and the top of the galley counter as a companionway ladder. In other words, finish detail of the Montego 25 is better than that of the O'Day 25, and you pay a price for the difference.

Interior accommodations of the two boats are remarkably similar, but the extra beam of the Montego 25 gives greater elbow room. Headroom of the Montego 25 is almost six feet under the main hatch. The O'Day 25 has five-foot, six-inch headroom.

With V-berths forward, two main cabin settees, and a quarterberth, each boat sleeps five, although a slide-out settee in each brings nominal sleeping capacity to six.

Do you really want to sleep six on a 25-footer? Unfortunately, the "how many does she sleep?" syndrome is alive and well in both boats—at the expense of both storage space and galley space.

Both boats are large enough to have separate head compartments—separate from the main cabin, that is. The head is really part of the forward cabin on both boats, a not unreasonable compromise in a five-berth 25-footer.

Small boat galleys rarely offer much except headaches for the cook, and neither of these boats is an exception. The O'Day 25's icebox is tiny, and the auxiliary box in the cockpit is really a daytime beer cooler, and is almost cut in half by the centerboard pennant trunk. While the O'Day 25 has a deep sink, it is almost directly underneath the companionway. Coming below with the boat heeled on port tack, you're likely to put your foot in the sink.

The Montego 25 has a larger icebox with an insulated lid. The insulation for the lid is styrofoam, however, and is exposed on the underside of the lid. It is likely to suffer a lot of abuse.

The Montego 25 has a slide-away two-burner alcohol galley stove which stores over the quarterberth. It is slightly easier to use than the same stove on the O'Day 25, which must be removed from a storage compartment and set on the galley counter for use. Since cooking under way is barely practical on a boat of this size, the lack of gimballing for the stoves actually is not a serious shortcoming.

Both boats have a reasonable amount of storage, as long as you don't want to unpack your seabag. Under-settee storage bins, found on both boats, would be far more useful with drop-in molded plastic trays, which are better for keeping things dry. O'Day offered the plastic trays as an option in the 25.

CONCLUSIONS

Both the Montego 25 and the O'Day 25 are good examples of the transition yacht (boats for owners wishing to move up from trailer sailers to small cruisers). Both retain some small boat features—outboard power, shoal draft options—while having many of the basic components of larger boats. These big boat features include deep draft options, sturdy cruising-type rigs, inboard power options, enclosed heads, and permanent galleys.

The shoal draft version of the O'Day 25 is still trailerable, but it is at the outside limit of size and displacement. The compromises in performance to make the O'Day 25 trailerable—short rig, less stability, keel-centerboard configuration—make the trailerable version of the boat more of a "small boat" than a "big boat."

Adding factory options to the O'Day 25, to make the boat comparable in equipment and features to the standard Montego 25, brought the price up to $19,400 from the base price of $18,600. The Montego 25 cost $23,900 with the same equipment.

Part of the difference in price was explained by the 500 pounds difference in displacement of the boats. Boatbuilding materials cost money, and it costs money to incorporate these materials into a boat. Until you get into exotic, lightweight construction, a heavier boat will always always cost more than a light boat. Much of the rest of the difference in the cost of the two boats was the result of O'Day's use of modular components, the efficiency developed in the large number of O'Day 25s built, and Montego's greater attention to finishing detail.

Equipped with an inboard engine and a deep keel, either boat will make a good coastal cruiser for a couple with two small children. Putting more people on such a boat for anything but daysailing will be more like camping out than cruising.

At about $23,500, fully equipped and with inboard engine, the deep keel, tall rig O'Day 25s represented just about the minimum investment you could make in a new, inboard-powered pocket cruiser. For a couple or small family moving up from a trailer-sailer, either the O'Day or Montego 25s provide a true transition from the weekender to the legitimate pocket cruiser at a minimum investment. Unfortunately, both boats are currently out of production, but they are boats that deserve serious consideration by the used-boat buyer.

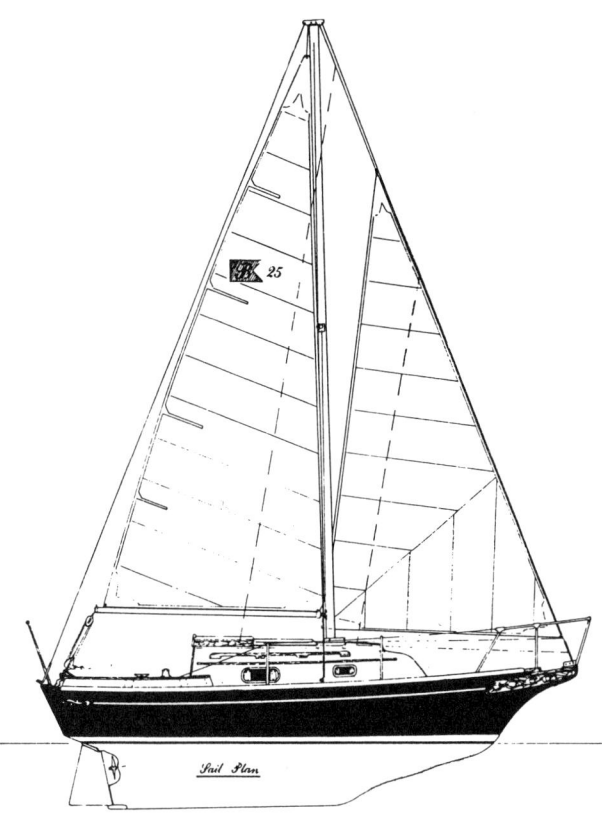

Specifications
Bayfield 25

LOA	25'0"
LWL	19'8"
Beam	8'0"
Draft	2'11"
Displacement	3500 lbs
Ballast	1300 lbs
Sail area	240 sq ft

Bayfield Boat Yard Ltd.
Box 1076
Clinton, Ontario
Canada NOM 1L0

Sail Plan

The Bayfield 25

THE BOAT AND THE BUILDER

It is rare when a boatbuilder, even a modest-sized one, builds a whole line of boats as identifiable as the Bayfield line. From 25 feet to 40 feet, the four models of boats built by Bayfield have almost identical proportions, styling, detailing, handling characteristics, and quality of finish, in a readily recognizable combination that has proven remarkably popular.

The styling of the Bayfield line may best be described as quasi-traditional: clipper bow with "carved" trailboards, raked transom, reasonable amounts of overhang, moderately low-aspect rig, a conventional cabinhouse profile, and squared ports. Underwater is a full length, relatively shallow keel with a cutaway forefoot and angled rudder.

All have displacement to length ratios that would be considered heavy. Moreover, with a generous solid fiberglass hull layup, molded headliners and hull liners, moderate ballast to displacement ratios (about 40%), there has been no apparent effort to keep displacement low.

The impression is thus of "solid" and "rugged" boats in keeping with their "seaworthy" traditional design. To some extent the impression is justified by reputation. The Bayfield boats don't seem to "break" and their owners, based on experience, seem to have considerable confidence in the ability of their boats to handle rough sea conditions.

With weight and tradition comes cost. The boats in the Bayfield line, compared to production boats of comparable size, are above average in price, a fact only partly ameliorated by the present favorable exchange rate of U.S. dollars versus Canadian dollars. Compounding this is the fact that the designated overall length of a Bayfield is a somewhat misleading figure. Because of the "artificial" way the clipper bow extends the length on deck, Bayfields are actually shorter than more "modern" boats with shorter overhangs; in spite of that fact, they have the interior space of other boats of their length overall.

Bayfield Boat Yard Ltd. is a family-type business with an impressive head in Jake Rogerson. He is a hearty, affable individual who has immense pride in his products and an uncommon enthusiasm in dealing with customers, potential and actual. Bayfield buyers are encouraged to visit the builder, call up with questions, and "keep in touch." There seems to have been a conscious attempt to control the growth of the Bayfield Yacht Yard to maintain this one-on-one relationship. As a result, owners and dealers alike report superb customer relations, no small reason why Bayfield has a better-than-average reputation as a builder.

Although we deal mainly with the smallest boat in the Bayfield line, the 25, much of what we see in the boat applies to her larger sisters. And what we see is an odd combination of good quality and mediocre details that may say much about cost, performance, livability, and construction of not just the Bayfield line, but a number of production boats touting their cruising features.

CONSTRUCTION

Amid the controversy over which smaller boats can be sailed offshore, many have tended to equate the Bayfield 25 with the Cape Dory 25D, a 25-footer we regard as capable of extended offshore passages. Superficially, the two boats do seem to resemble each other—more closely, that is, than more "modern" boats. They share a full length keel, traditional appearance, and reputation for rugged construction. But there are some notable differences.

The Bayfield 25 is 1,500 pounds (32%) lighter, carries 20 percent less nominal sail area, and has seven inches less draft. Actually the Bayfield 25 is not really a 25-foot LOA boat; subtract the clipper bow that in effect is merely a bowsprit

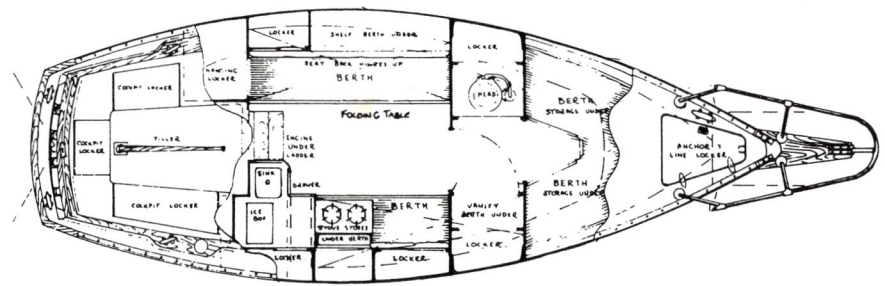

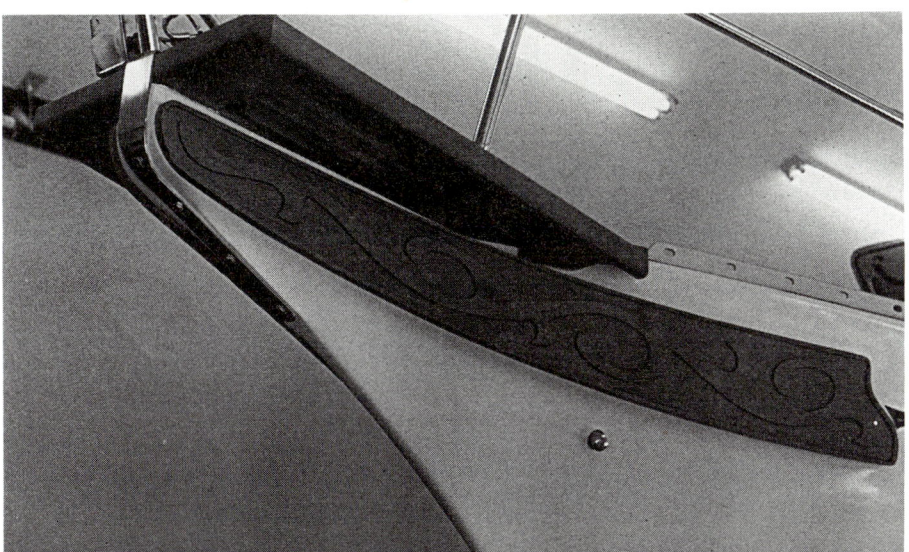

Trailboards give a distinctive traditional look to the Bayfield bow under a truncated platform/bowsprit.

and the 25 feet shortens to less than 24 feet. And that is what the Bayfield 25 is: a nominal 25-footer with the scantlings, performance, accommodations and proportions of a smaller boat.

But comparisons aside, the Bayfield 25 is built adequately for the use the majority of buyers have in mind when they look at her. Most mention coastal or Great Lakes cruising. The spaciousness of her cockpit, the lack of space for stores, and her modest overall size to our mind precludes offshore passages of any duration, but owners should find they have a boat built strongly enough for normal use of a 25-footer.

The full keel does afford a strong hull. As long as it is, the keel gives unsurpassed rigidity to the hull fore and aft. The keel also should have good resistance to grounding and facilitate hauling and storage in contrast to modern fin keel configurations.

The debate over the pros and cons of internal versus external ballast is waged throughout the boating world. There is no question that an external lead keel offers shock absorbing characteristics in the event of a hard grounding and damage from a grounding is usually easier to repair. On the other hand, in a sturdy full keel design like the Bayfield, the strength of hull, smoothness of bottom and lack of keel-bolts to leak and work loose make encapsulated ballast an advantage.

The deck is joined to the hull at the inward-turned hull flange at the sheer. The joint is bonded with a flexible adhesive sealant. The joint is then mechanically connected with stainless steel bolts through the aluminum toerail, the deck and the flange.

The deck is balsa-cored and stiff underfoot. The high crown of the large cabinhouse provides structural stiffness; the sidedecks are narrow and the small foredeck is stiffened further by the anchorwell. Upright structures such as the seat risers in the cockpit do have some flex. Similarly the interior liners are thin, unsupported laminates that serve a largely cosmetic function. However,

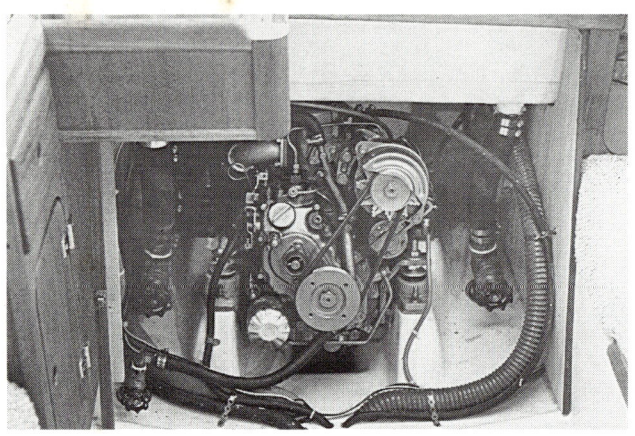

Engine accessibility in the 25 is no better, no worse than in the average boat. In short, wretched.

interior structural components such as bulkheads seem well tabbed to the hull and we detect no tendency of the hull to "oil can" or flex.

The deck-stepped mast is supported by a beam that carries the downward thrust to the main structural bulkheads. In boats under 30 feet or so, we see nothing inherently wrong with such a system, provided that the engineering properly distributes the loads, as it appears to do in the Bayfield 25. The arrangement has the significant advantage of leaving the interior, where space is at a premium, unobstructed by mast or mast support structures. The single chainplate for the upper and lower shrouds on each side is carried by the main bulkhead.

The cosmetic finish of the Bayfield 25 is average. There is noticeable print-through of the underlying glass roving in the topsides, a shallow (and barely adequate) stippled pattern as non-skid on the deck and cockpit, and a good deal of unrelieved white surfaces in cockpit, coamings, cabin sides, after cabin bulkhead and interior that strike us as needlessly antiseptic. We'd opt at least for a "non-standard" deck color in a pastel.

Exterior trim is teak, notably the slatted bowsprit and a taffrail supported by turned spindles. Add to these the capped coamings, half-round cabin trim, handrails on the house roof, and the trailboards, and the Bayfield sports enough wood trim to carry out the traditional styling theme. What is less attractive is the angled perforated aluminum toerail that is a conspicuous concession to modernity. We'd like to see a teak toerail offered as an option.

For all of the positive features of what is basically a tidy package for a 25-footer, there are some disturbing flaws. The rudder seems flimsy and poorly fitted with evident play at the tillerhead. The through-hull fittings are fitted with gate valves instead of seacocks. The sliding companionway hatch has a half-inch of athwartships play and is the worst we have seen on a production boat. The space in the lazarette is woefully obstructed with the likes of the bilge pump, hoses, the backside of the engine control panel, and too-long bolts

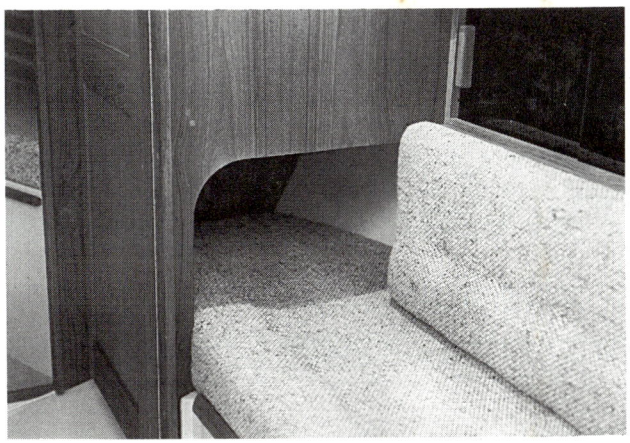

through the backstay chainplate. Likewise, the starboard seat locker is cluttered with batteries and engine controls, with nothing but the fuel fill hose to prevent its contents from sliding into the engine space under the cockpit. These are, of course, not serious complaints; rather they are curious—and obvious—weaknesses in a boat that other-

The starboard settee berth extends through the main bulkhead and under the sink in the head to give length as well as a nifty place to stow bedding.

wise seems better thought-out than many boats on the market.

PERFORMANCE

Handling Under Power

The 25's 7.5-horsepower Yanmar diesel turns a fixed three-blade prop in the aperture at the after end of the keel, assuring no problem with power or maneuverability in normal use. It will get the boat in and out of a harbor, home in light air, and even to windward in reasonable wind and seas.

Where owners complain is in backing down. Props in apertures are at their worst in reverse as they are operating in a confined space rather than in open water. Moreover, until the boat gains sternway so the rudder can be used to steer the boat, the torque in the prop dictates the direction the boat will turn, a problem compounded by the not inconsiderable windage of the hull and rig. Powering the 25 into a confined area such as a marina slip takes practice and care.

The weight and bulk of the Bayfield 25 plainly call for inboard power, which is consistent with its intended primary use as a cruising boat. Early models had tiny Vire gasoline inboard engines that are quieter and more compact than the present Yanmar diesels. Neither the Vire nor the Yanmar boasts accessibility. The engine is only accessible from the forward end through a removable panel/bulkhead at the companionway. In a timed experiment it took us 10 minutes to remove the panel, work the oil dipstick free of the engine, replace it (the hardest part of all) and put the panel back in place. As with many boats with poor accessibility, such a configuration hardly encourages monitoring the oil level.

Handling Under Sail

In these pages we have debated at length the issue of where performance under sail should fall in a list of priorities for a desirable boat. We maintain it should be at or near the top. That said, we will point out the most serious drawback we see in the Bayfield 25 (as well as the other boats in the Bayfield line): mediocre sailing performance. We are not impressed by the assertion of both the builder and owners that performance is not why they built the boat or why they own her. The point is that performance and displacement, comfort, aesthetics, and construction need not be mutually contradictory priorities.

The performance of the 25 is compromised in a variety of ways in a variety of conditions: in light air by excessive wetted surface and a three-bladed prop; to windward by a shallow keel and low aspect rig; in a breeze by her generous beam and considerable windage; and in choppy conditions by modest sail power.

Clearly, owners have decided—or learned—not to race. When they have raced under PHRF they sailed with a rating about the same as a Catalina 22, a clear indication that whatever are the Bayfield 25's virtues, good performance is not one of them.

Underwater, the drag of the excessive surface area is compounded by protruding through-hull fittings, an only partially faired prop aperture, a rudder with a blunt trailing edge, and an unfaired rudder heel fitting (the nuts on both sides protrude completely). It seems one thing to regard performance as a low priority; quite another to eschew the rather simple and inexpensive ways to improve it.

Clearly this is a boat that can benefit from a headsail of generous size to go with the small working jib that comes as standard. She can also benefit from slab reefing (standard), made quicker and easier by leading the halyards and reefing lines to the cockpit. Owners report adequate stability as the breeze increases but a disconcerting weather helm. Given the Bayfield 25's beam, the outboard trim of her jib, and her shallow draft, we can understand why she quickly acquires a strong weather helm. The best solution is to reef the mainsail as soon as the weight on the tiller becomes uncomfortable. Reefing plus the wide roller traveler (stock equipment) plus a well-cut genoa should do much to alleviate the weather helm and improve all-around performance.

Handling the Bayfield 25 under sail can be made easier in a number of other ways. First of all, do not bother with the stern pulpit option. The cockpit is deep enough to be quite snug without lifelines extending beyond the after end of the cabinhouse. If a stern pulpit is fitted, end the lower lifeline forward of the cockpit; further aft it interferes with the jib winches.

Run all halyards aft to the cockpit. The narrow sidedecks further obstructed by shrouds make going forward at any degree of heel more than a chore. When anchoring, position ground tackle in the bow roller chock before lowering he jib; horsing it out of its foredeck well and through the bow pulpit will be next to impossible with the jib on deck (perhaps a good argument for roller furling if the furling drum wouldn't present a different but equal impediment).

Because the question is sure to arise, we might do well to examine briefly the capabilities of the Bayfield 25 for offshore passages. Apart from the normal limitations on any boat of this size, there are some special concerns. One is the cockpit. It is large, carried well outboard, and well aft. Filled by a wave, it would probably make the 25 unmanageable, inviting further waves aboard. Worse still is the low sill at the companionway; regardless of its inconvenience, we would permanently seal the companionway to the height of the seats. Commendably the relatively narrow companionway has vertical sides to discourage the hatchboard from floating loose, and the after cabin bulkhead is vertical, discouraging rain and spray from getting below.

Regardless of the size of the boat, when sailing offshore a rig should have fore and aft support in mid-span (forward and aft lower shrouds) to prevent pumping in a heavy seaway. The single pair of lowers on the Bayfield rig terminate at the same chainplate as the uppers athwartships of the mast, thus giving no such support. This should only be considered a problem offshore. We are otherwise impressed with the spars and the 25's rigging.

LIVABILITY

As often as owners downplay—or ignore—the Bayfield 25's so-so performance, they extol her livability. Many report that her interior and cockpit space are the reasons they bought the boat. The 25 is a clear example of a larger yacht scaled down (as opposed to an enlarged daysailer).

Like most boats in this size range, livability has some limits. In a 25-footer with a generous beam, heavier displacement (hence "deeper" hull form), fair amount of freeboard, and large house, there can be spaciousness. Yet, the hull is only so long, regardless of its other dimensions, and the premium is on fore and aft space: it is hard to get full-length berths, an enclosed head, a galley, and a good-sized cockpit in a boat of this overall length. In the Bayfield 25 the problem is made worse by the loss of usable interior in the clipper bow.

As a result the forward V-berths come together in a sharp point; foot room for two people taller than about five feet is of the overlapping sort. The starboard settee berth offers foot room in the form of a niche that extends under the head sink. And the cockpit seats are barely over five feet long, too short for most adults who might yearn to sleep under the stars or nap on the leeward seat underway. For a young family the accommodations are satisfactory. For two couples they are too tight. And for one couple there is all the wasted space of unusable berths in the forward cabin.

There are additional, more subtle limitations. The athwartships head closes off from the main cabin with a hinged door, but not from the forward cabin. The "portable" galley stove, which stows under the starboard settee and fits into bulkhead-mounted latches when needed, reduces the settee to one seat when in use. Most objectionable of all is that stowage space, especially for clothes and food, is sorely lacking. There is less stowage space in this 25-footer than in any production boat we have examined.

The dearth of stowage is partly due to the arrangement of the two settee berths. Both extend outboard to the hull liner (a commendable width for sleeping) with a fold-up backrest and "molded" cushions for sitting comfort, but

A Glance at the Rest of the Bayfield Line

As we noted at the outset of the description of the Bayfield 25, the line of Bayfield-built boats are all readily identifiable as sisters. Most of the virtues and vices of the 25 are repeated throughout the line. The following is a glance at the three other Bayfield offerings.

The Bayfield 29

In a number of ways this is the most interesting member of the Bayfield fleet. In fact, the first inclination to do the full evaluation on the 29 was resisted because she is also the most unusual.

With no berths forward of the head, the Bayfield 29 has the best accommodations for a crew of two. Instead of berths, the forward "cabin" has a large head/dressing room plus what is sorely needed in the Bayfields, good stowage space. In boats under 30 feet where forward berths become too cramped, this is a superb way to save space.

As a "consolation prize" for giving up the forward berths, the 29 has been endowed with a pair of quarterberths. Though there are fans of such berths, they further restrict the amount of room in cockpit seat lockers. Similarly, the 29 has a chart table (combined with the icebox) for fans of sit-down navigation although non-fans realize that there may be better uses to which this space can be put, given the limited need for a nav area on most boats under 30 feet.

The built-in dust bin/drip pan with teak grate at the base of the companionway is a neat touch. So too is the engine access hatch built into the sole of the cockpit. This hatch, though, needs to be cored with balsa as it acts disconcertingly like a small trampoline in the boat we looked at. Still, with a good watertight fit, such a hatch is safe and permits working on the engine, or even removing it, and is a splendid addition to the normal access (or lack of it) under the companionway. In a boat of 29-feet LOA

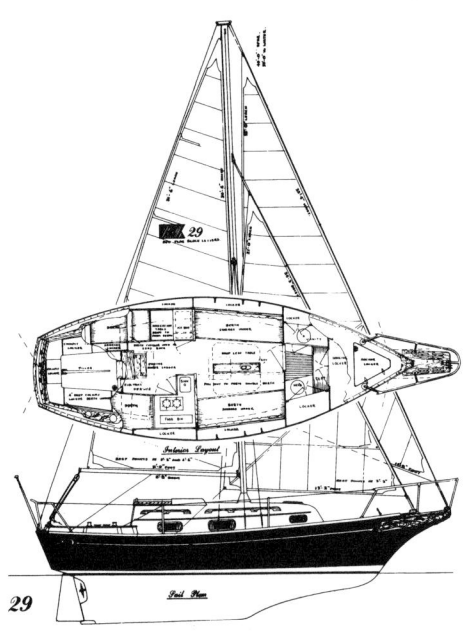

Bayfield 29

we can see no justification for a cutter rig. A boat as heavy as the 29 (7,100 pounds with a displacement to length ratio of over 300) needs all the sail power she can get. We would opt to do away with the staysail and stay (or make the stay removable and use the staysail only as a storm sail) to free up the foretriangle for a large genoa.

Proportions of the 29 are more attractive than those of the 25; she is not as stubby looking. At $50,000 equipped, the Bayfield 29 is pricey for a boat with less than 22 feet of waterline.

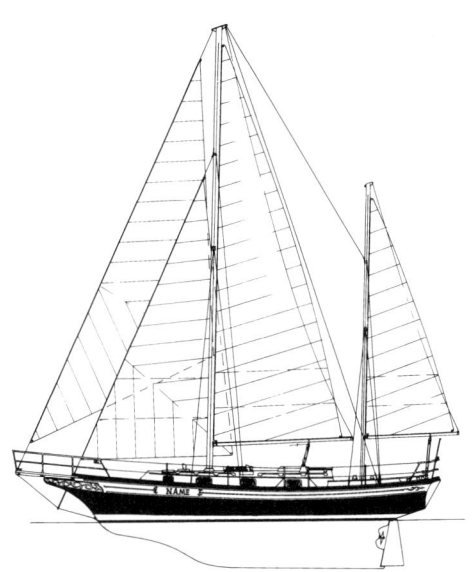

Bayfield 40

The Bayfield 32 and 32-C
The Bayfield 32 was the second boat in the Bayfield line after the 23/25 (now the 25). The 32 was upgraded as the 32-C with a taller rig (4'), a bowsprit (3'), more sail area, and, for looks, wider hull striping. At this size, the interior can have a double berth, U-shaped galley, and a practical chart table/nav area. The cockpit features wheel steering (that we would mount forward to avoid the mainsheet). For normal coastal cruising we certainly would elect the larger sailplan of the 32-C. This is a rig in which the cutter's double headsails begin to be worthwhile. Only the 32-C has the proportions of a cutter (with the jib topsail fitted with roller furling for relative ease in tacking). We would do away with the staysail on the short rig just as we would on the 29.

The Bayfield 40
The latest addition to the Bayfield line was the ketch-rigged Bayfield 40. As might be anticipated, this is the best proportioned and does the best job of making traditional styling "work" aesthetically. At this size, the ketch rig makes some sense as does a double-headsail rig (with provision to set a large genoa). Sail size is kept within manageable limits although the cockpit does get cluttered with the mizzenmast. It will be interesting to see how this larger yacht fares in the marketplace against the plethora of more modern looking boats in this popular size.

there is no stowage space outboard of the berths, only relatively small shelves and lockers above. Underberth scuttles, not the driest or most convenient stowage space, are reduced by the holding tank forward, the water tank under the port settee, and the stowed stove under the starboard settee.

Stowage space, then, consists of a hanging locker of sorts behind the head, room for toiletries behind the head sink, dish compartments outboard of the galley counter/icebox, a small cuddy and cutlery drawer under the galley counter, and a large locker aft of the port settee extending under the cockpit seat. This locker seems intended as a hanging locker or a wet locker, but we'd prefer to see it fitted with shelves for more effective stowage. A true hanging locker in a 25-foot boat seems a waste of space. Besides, the similarly tall locker outboard of the head could be better used for either purpose.

Having dwelt on the deficiencies of the accommodations of the 25, we should look at her strengths. Start with the main cabin: by extending the cabinhouse as far outboard as possible and separating the settees by plenty of cabin sole, there is little of the sense of claustrophobic confinement that typifies "pocket cruisers." A cook can tend the stove and still leave room for anyone to pass fore and aft or get through the companionway. Sitting upright on the settee is not a frustrating exercise in where to put the back of one's head to avoid a crick in the neck. The head is fully usable standing or sitting, provided the V-berth is not filled with spectators. Above decks, the cockpit has high enough coamings to support the backs of those who sit there and plenty of leg room (too much, in fact, to brace one's feet on the opposite side).

We like the portable stove; cooking is too uncommon an activity to take up valuable space on this size boat. The icebox is certainly adequate (aside from its tiny drain) and well insulated, including the lid.

Headroom belowdecks is, to our way of thinking, quite adequate for 25 feet although we must chide the builder for boasting she has six feet. Only under the companionway does headroom approach six feet; otherwise there is barely five feet, eight inches in the center of the main cabin and less than five feet, six inches through the head. The height of the topsides and of the cabinhouse already border on making the 25 look chunky and if headroom is thereby curtailed, so be it.

The decor below is what might best be described as Production Boat Functional. It combines Operating Room white gloss with dark teak bulkheads (plywood) and trim and patterned white overhead. It is, in short, "traditional" only insofar as fiberglass production boats established a "tradition" in the early 1960s and have steadfastly maintained it ever since. Given the imaginative and attractive interiors using light woods, fabrics, and laminates in a number of boats now being built, we cannot give the Bayfields high marks.

CONCLUSIONS

If we wanted maximum space, a distinctive appearance, good construction, and proven resale value in a 25-footer, we'd look seriously at the Bayfield 25. If we wanted good sailing performance, stowage space, a light and airy interior, and accommodations better suited for a couple, we'd look elsewhere. At a total of close to $30,000 we are confident that we could find suitable alternatives.

At the same time, the enthusiasm of Bayfield owners is understandable. They see their boat, justifiably, as a small yacht. They have been treated well by the builder and his dealers. They boast an uncommon involvement with their boats, citing extensive and comfortable cruising, and a concern for their boats. Most understandably plan to "trade up" to larger boats from the same builder, perhaps the ultimate compliment.

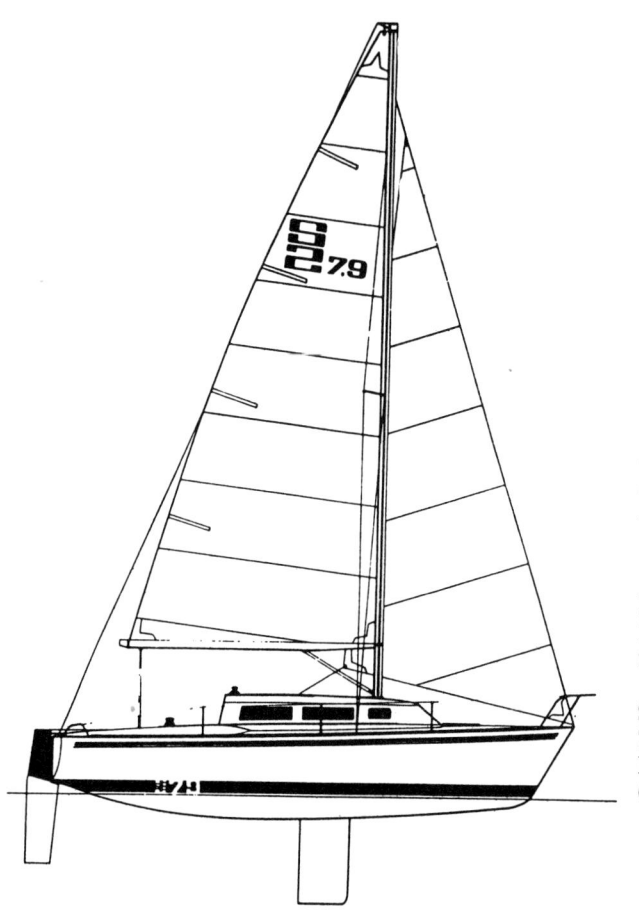

Specifications
S2 7.9

LOA	25'11"
LWL	21'8"
Beam	9'0"
Draft	
board up	13"
board down	5'0"
Displacement	4250 lbs
Ballast	1750 lbs
Sail area	329 sq ft

S2 Yachts Inc.
725 East 40th Street
Holland, Mich. 49423
(616) 392-7163

The S2 7.9

THE BOAT AND THE BUILDER

After Leon Slikkers sold Slickcraft, his powerboat company, in the early 1970s, he built a sailboat factory the way a sailboat factory should be built. Then for 15 years Slikkers, with the name S2 Yachts, built a line of sailboats characterized by an uncommon attention to detail, top-of-the-line construction, and superb customer relations.

Originally S2 produced a number of what were basically cruising boats before opening its second decade in the sailboat business by turning to higher performance models. Initially the racy models were call the Grand Slam series, but that name was soon dropped. The S2 7.9 looked at here was the first in that series. Finally, recognizing that the bloom was off the production sailboat market in 1987, Slikkers went back to building powerboats, continuing to build his sailboats only to order.

Such a status might normally disqualify an S2 from inclusion in this book, but the continued availability of the 7.9, albeit on a limited basis, and the special nature of not only the 7.9, but other S2 boats seems to warrant an exception. By the time you read this, the 7.9 may no longer be available on the new boat market, but she will remain an interesting and informative example of a solidly performing smaller boat with the capability of being trailered, raced, or cruised, all with equal facility, as well as being a sturdy, well-finished craft.

Designed by Chicago-based naval architects Scott Graham and Eric Schlageter, the 7.9 (the metric equivalent of her LOA of 25'11") from the outset did well in MORC and PHRF racing as well as in her own one-design fleets. With well over 400 built since 1982, the 7.9 was relatively successful during a time when, with the notable exception of the J/24 and Olson 25, not many performance-oriented production boats of her size were selling.

Such success and quality does come at a price. The 7.9 is a pricey boat for her size. Equipped with sail handling gear, four sails (mainsail, small jib, genoa jib and spinnaker), outboard motor, speedometer, and compass, her price in 1986 was almost $30,000, close to $10,000 higher than a comparably equipped J/24. Add an inboard engine, a trailer, and miscellaneous gear and the cost could easily climb to over $36,000, a hefty tab for a 26-foot boat.

CONSTRUCTION

The hull and deck of the 7.9 are hand-laid fiberglass, cored with end-grain balsa. S2 brags about its glasswork, and the company has a well-deserved reputation in the boatbuilding industry for both its excellent tooling and hand layup.

Beginning somewhere around hull number 400, S2 switched from conventional polyester resin to a modified epoxy resin—AME 4000. The company claims the epoxy resin is stronger, lighter, and less subject to blistering.

The hull is fair with no bumps or hard spots evident—partially the result of the company's practice of installing most of the interior before removing the hull from its mold. The gelcoat appears to be thicker than is usual in production boats—a good feature since minor scratches and dings can be "rubbed out" without penetrating to the glass laminate.

For their standard hull to deck joint, S2 uses an inward turning flange onto which the deck molding is set—a desirable design, especially when bedded in flexible adhesive (such as 3M 5200) and through-bolted at close intervals. However on the 7.9, rather than being through-bolted, the deck is mechanically fastened to the hull only with screws through the slotted aluminum toerail, a detail that indicates the boat is not intended for heavy-duty offshore work.

The boat comes with a one-design "package" of good quality deck hardware. All hardware is though-bolted, with stainless backing plates on the lifeline stanchions, but with only washers and nuts on all other hardware. This would seem to be problematic with the balsa core, but we have heard no reports of problems so far.

The S2 7.9 Meter
107

Although the company has offered the boat in a fixed-keel version, the vast majority of boats sold have a lead-ballasted daggerboard.

The advantages of a daggerboard are, first, that it retracts to be flush with the bottom of the hull to make the boat trailer-launchable; second, that you can float the boat in a mere 13 inches of water (although she will have no directional control with the board totally up—you'll need at least a foot of board showing for control under sail or power); and third, with the board totally down, the boat has a five-foot deep hydrodynamically efficient keel, a depth that would be extreme on a fixed-keel boat this size.

The disadvantage of the daggerboard will come in a hard grounding. Whereas a centerboard would kick out of the way, the board is likely to bash around a bit in its trunk. A nice detail by S2 is that the bottom opening of the trunk is surrounded by a strong weldment which will mitigate the potential damage to the hull from a grounding. Another potential disadvantage is that, on many boats, the daggerboard trunk messes up the interior, but the designers have done a good job on the 7.9, incorporating the daggerboard into a centerline bulkhead.

Nearly one-third of the 1,750 pounds of ballast is in the board, with the remaining two-thirds glassed to the interior of the hull. When the board is fully lowered, it fits snugly in a V-shaped crotch—a good design detail—but when it is raised out of the "V" using the three-part tackle and winch, it will bang about loosely in the daggerboard trunk. There is no way to pin the board down—an obvious potential problem in severe conditions.

The boat, however, has passed the MORC self-righting test with the daggerboard in the fully raised position. In the test, the mast-head is hove down to the water, the bagged mainsail and genoa are tied to the masthead, and the whole shebang released. If the boat returns upright, she has adequate stability to pass the test. This is not a test of ultimate stability, since other boats which passed the test have turtled and sunk, but it is reassuring. However, the design is clearly dependent mostly on its beamy hull form for righting and not on its ballast—another indication the boat is intended for close-to-shore sailing.

The transom-hung rudder—pivoted for trailering—is of foam-cored fiberglass (the foam gives it neutral buoyancy in water). We like the idea of a transom-hung rudder: it's accessible for inspection and service, it lessens the

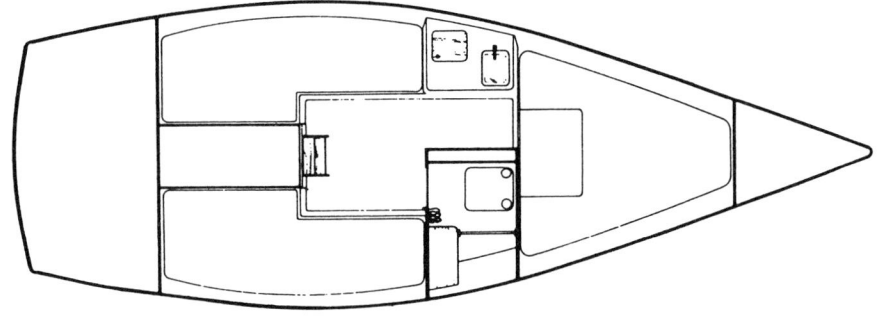

potential damage to the hull that can occur when a rudder smashes into something, and it gets the rudder farther away from the keel to give the tiller a more responsive feel.

The fractional rig—with mast and boom made by Offshore Spars—is dinghy-like, having swept-back spreaders which make the upper shrouds function as backstays. The actual backstay does virtually nothing to support the rig; instead, its primary function is to bend the mast to control mainsail shape. Although the mast is easily bendable, it's a surprisingly heavy section for a modern racing

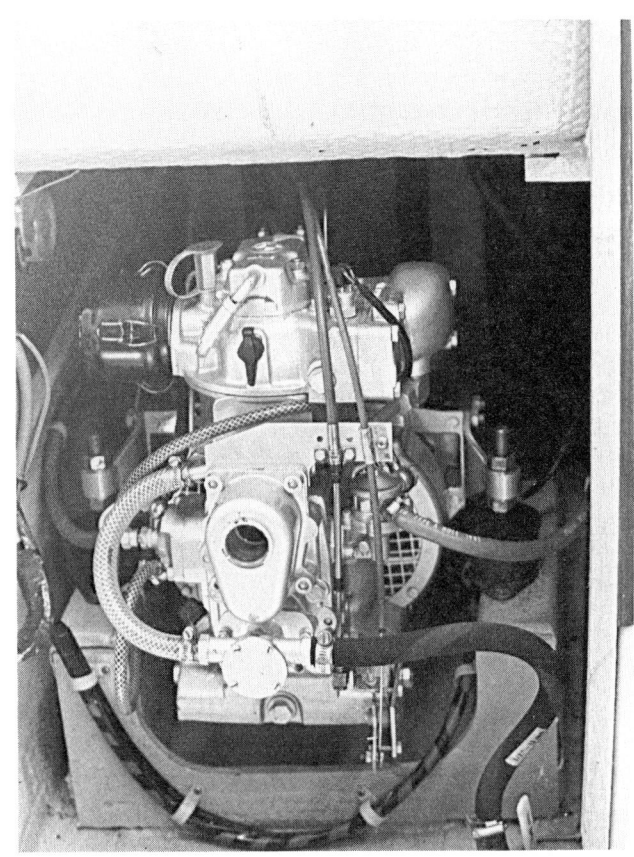

Companionway steps swing open to give good engine access. Installation is workmanlike and tidy.

rig—it's also untapered. Everything is internal in the mast and boom, with all lines eventually coming back to the cockpit in typical modern racing style.

Upper and lower shrouds attach to inboard chainplates. The starboard chainplate is attached to a well-bonded plywood bulkhead, but the port chainplate is longer, attached to the fiberglass structure which forms the front edge of the galley. Since there is a two-foot "free span" of unsupported chainplate between the galley and deck, the chainplate in the highly-loaded rig works a lot, and one of the most common owner complaints about the boat is the leaking port chainplate that results.

A fiberglass pan makes up the berths, cabin sole, and galley area. Instead of a ceiling, S2 uses carpeting for interior covering of the hull. One good detail about the carpeting is that Velcro will stick to it—you can hang anything anywhere—but we have to wonder how the carpet will stand up to salt accumulation. There is virtually no bilge, so water inside will turn everything soggy.

Generally, the boat is well constructed with good detail work and hardware.

The S2 7.9 Meter
109

While we believe that every "racer-cruiser" should be designed and built to handle extreme conditions offshore, the hull shape, the daggerboard design, and the hull to deck joint show us that S2 expects this boat will not be involved in those extremes.

PERFORMANCE

Handling Under Power

The standard 7.9 will be outboard powered. The option has been a BMW 7.5-horsepower, one-lung diesel with the shockingly high price tag of $5,400. With BMW getting out of the marine business, S2 will be offering the boat with the 7.5-horsepower Yanmar, probably a little noisier than the BMW, but with a much better dealer and service network throughout the country.

The little diesel handles the boat well, although owners report that it will not punch through a heavy head sea. This may be more the result of the folding Martec prop which comes as part of the inboard package rather than any lack of power in the engine.

The inboard installation is well done. The plywood stringers glassed to the hull support vibration-damping mounts for the engine. Standard installation includes a stainless steel eight-gallon fuel tank, properly grounded, a heavy duty Purolator filter/water-separator, a waterlift muffler, and single-lever shift/throttle controls.

Both the fuel shutoff and the fuel filter are difficult to get to—through an inspection port in the port quarterberth—but access to the engine is otherwise good, with hinged companionway steps opening out of the way so dipstick, decompression switch, engine controls, and water pump are easy to get at. For more serious work on the engine, the quarterberth panels are removable for virtually total access. One good feature of the BMW is that it is the only engine we've ever seen that is actually easy to start by hand-cranking. It made S2's one-battery installation workable. With the Yanmar, owners may want to seek a place to stow a second battery; offhand, there's no obviously good location.

As you might expect on a 4,400-pound boat, the outboard is minimally adequate in any wind or sea conditions; that is to say, the outboard is ordinarily inadequate. We would normally recommend the inboard for the 7.9, but there are two major problems. First is the extreme price. Second is the underwater drag of the shaft, strut, and propeller for which rating rules give inadequate credit—an important consideration for the racer.

Our conclusion is that the serious racer should probably buy the outboard model and just suffer the poor performance under power. If you will be primarily daysailing, weekending, and cruising, we recommend gritting your teeth and writing a check for the inboard. If you're planning a combination of racing and cruising, you'll just have to make a judgment as to which aspect deserves a higher priority.

Handling Under Sail

The 7.9 is a proven performer under sail, being not only a fast boat for her size,

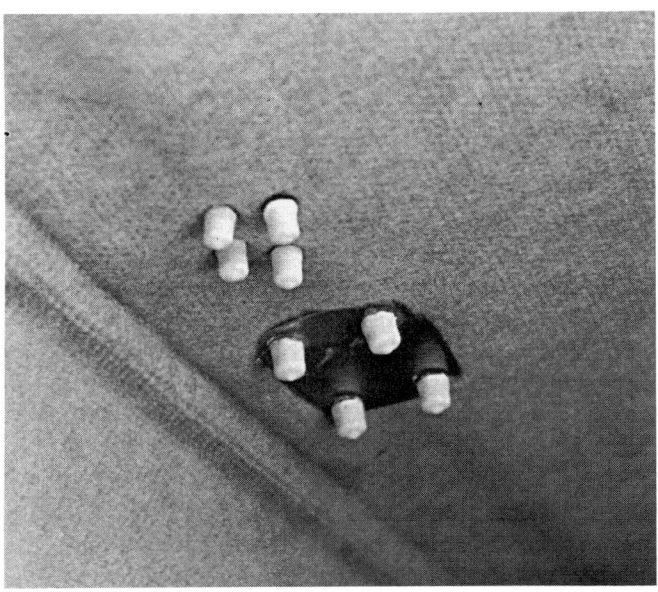

but also competitive in handicap racing under the MORC and PHRF. Her PHRF rating of 168 says that she's about the same speed as the J/24, Merit 25, and similar current racing boats, and about the same speed as such older racer-cruisers as the Pearson 30, Cal 34, Catalina 30 tall rig, or the Irwin 30.

Stainless steel plate backs up the stanchion base, but not a deck-mounted cam cleat beside it, which, like all other deck hardware, has only plastic-capped nuts and washers.

With her narrow entry forward, a big fat rear end, and a fractional rig with most of the power in the mainsail, she will be better behaved than her high-performance cousins designed to the IOR rule. Owners report that her one bad habit is to wipe out in the heavy puffs when beating. Her dinghy-shaped hull means she'll have to be sailed flat for best performance, which in turn means lots of lard on the rail when the wind pipes up. Five people, the heavier the better, is *de rigueur* for heavy-air racing. For daysailing and cruising, she's got plenty of reefable sail area, and she should perform well with the four standard class sails: mainsail, 150-percent genoa, 105-percent jib, and spinnaker.

Peak performance will take lots of tweaking and fiddling with the rig. This will be no problem for the high-performance dinghy sailor graduating to a cruising boat, but it will take a lot of learning about mast bend and sail shape for the newcomer. Nonetheless, even when not tuned to perfection, she should perform well enough to be a pleasant daysailer.

LIVABILITY

Deck Layout

The 7.9's inboard shrouds, wide decks, and big cockpit make for pleasant moving about on deck. The non-skid is good—among the best we've seen on a production boat. It will remove skin from bare knuckles.

The boat will be sailed from the cockpit, and she's well laid out for sail handling. The primary winches are, if anything, oversize—a true rarity these days—and the secondary winches on the cabin top are adequate for halyard and spinnaker work. (Note, though, that the daggerboard is raised and lowered using the starboard secondary winch. One owner reports blowing up the winch; another says, "The #16 winch is inadequate for a woman or small man to handle the board.")

Like the J/24 and other performance boats, the helmsman and crew will sit on the deck rather than in the cockpit when racing. However, unlike the J/24, the 7.9 does have a true cockpit, and it's comfortable. The seat bottoms are slightly concave, the seat backs are nearly a foot high and contoured to support the small of the back, and the seat-to-sole distance gives comfortable leg room. The mainsheet traveler is smack in the middle of the cockpit and will prove a shin ravager until you get used to it. But, the cockpit will comfortably daysail six and drink eight at dockside and is definitely a strong point for the boat.

There are two substantial cockpit lockers for stowage. Several owners report that the lockers leak—a nuisance in what appears to be an otherwise dry boat.

Belowdecks

As one owner puts it, "The interior does the best it can." With about five-feet, four-inches headroom, the cabin will require stooping for most people. Still, we admire S2's restraint—they could have easily added six inches to the cabin-house to get "standing" headroom. And to get a boat that would be as ugly as some of S2's early cruising models.

S2 was not suckered by the how-many-does-she-sleep syndrome for this model. Both quarterberths are long and wide, and the forward V-berth is truly sleepable with the boat dockside or at anchor. The only drawback to the arrangements is that the space between berth and side decks is so short that sitting upright will be uncomfortable for anyone over six feet or so.

The galley (or, more accurately, the galley area) is minimal, with a shallow sink and small icebox. There's a tiny counter area—either for counterspace or for a one-burner alcohol stove—but anyone wanting to weekend or cruise with more than PB&J's will have to revamp the galley.

The daggerboard trunk is well disguised, forming one wall of the head. The head itself is cramped, to say the least—you can sit on the Porta Potti, but your knees will stick out through the privacy curtain. Still, the head location is preferable to the all-too-common position under the V-berth.

Ventilation below is nonexistent. Opening ports are available as options. A small quarterberth opening port might be a possibility, and a forepeak vent would be desirable.

Compared to a larger boat's "yacht" finish or even to a 25-foot cruising boat, the 7.9's interior will seem plain and functional. On the other hand, it's luxurious compared to a J/24, J/27, Merit 25, or Evelyn 26. The boat can be weekended in comfort. If you can stand camping out, the boat can even be cruised.

Trailerability

With a nine-foot beam, the 7.9 is not legally trailerable in any state without special wide-load permits. Yet most of the boats have been sold with trailers, and the company boasts of its trailerability and easy launchability. How is this possible?

The consensus is that, with the daggerboard retracted, the boat sits so low on the trailer that she doesn't look that wide. A keelboat on a trailer—a Merit 25, for example—looks much bigger and a bored cop is more likely to stop and measure a keelboat than a 7.9.

At any rate, 7.9s are trailered, and we know of none ever being ticketed or, for that matter, even questioned.

CONCLUSIONS

S2 has done a good job of aiming the boat at a variety of sailors: racers, daysailors, and weekenders. For racers interested in a one-design boat, the class is not yet strong outside the Great Lakes. But for the sailor into handicap racing, the boat seems a good possibility. She is definitely competitive in MORC and PHRF fleets. And unlike other high-performance boats her size— the Olson 25, J/24, Merit 25, Evelyn 26, or Capri 25—the 7.9 is a boat you could stand sleeping aboard or taking on a rainy overnight race.

For the sailor primarily interested in daysailing and weekending, the 7.9 will also be worth serious consideration. She is definitely on the pricey side for 26-foot boats, but her quality construction and equipment are what you get for the extra money. She may be a little on the high-performance side for the real novice, but her four-sail class package should be fairly easy to handle even for the newcomer.

We really cannot recommend her as a cruiser. Well, maybe as a pocket cruiser. S2 clearly didn't intend her for cruising or offshore sailing; still, she's well made, a fast boat, and . . . maybe if our seamanship were good enough . . . but no!

If it's a fast cruiser we were looking for at 25 feet or so, we'd keep looking. For the racer, daysailor, and weekender, however, she's a good boat from a good company—a combination we don't see every day.

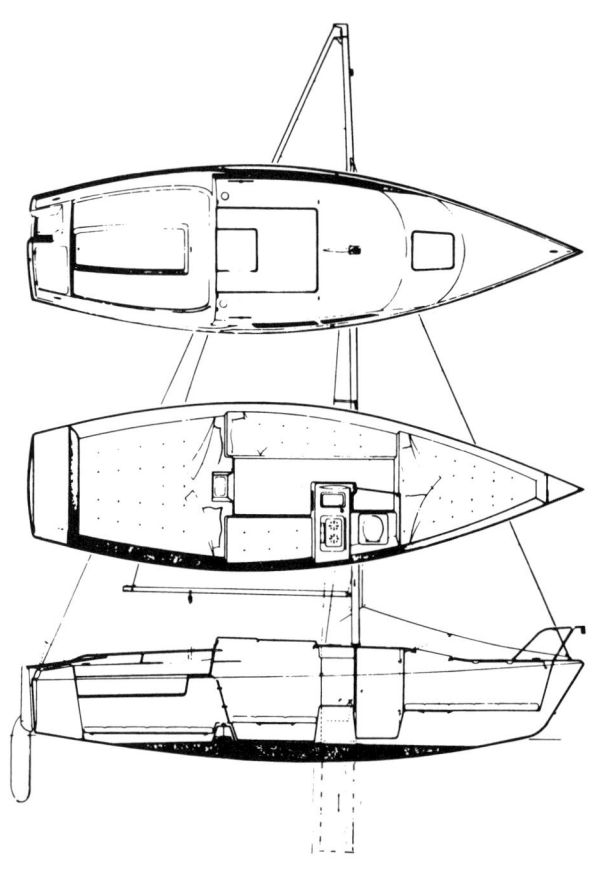

Specifications
MacGregor 26

LOA	25'10"
LWL	23'6"
Beam	7'11"
Draft	
board up	1'3"
board down	5'4"
Displacement	
tank empty	1650 lbs
tank full	2850 lbs
Sail area	236 sq ft

MacGregor Yacht Corp.
1631 Placentia
Costa Mesa, Calif. 92627
(714) 642-6830

The MacGregor 26:
A Water-Ballasted Trailer Sailer

THE BOAT AND THE BUILDER

The MacGregor Yacht Corporation is a survivor. It stands as one of the few boatbuilders from the 1960s still in business and still making money. It also stands on a street in Costa Mesa, California that once housed now-defunct builders like Islander and Westsail. While other builders are struggling to survive, MacGregor is back-ordered for more than six months.

MacGregor is, and always has been, a one-man show; in this case the man is Roger MacGregor. He founded the company in 1964 to prove the validity of his Stanford MBA thesis, the hypothesis of which was that boatbuilders would be more successful if they were more efficient. A "hobby" at first, with only 26 employees, MacGregor decided in 1967 to "really go at it" and build the company to its present size of over 100 employees.

Through the years, MacGregor has produced a number of boats, first under the Venture trademark, and for the last ten years, under the MacGregor name.

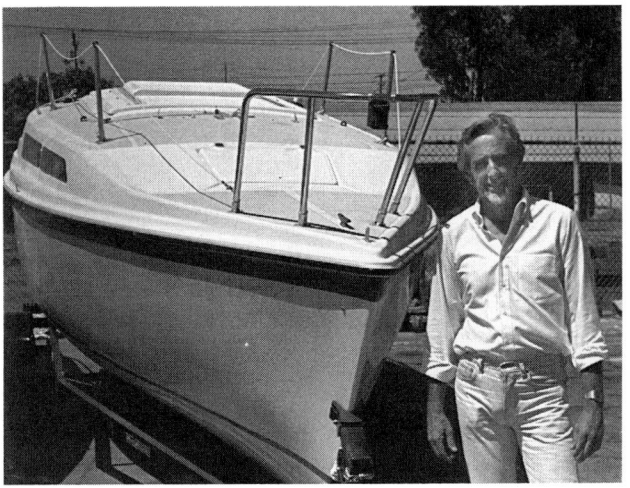

The thrust of the line has always been aimed at the first-time sailor. Roger MacGregor has a better handle on that market than anyone else in the industry.

The first boat the company built was the Venture 21; it was discontinued in 1986, after 22 years in production. In the interim, a number of small boats were produced, like the Venture 22, 222, 23, 24, and 25. The only deviations from the trailerboat theme have been a 36-foot catamaran, and a 65-foot ULDB "sled," which is the only boat still in production other than the new MacGregor 26.

Roger MacGregor with his new 26-footer: a one-man show.

Of the 24,000 boats built to date by MacGregor, 17,000 of them are MacGregor 25s. From this statistic, MacGregor learned that the trailerboat market prefers bigger boats, so he replaced the 25 in 1986 with the 26, a new, but similar design.

To get around the problem posed by smaller and smaller automobiles, the designer eliminated the 25's swing keel, which weighs 600 pounds. This leaves the 26 weighing only 1650 pounds (2200 pounds with trailer), light enough for most mid-size cars. The lack of a keel also puts the boat lower to the road for less windage.

To provide stability lost by removing the keel, the MacGregor 26 was designed with a slight "V" to the bottom, which houses a water ballast compartment. The compartment holds an additional 1200 pounds of water, to bring the total sailing weight to up 2850 pounds.

Roger MacGregor says he knows why the boatbuilding industry has gone sour, and has found, in the MacGregor 26, the secret to success. He cites the common explanation that the market has dried up, that fewer people are interested in sailing at the introductory level because of the cost and complication. He has overcome those objections by making his boats very uncomplicated, writing lengthy instruction manuals in non-nautical terminology, and by having a dealer network that caters to the first-time sailor.

One-half of MacGregor owners are beginning sailors, and the dealers know it. Most dealers go so far as to show the new owner how to rig and sail his boat, or arrange for sailing lessons, says MacGregor. Of the 40-odd *Practical Sailor* boatowner evaluations returned on the MacGregor 25, not one reader had anything but kind words to say about his dealer. This is an exceptional record.

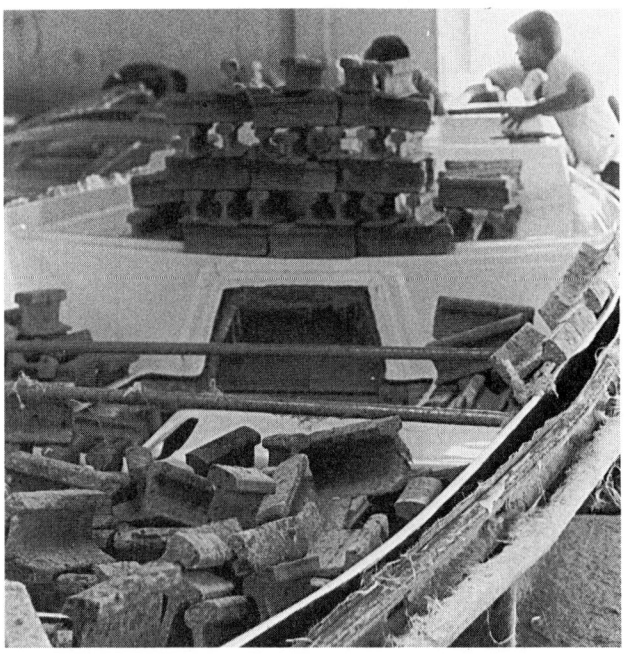

Iron weights hold the overhead liner against the deck molding while it is still in its mold, until the glue dries.

Another pitfall of modern boatbuilding that MacGregor has conquered is the prohibitive cost of compliance with environmental regulations. Because he owns his plant, Roger MacGregor says he can support the expense of compliance, while builders trying to get on their feet in rented property cannot.

MacGregor says many boatbuilders were closed after being purchased by conglomerates, because the conglomerates weren't willing to weather a sustained period of operating in the red. Roger MacGregor says he'll never sell his company; that's why he changed the name of his boats from Venture to MacGregor.

The biggest reason that builders fail, says MacGregor, is inefficiency. This is where MacGregor Yacht Corporation shines. The MacGregor 26 has only three options: cockpit cushions, bottom paint and surge brakes on the trailer. The boat comes complete with trailer, sails, lifelines and pulpits, battery and lights. The only major item you have to buy is an outboard.

Making the boat relatively complete accomplishes two things. First, it helps satisfy the most common owner complaint about the MacGregor 25—that the boats required too much additional equipment. Second, it simplifies the "tracking" of boats through production. There is no need to keep track of which boat goes to which dealer while in production. If a dealer's sale falls through, he isn't stuck with an odd boat, because all boats are the same. Red tape and paperwork are drastically reduced. Making all boats alike has allowed MacGregor to "jig" almost every step in production, saving time. MacGregor says this saves about $800 per boat.

MacGregor also saves money by owning and maintaining a company fleet of 12 trucks, complete with drivers and mechanics. The outside dimensions of MacGregor 26 were determined by the space required to fit four of them, with trailers, on a company-owned truck. The cost of shipping to the East Coast is only $900.

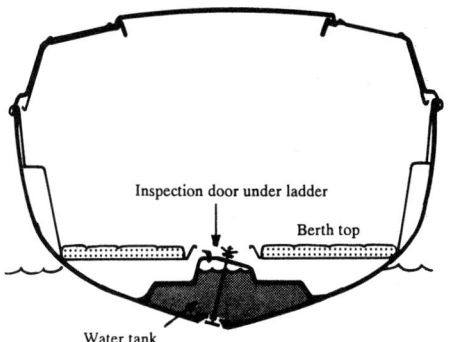

Inspection door under ladder

Berth top

Water tank

MacGregor 26's innovative water ballast system can be opened and closed from inside the cabin.

MacGregor has individual shops to build trailers, spars, and upholstery. While other builders usually farm out these tasks, MacGregor says they save money by doing them "in house." We can't argue with that; the MacGregor 26 retails for only $8900, and that's after giving the dealer a 30% markup.

CONSTRUCTION

Hull and Deck

The best way to describe the construction of the MacGregor 26 is "quick and dirty." The plant finishes four boats a day, five days a week. A hull is in the mold for only 13 hours. There's a timetable to be met at every step of production. Production hangups are not allowed. If the work gets a little behind, the workers work a little faster. Sloppiness is inevitable.

The construction flaws caused by this sloppiness are hidden from view, but the finish details are not. The MacGregor 26 will appear somewhat crude to the experienced sailor, but the "rough edges" may not be so apparent to the inexperienced sailor for whom she is intended. This isn't to say that the buyer of a MacGregor 26 is getting a bad deal. On the contrary, the MacGregor 26 is a lot of boat for the money.

The MacGregor 26 hull is a solid fiberglass laminate, and a not particularly thick one; the laminate schedule calls for a total of 54 ounces of glass fiber per square yard (cloth and roving) below the waterline, and 30 ounces above the waterline—but remember that this is a lightweight boat.

MacGregor's immigrant work force lacks the skill needed to operate a chopper gun, or to trim the fiberglass to size by first rolling it onto the mold. To avoid mistakes—and improve efficiency—the fiberglass is cut to a table pattern, then folded and boxed, one box to each step of the lamination.

The flat areas of the deck are cored with plywood, which is pressed into the wet fiberglass mat by laying dozens of weights on top of the wood. The overhead liner is installed in the deck in the same manner.

To save time, the fastening holes for all of the deck fittings are made by dropping a single jig onto the deck and drilling the patterns of holes. Then the interior side of each hole is bored to 5/8" diameter, to countersink the nuts and washers. Finally, the nut is hidden by a plastic cap; this gives access to the fastenings should you want to replace deck hardware.

Small backing plates, made of scraps of fiberglass, are used on the bow cleats, but not on any other fittings. While the plywood core in the deck reduces the need for backing plates, the practice of countersinking the washers and nuts reduces the strength of the attachment. In addition, plywood is more

The MacGregor 26
117

likely than balsa core to absorb water and delaminate should the deck fittings leak.

The hull to deck joint, fashioned by a deck flange overlapping the hull and hull liner, appears to be adequate. A rubrail is bolted through the joint with #10 bolts on 6" centers. Foam weatherstripping forms the bedding for the joint, but adds no strength. Final waterproofing is achieved by running a bead of 3M 5200 adhesive sealant around the edge of the deck flange. The same 5200 is also used to bed deck fittings.

The hull liner is pressed into wet mat laid on the keelson. Then vertical surfaces of the liner, where accessible through holes cut in the liner for lockers, are glassed to the hull. To save time, no filleting is used; the tabbing of the liner is done with roving 8" wide. This is not a clean or particularly strong method, but it's adequate for the use for which the boat is designed.

The chainplates are bolted directly to the hull, at the outboard edge of the gunwale. The hull in the area of attachment is reinforced with additional fiberglass at the rate of 150 ounces per square yard.

The cabin house extends to the edge of the deck, and there are no structural interior bulkheads save those formed by the hull liner. This design gives less support for loading from the rig than would be advisable when sailing in heavy weather. While none of the MacGregor 25 owner surveys we received mention structural problems, we have personal experience with a MacGregor-built boat splitting open at the stem in heavy weather.

MacGregor 25 owners complain of cockpit floor flexing and resultant gelcoat crazing. MacGregor says that they have solved this problem on the 26 by adding extra fiberglass around the corners of the cockpit floor.

Rig

Our owner surveys did register complaints about the MacGregor 25's rig, which is virtually identical to that of the 26. Made by MacGregor, the mast is anodized but untapered.

The rigging is minimal, external and crude. The rig is fractional with swept-back upper and lower shrouds. The spreaders are tubes that swing freely on small, U-shaped brackets. If the spreaders were fixed they would add stiffness to the mast and safety in heavy air. With freely swinging spreaders the mast looses athwartships support when it bends excessively. Shroud tangs are external, but through-bolted. Halyards are external as well, and they cleat on the mast.

The shrouds terminate with Nico-pressed eyes, rather than swage fittings. While MacGregor says they've never had a failure, our owner surveys contradict this contention. Plate adjusters are used instead of turnbuckles on the shrouds.

Daggerboard/Rudder

The MacGregor 26 has an unballasted daggerboard, housed in a trunk running from bilge to deck just aft of the mast. The trunk acts as a compression post for

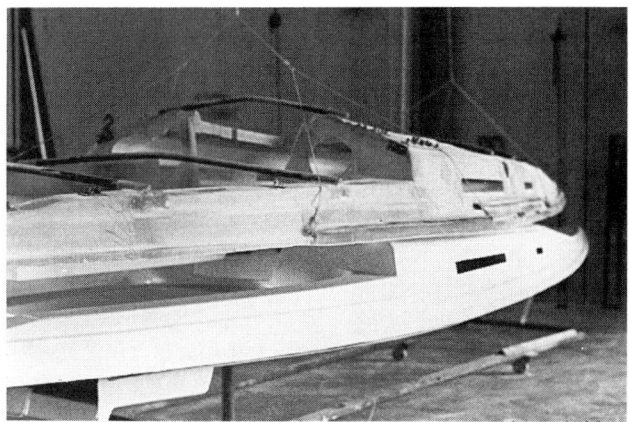

the deck-stepped mast. The trunk also bisects the water ballast tank, which is both good and bad. If you were to fracture the trunk in a hard grounding, the ballast tank would leak, not the hull; but if the ballast tank leaks, you could lose the ballast required to keep the boat upright. To solve this problem, MacGregor

Jig placed over the deck serves as a guide for drilling holes to fasten all the deck hardware and rigging.

says, the daggerboards are designed to shear off in a hard grounding. Replacement boards are $125.

The innovative board and rudder are nicely shaped airfoils. Holes are drilled in them so they will fill with water when sailing. In the daggerboard, this is a good idea. It leaves it lightweight for trailering, yet allows it to have negative buoyancy so it won't float up when sailing.

In the rudder, however, it only makes the helm feel heavier and more sluggish. Rudder action is further aggravated by a sloppy pintle-to-gudgeon fit and play in the rudderhead. The pintles, like all of the MacGregor 26's rigging, are underbuilt.

The daggerboard is short enough to be self-contained inside the trunk when trailering. This means that there isn't much board inside the trunk when it's lowered for sailing; this adds to the loads placed on the trunk. However, the ballast tank gives the trunk some extra support.

The fit between the board and trunk is not particularly tight; we expect you might hear it "thunk" as the boat rolls in waves.

Ballast Tank/Flotation

The most unique feature of the MacGregor 26 is her water ballast system. Water ballast in sailboats is usually restricted to singlehanded offshore racers, where ballast tanks are mounted under the gunwale to add stability. Their system requires that the leeward tank be filled, and the weather tank emptied, before each tack.

MacGregor's system is different. Patterned after European trailer sailers, it uses a single ballast tank running the length of the bilge. This configuration doesn't provide the leverage of a lead keel of similar weight, nor of a gunwale-mounted ballast tank, but it does make the boat self-righting. It takes 125 pounds to hold the tip of the MacGregor 26's mast in the water, says her builder, compared to 75 pounds for the MacGregor 25.

The MacGregor 26
119

The ballast tank can be opened and closed, and the water level inspected, from inside the cabin. The tank is closed by drawing a rubber-backed plate up into a recess in the keelson. The rubber must be kept clean of fouling or the tank could leak ballast when the boat heels. The tank has a fiberglass baffle to keep the water from sloshing around when sailing. It takes about six minutes to fill or empty the tank when launching or hauling.

The MacGregor 26 has positive flotation when swamped, a commendable feature, especially in a lightweight trailerable sailboat. The flotation is provided by blocks of styrofoam under the V-berth, aft berth, over the galley, and under the cockpit.

Styrofoam is preferable to sprayed-in urethane foam, because it's less likely to absorb water and doesn't expand when exposed to heat. On the other hand, sytrofoam blocks don't fill the compartments as completely as pour-in-place polyurethane foam would, so some of the flotation space is wasted. For example, the styrofoam in the MacGregor 26 only fills one half of the space under the V-berth, yet the berth is completely closed off.

The waste is less serious than it might be, however, as the MacGregor 26 needs only 14 cubic feet of flotation because her water ballast is neutrally buoyant. The MacGregor 25 has 25 cubic feet of flotation.

PERFORMANCE

Handling on the Water

The MacGregor 26 is not a performance boat. She is hampered by a rig which is too small for light air and too flimsy for heavy air. The standard boat comes equipped with a main and working jib from Gaasta, a quality Hong Kong sailmaker. The cloth weight is on the light side, but the workmanship and sail shape is above average for OEM sails.

Adding a genoa to the inventory would improve her reaching, but not her upwind performance. That's because the genoa has to sheet around her gunwale-mounted shrouds. The working jib sheets inside the shrouds, which reduces the sheeting angle and allows the boat to point higher.

The MacGregor 26's rigging is too simple to make her handle well in a strong breeze. There is no traveler; the four-part mainsheet is fixed on the bridgedeck. There is no boom vang. The deck-stepped mast is light and bendy, but there are no backstay adjuster or turnbuckles on the shrouds to control mast bend. No tiller extension, either.

The jib leads are fixed bull's eyes. Lewmar #6 single-speed winches are standard. While adequate for the working jib, they are too small for a genoa. The cam cleats for the jib sheets are cheap and poorly angled. On the boat we looked at, the bedding compound had gotten into and gummed up one of the cam cleats.

Halyards cleat on the mast, and reef lines and outhaul cleat on the end of the boom. The standard mainsail has two reefs. At least the MacGregor 26 is rigged for slab reefing; the 25 has roller reefing on the boom, which works poorly. The gooseneck and the reefing hook for the tack are lightly built.

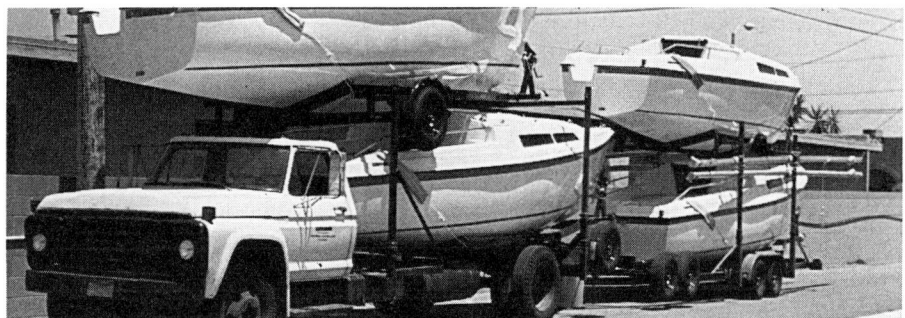

MacGregor maintains its own fleet of trucks to keep shipping costs low. The outside dimensions of the MacGregor 26 were determined by the space requirements of getting four on the truck at a time. Coast-to-coast shipping charge is only $900 a boat.

The 1220 pounds of water ballast sitting in the bilge is also a detriment to the performance of the MacGregor 26. Because the ballast runs for two-thirds of the length of the boat, she is heavy at the ends. Combined with the sloppy rudder assembly, this makes her steer sluggishly and turn slowly. We also expect it will make her pitch more in a seaway. With the ballast in the bilge instead of hung from a keel, the boat is initially tender.

The outboard motor mounts directly on the transom, as it would on a dinghy. There is no external transom bracket. When tilted up, the head of the motor lies in a recess molded into the afterdeck. This doesn't make the outboard any more secure, but MacGregor says that it allows you to trailer with outboard attached because it doesn't hang far off the stern.

The MacGregor 26 has an afterdeck almost 3' long. This makes for a long reach to the motor controls. It's a good thing that the motor isn't mounted on an external bracket. The afterdeck also houses a large lazarette that has more than enough space to stow the outboard and tank. The cockpit drains obstruct the lazarette, though, and are fabricated of unreinforced hose and fastened with single hose clamps. You'd have to be careful when stowing the motor.

Handling Off the Water
The boat comes equipped with a MacGregor-built trailer. Surge brakes are optional and recommended if you don't want to wear out your car brakes on lengthy road trips. The trailer is painted steel; a galvanized finish is not even offered, because California environmental laws make it cost-prohibitive, says MacGregor.

The trailer is made of steel channel with only a short section of the tongue made from steel box. Channel can be kept from rusting because all surfaces are exposed and can be scraped and repainted. Box will eventually rust from the inside out.

MacGregor builds the trailers on a jig which rotates so all of the welds can be horizontally applied. The welding appears clean and completely encompasses the joint. In preparation for welding, the metal is only wire brushed, not ground or degreased. In preparation for painting the metal is, again, only wire brushed. Although a zinc chromate primer is used, we suspect that the trailer will need to be repainted every other season if kept near salt water.

The MacGregor 26 sits low on her trailer because she has no external center-board or swing keel. MacGregor owners complain that a tongue extender is often needed to float their boat off the trailer. MacGregor says that the 26 will float off when the wheels are in 2'3" of water—9" less than the depth required for the 25. A jack stand would be useful, but the trailer does not come with one.

Because the mast is deck-stepped on a tabernacle, raising it simply requires that you walk it upright and attach the headstay. The swept-back shrouds only come taut when the mast is upright. To keep the mast from swaying sideways before the shrouds come taut, an extra set of in-line lower shrouds is rigged. To give you extra leverage when raising the mast, there is an optional "mast raising pole" which runs from the base of the mast to a tackle at the base of the headstay.

LIVABILITY

Deck Layout

To make space for the double berth under the cockpit, the cockpit sole had to be raised. This makes for cramped legroom and almost non-existent cockpit seatbacks. MacGregor made an attempt to solve the seatback problem by in-stalling stainless steel handrails along the cockpit coaming. The optional cock-pit cushion package includes cushions for the seatbacks which attach to the handrails. This makes for comfortable sitting in calm conditions, but the cush-ions could be torn from under their straps and washed overboard when water comes over the rail while sailing in a strong breeze.

The boat comes equipped with a bow pulpit and a set of stanchions and lifelines on each side of the cabin house. The lifelines are needed to go forward in safety because the house extends all the way to the gunwale. The stanchion bases have extra bracing and seem adequately attached to the boat. The life-lines are run to the base rather than to the top of the bow pulpit. This makes for less wear and tear on the foot of the jib at the expense of a proper handhold ot the bow.

Belowdecks

For a trailer sailer, the MacGregor 26 is spacious belowdecks; but compared to most 26-foot sailboats, she is cramped. The requirements for trailering require the boat be light, narrow and shallow. This doesn't leave a lot of interior volume.

The 26 is just big enough so that the daggerboard trunk is relatively unobtrusive, being used to form one side of the galley. The first thing you notice when going below is the huge, 9-square-foot mirror over the galley. MacGregor says the mirror adds the illusion of space. Even if the mirror were of better quality, so the reflection wasn't distorted, we'd still think it rather gaudy.

The galley is barely adequate, even for weekending. There is a molded sink with a collapsible 5-gallon water tank, removable for refilling. There's counter space, but no stove; mounting one would use up most of the counter. There's no table or icebox. There is no space for a portable ice chest; it would have to live on top of a berth or in the middle of the cabin floor.

There is an enclosure for a head, but no head is provided. The enclosure is designed to fit a portable toilet, but you might be able to squeeze a permanent head into it.

The V-berth is very narrow at the foot. The settees are narrow, too, but they have seatback cushions and the port settee is 7' long. Under the cockpit is a queen-size berth, a feature growing in popularity, even on boats this small.

There is plenty of sitting headroom, and a "pop top" for standing headroom. A dodger for the pop top is standard. The hatches are made by MacGregor and use weatherstripping for watertightness. We doubt that they would remain watertight with green water on deck. The cabinhouse windows are bedded in silicone sealant with a few mechanical fastenings.

The boat is equipped with a battery, running lights, and two small cabin lights. Interior joinerwork is sparse and cheaply done. All pieces are cut by a pattern router to save time, and finished with imitation wood plastic veneer. The plastic peels off easily; we doubt it will stay on the facings of the joiner-work for very long.

There is almost no interior storage, save that inside the head compartment. There are small bins under the settees and aft berth, but much of that space is filled with flotation.

CONCLUSIONS

At $8900, the MacGregor 26 is a good deal. The water ballast makes her truly trailerable. For weekending on inland lakes, she is an excellent choice. She's also a good choice for daysailing in protected waters if you cannot afford dock space or a mooring.

The boat has certain limitations, however. While she is simply rigged, that simplicity hampers her sailing ability and her seaworthiness. While there are no glaring structural flaws, the entire construction is just slipshod enough to make her unsuitable to sailing where you might get caught in heavy weather.

We're sure that many passages have been made to places like Catalina Island in 20 to 25 knots of wind and healthy seas, but doing that on a regular basis in a MacGregor 26 is, in our opinion, asking for trouble. Don't ask her for more than she was intended to do.

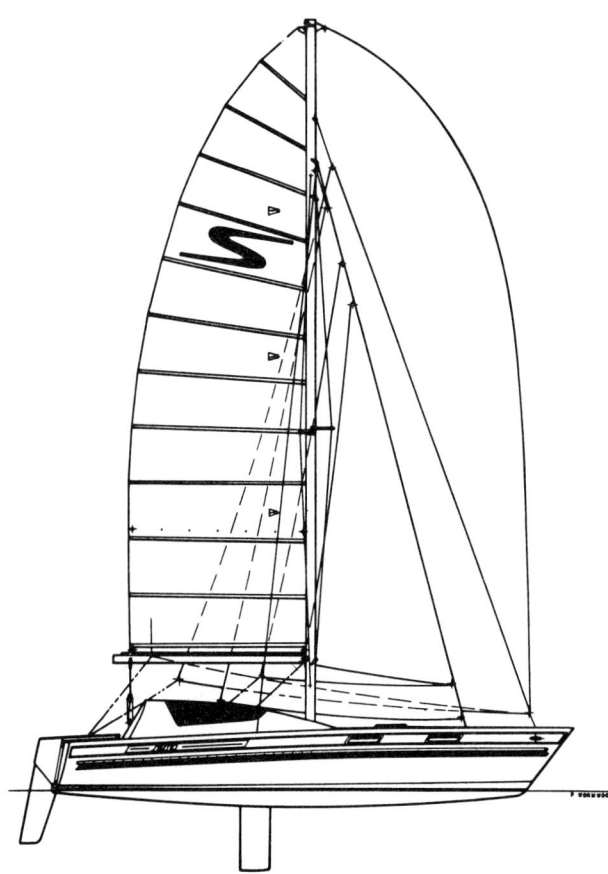

Specifications
Stiletto Catamaran

LOA	26'10"
LWL	24'0"
Beam	13'10"
Draft	
board up	9"
board down	4'0"
Displacement	
	1100-1570 lbs
Sail area	
Main	230 sq ft
Jib	106 sq ft
Reacher/	
drifter	265 sq ft

The Stiletto Catamaran: Performance at a Price

THE BOAT AND THE BUILDER

Many sailors consider multihull sailing to be on the fringes of the sport. If this is true, then the Stiletto catamaran is dangling one hull over the edge. It's hard to mistake her appearance, with blazing topsides graphics, aircraft styling, and pop-top companionway hatches. It's also hard to appreciate the sophistication of the Stiletto's construction—epoxy saturated fiberglass over a Nomex honeycomb core.

The 26-foot, 10-inch Stiletto is anything but conventional. Multihulls larger than 20 feet can usually be divided into one of two classes. The larger group is that of the "cruising" multihull, characterized by beamy hulls, with a cabinhouse across the bridgedeck, stubby undercanvassed rigs, and monohull-like displacements. They often display mediocre performance, and are sometimes regarded with embarrassment by multihull enthusiasts.

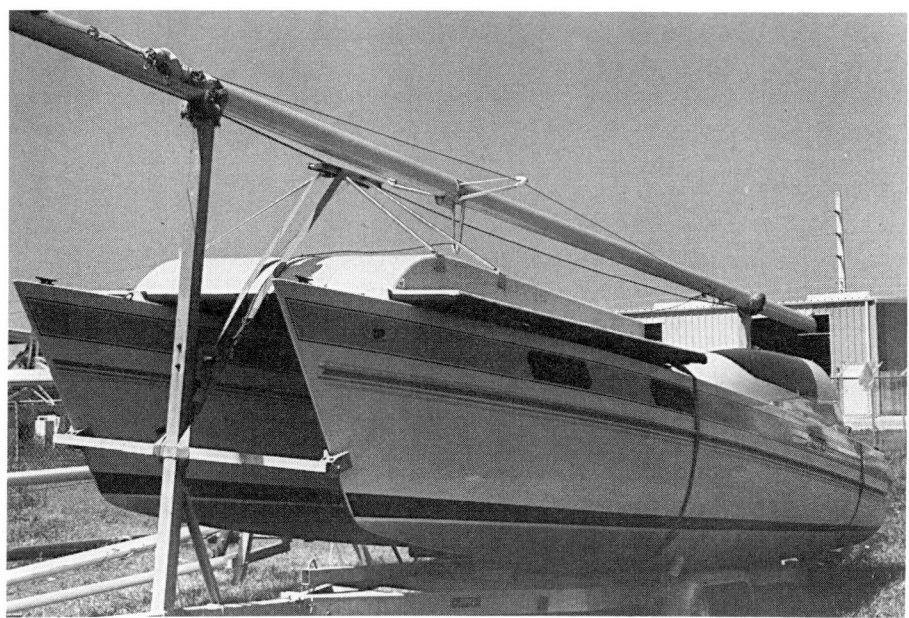

The other type of large multihull is characterized by light displacement, powerful rigs, and lean interiors. Custom ocean racing multihulls fall into this category, as do a very few production catamarans—like the Stiletto.

The Stiletto's builders touted her trailerability, "scorching performance," and "cruising comforts." She was supposed to be the next step up for the sailor weaned on small, high-performance catamarans. In fact, three of the five owners we spoke to were former Hobie Cat sailors.

Almost anyone can understand why catamarans, like the Hobie 16, are so popular. They offer breathtaking performance without making great demands on a sailor's expertise—or his pocketbook. To step up to a Stiletto was expensive, however. She came in three versions. For $17,950 (in 1982), the standard Stiletto came with a mainsail and a jib, but a stripped interior and no options. The racing version (called the Championship Edition) came with such options as deck hatches, rubrails and removable berths—plus extra racing sails, winches and a knotmeter. This version cost $22,900. Then the "cruising" version, called the Special Edition, cost $24,900. That healthy chunk of cash bought a boat equipped with the options needed for pocket cruising—such as galley, head, berths, carpeted interior, and running lights. The builder reported that 75 percent of Stilettos sold were Special Editions, while 20 percent were Standards, and 5 percent the Championship model.

Force Engineering, a small, high-tech outfit in Sarasota, Florida, was formed to build the Stiletto in 1978. Subsequently, they produced more than 300. Before he joined Force Engineering, co-owner and marketing director, Larry Tibbe, was an aircraft-account salesman for Ciba-Geigy, a manufacturer of Nomex. Nomex coring is used in a variety of aircraft parts (e.g. helicopter

The Stiletto Catamaran
125

blades). Force made several non-marine products from Nomex, which helped them to survive (temporarily) the recession of 1981. Force employed 35 people when business was booming, but most were laid off in 1981. When we visited the plant in March of 1982, Force had only 17 employees. Tibbs said orders were beginning to roll in, and he was planning to hire more help. But, he admitted, Force couldn't have survived a spring as bad as that winter. Apparently, another bad spring came in '85, because Force is no longer on the rolls of Sarasota businesses. Used Stiletto catamarans, depending on year, model, and accessories, run today from $25,000 to $30,000.

The boat owners we talked to had no negative comments about dealer/ builder service. One Stiletto sailor from New Jersey's Barnegat Bay reported that his dealer serviced a broken chainplate eye, even though his boat was out of warranty. The dealer shipped the boat to Florida, where it was repaired and shipped back, all free of charge.

The Stiletto class organization holds a national championship each year. Class organizations help to maintain interest which enhances resale value, and owners report that their boats have appreciated. Probably due to shipping costs, most of the boats were sold to East Coast sailors. The biggest fleet, 44 boats, is in Annapolis, Maryland.

CONSTRUCTION

Very few boats are cored with Nomex honeycomb as are the Stiletto's hulls and bridgedeck. Sandwiching a core material between two layers of fiberglass laminate is not a new technique; many boatbuilders use cores of balsa, Airex or

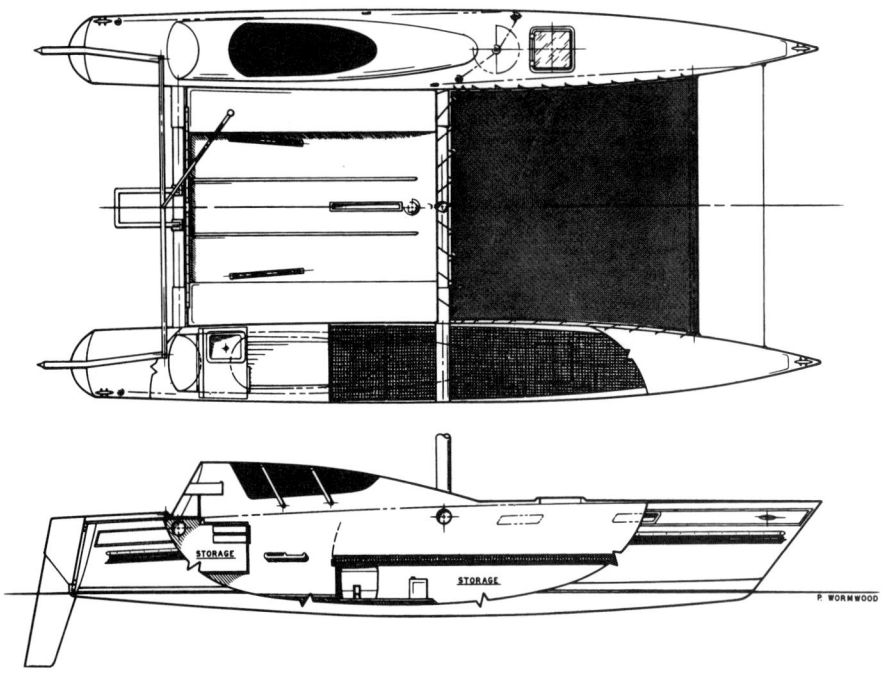

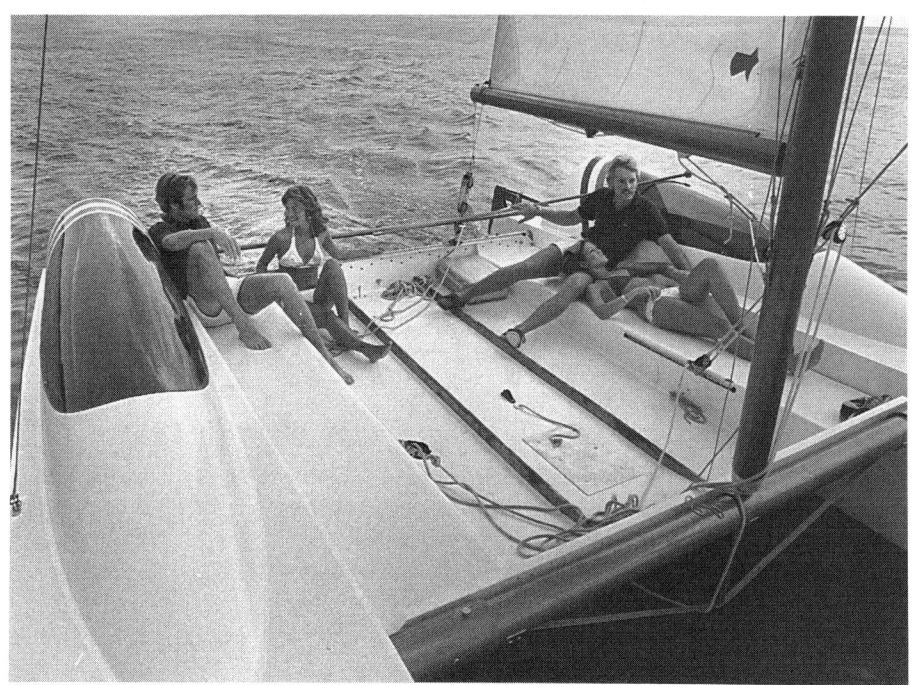

Klegecell foam. Core construction offers several advantages over single-skin construction. It is stiffer for a given weight, lighter for a given stiffness, makes the boat quieter and reduces condensation.

Honeycomb is rarely used for boatbuilding because the molding procedure is far more sophisticated (and expensive) than with balsa or foam cores. Honeycomb can be made of several materials. We question the use of paper or aluminum honeycomb in boats, because of their susceptibility to water damage should the outer laminate of the core be ruptured. The Stiletto's Nomex honeycomb core is made of nylon.

Force Engineering claims that a Nomex honeycomb-cored panel, for a given weight, is stronger, stiffer, less brittle and more puncture resistant than foam or wood cores. Nomex is also said to be impervious to water, so there would be no water migration between the honeycomb cells should the outer skin be ruptured.

These grandiose claims depend on a sophisticated and expensive molding procedure. Getting the honeycomb to bond to the fiberglass skins isn't easy. First, Force Engineering buys its fiberglass cloth pre-impregnated with epoxy resin. Most boatbuilders use polyester resin, which is an inferior adhesive, and saturate the fiberglass after it has been laid into the mold—a messy and inexact procedure. Pre-impregnated cloth, or "prepreg," has an exact resin-to-cloth ratio, which means that the builder always has the optimum strength to weight ratio. Most boat builders err on the resin-rich side when saturating cloth, which increases weight but not strength.

The Stiletto Catamaran

To keep the prepreg cloth from curing before it is laid into the Stiletto mold, it must be shipped and stored in a refrigerator. To completely cure the prepreg after layup, the mold is placed in a long, modular oven and baked at 250 degrees for 90 minutes. At the same time, the fiberglass skins are vacuum-bagged to the honeycomb to ensure proper adhesion. Vacuum-bagging cored hulls is also not a new technique, but for many builders it simply means laying a sheet of plastic into the mold and sucking the air out with a single pump. Force Engineering uses a blotter to absorb any excess resin and 15 spigots to pull the vacuum, a more effective technique. When finished, each of the Stiletto's hulls weighs only 220 pounds and is impressively strong and stiff.

The Stiletto's hull and bridgedeck may be state-of-the-art, but the rest of her rig, like her aluminum mast and crossbeams, is built with conventional (and relatively heavy) technology. All-up, the Stiletto weighs 1100 to 1570 pounds, depending on optional equipment. By comparison, an Australian-made, single skin imitation of the Stiletto has hulls that weigh more than double the Stiletto's, but the all-up weight of the boat is only 2000 pounds.

All of Force Engineering's business revolved around the molding of Nomex products. They were the leading proponent (and salesman) of honeycomb to the marine industry. They fervently believed that it is the material of the future for tomorrow's weight-conscious boatowner. We wonder whether building the Stiletto of Nomex is worth the extra trouble and expense, or if she is being used as a platform to prove the material's viability.

Gelcoat cannot be used in the Stiletto's molding process. Instead, each boat must be faired with putty and painted with polyurethane. Paint has the advantage that it will not chalk like gelcoat, but it is more susceptible to nicks, scrapes and peeling, especially if improperly applied. The Stiletto's optional hull graphics are adhesive-backed vinyl. Both the paint and the graphics were chipping on one five-year-old Stiletto we looked at.

The spars and the crossbeams are also painted with polyurethane. Although Force said it carefully sands and primes the spars, several of the masts we looked at had adhesion problems. The fittings were unbedded. The crossbeams were not anodized, and were only painted on the outside. Water can get inside the beams and accelerate corrosion.

The deck rests on an inward-turned hull flange, a common, safe design. But the deck is only epoxied to the hull without screws or bolts, inviting separation in the event of a catastrophic collision. Epoxy is undoubtedly stronger than polyester. However, we prefer mechanical fastenings in addition to a flexible adhesive like 3M 5200.

The Stiletto has a single daggerboard that is mounted on centerline through a slot in the bridgedeck. It is held snugly in place by a latticework of stainless steel tubes extending downward from the underside of the bridgedeck. This daggerboard frame is designed to collapse in the event of a hard grounding. A new frame costs under $200. There is no chance of the hull rupturing, as there would be with a daggerboard trunk built into the hull itself. The Stiletto's single board is not as efficient as the dual boards found on other catamarans, and the board's support frame does tend to drag in the water while sailing. To keep water from squirting through the bridgedeck slot, the slot is covered by cloth gaskets. The gaskets occasionally jam.

The Stiletto has an airfoil daggerboard. Older models were made of wood, and chipped trailing edges were a common problem. Newer boards were molded of fiberglass and more resistant to minor damage.

The Stiletto gets high marks for her rudders. They have strong aluminum heads and double lower pintles. To be beachable, a catamaran must have kick-up rudders; these kick-up systems often refuse to work when you need them most. The Stiletto's rudders, however, work smoothly and positively.

PERFORMANCE

Trailerability

Force Engineering emphasized the Stiletto's trailerability. True, she is light enough to be pulled by a modern automobile of modest power. But all of the owners we talked to said they rarely, if ever, trail their boats. Force says 80% of the boats are sold with trailers, but it appears that most are used only for winter storage.

Rigging and launching the Stiletto is not a simple chore, despite the fact that the builder claimed a man and woman can do it in only 45 minutes. Owners say it takes at least several men well over an hour to do the job. The Stiletto has a beam of 13'10"; legal highway trailering width in most states is 8 feet. To solve this problem, both the Stiletto's crossbeams and the trailer collapse to legal width. The compression tube that spans the bows must be removed for trailering, as must the dolphin striker beneath the mast step, and the 125-pound bridgedeck.

To raise and lower the mast, the headstay is shackled to a short, pivoting gin pole mounted just aft of the trailer winch. The winch is used to pull the gin pole, which in turn provides leverage to hoist the heavy mast. Owners say that lifting the bridgedeck and manhandling the spar is next to impossible with just a man and woman. The Stiletto assembly manual points out, "...she never fails to draw a crowd, so help is usually available if you are shorthanded." As long as you have the muscle, this clever system does work.

Handling Under Sail

The Stiletto is a performance catamaran. In a breeze, owners report, she is as fast or faster than a Hobie 16, but a bit undercanvassed in light air, especially with her 106-square-foot working jib. This is preferable to overcanvassing; a catamaran of the Stiletto's size cannot afford, for safety's sake, to be a bear in heavy air.

According to owners, the Stiletto does not have some of the bad heavy air habits of smaller catamarans. They say she is relatively dry to sail, does not "fly a hull" too easily, has no tendency to pitchpole, and does not get "light' as she comes off a big wave sailing upwind. Like most catamarans, the Stiletto has a fully-battened mainsail. The advantage of these sails is that they can have a much larger roach, and because the battens dampen luffing, the sail will last much longer. However, this inability to luff can present a real safety problem in a sudden squall. The builder says it is prudent to reef when the wind reaches 20 knots. A smaller roached, short-battened cruising mainsail is available as an option for offshore cruising. The sails that come as standard equipment seem to be of better than average OEM quality.

Stiletto sailors told us that they sail very cautiously in a strong breeze, knowing the dangers of capsizing so large a multihull. Once capsized, a catamaran turns turtle (completely upside down) very quickly. A turtled multihull with a mast full of water is nearly impossible to right. The Stiletto's builder offered a self-righting kit as an option, but they sold very few. The kit consists of a bulky foam float permanently mounted to the masthead, and a 17-foot

---

The Price of Performance

Multihulls are separated from the monohull mainstream by several things (in addition to the number of hulls). The first is performance. Multihulls, particularly catamarans, are lighter, more easily driven and hence far more exhilarating to sail than most monohulls. Yet even a novice can enjoy catamaran performance in most wind conditions because of the tremendous initial stability that a catamaran's beam offers.

The flip side of this hot performance is safety. Catamarans also have tremendous stability after they have capsized and turned turtle. All but the smallest catamarans are nearly impossible to right after they have gone completely upside down, especially if the mast is not airtight.

When reaching in strong winds, many catamarans have a nasty tendency to bury the leeward hull and pitchpole. Some cats can even be blown over backwards if a very strong puff catches the underside of the trampoline. Nearly all trimarans that are raced offshore have watertight hatches on the *bottom* of the main hull to allow the crew to escape if the boat flips over.

Another price of performance is comfort. Multihulls tend to be wet. When you're flying along at 20 knots, even a light spray can feel like a firehose. It's harder to find a comfortable spot to relax when you're sailing. The trampoline/bridgedeck separating the two hulls of a catamaran is usually flat—you sit *on* it, not *in* it. Moreover, the hulls of a thoroughbred multihull are narrow, so there is little space in which to put creature comforts. The wide-hulled "cruising" catamarans with a deckhouse spanning two hulls are usually no more sprightly than a monohull of similar displacement.

Multihulls are also less maneuverable than monohulls. They can be difficult to tack without getting into irons, and they have a much wider turning radius. Sailing in a crowded harbor requires greater care.

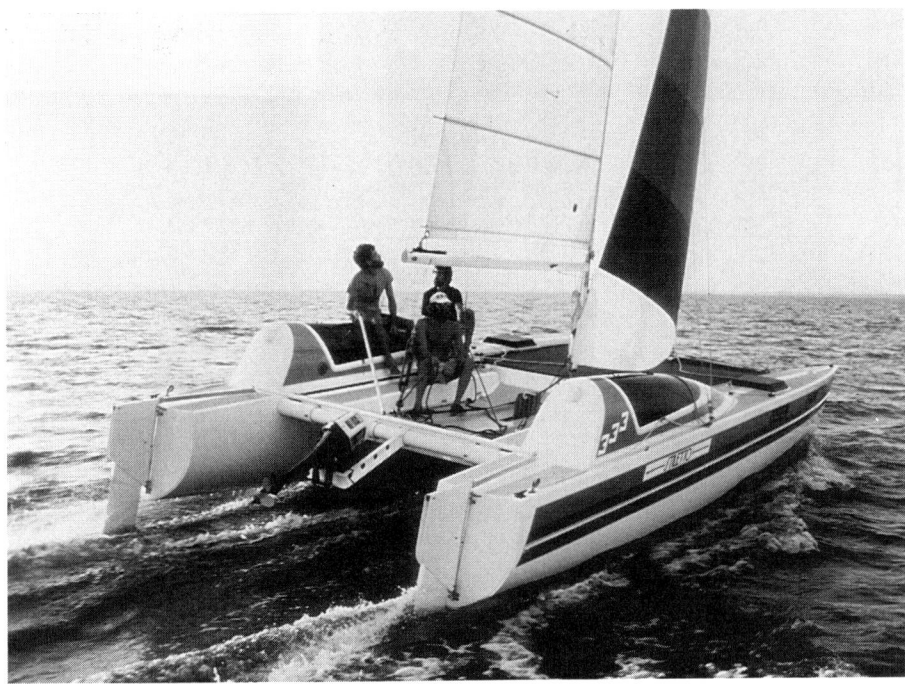

righting pole stowed under the bridgedeck. The float is supposed to prevent the boat from turning turtle, but when it *does*, the righting pole is extended outward and its three stays are rigged to the underside of the boat. Then two crew members swim out to the ladder dangling from the end of the pole, climb up (righting the boat), and swim like the dickens to avoid having the ladder drag them down 17 feet into Davey Jones' locker.

Force Engineering pointed out that the air cells of the Stiletto's honeycomb construction make her unsinkable in the event of a holing or capsize. However, they did not point out that once the hull is flooded, the boat cannot be sailed or motored home without inviting the flooded hull to submerge and capsize pitchpole the boat.

The Stiletto, like most high-performance catamarans, has a rotating mast. Owners say they have not had problems with the mast popping out of rotation while sailing upwind. The older masts have only athwartships diamond shrouds; newer masts have an added third diamond extended forward to control fore-and-aft bend in a strong breeze. This three-diamond system is strongly welded together and a real plus for heavy weather sailing.

LIVABILITY

Deck Layout

The Stiletto has a solid bridgedeck stretched between the two hulls aft of the mast, and a polypropylene cloth trampoline forward of the mast. Those few sailors planning to venture offshore might want to remove the trampoline lest it collect water in heavy seas. On early Stilettos, the trampoline was attached with a series of hooks. On later boats, the trampoline has bolt-rope edges, and slides into tracks on the hull and crossbeams—a simpler and cleaner system. The bridgedeck, which is where you spend most of your time, has no seats and is said by several owners to be uncomfortable. Because of this, the temptation when sailing is to sit on top of the flimsy companionway hatches. We feel that a cruising catamaran should have proper seats with angled backs.

A wire, stretched between the bows, forward of the headstay, acts as a traveler for the optional reacher/drifter. Most sailors opt for this sail before they buy a cruising spinnaker. Poleless cruising spinnakers are more effective on a catamaran than on a monohull, because they can be tacked on the weather hull, away from the blanketing effect of the mainsail. A roller furling headsail with a Hood Seafurl system was a $777 option. Headsail winches were standard on the Championship Edition, a $160 option otherwise. The main halyard winch, which owners recommend, was a $133 option.

The Stiletto has a ball-bearing mainsheet traveler, a worthy item rarely found on catamarans. But the mainsheet has only a 6:1 purchase, which owners say is insufficient in a breeze. The tiller extension passes behind the mainsheet, and the tiller crossbar is adjustable so you can align the two rudders. The jib sheets are led to Harken ratchets to make trimming easier. The outboard engine bracket is hung off the aft cross beam.

Interior

Those of you who have peeked below on the Stiletto might ask, "What interior?" It's a valid question. The Standard Stiletto version is nothing but an empty shell below. Depending on the care that was taken during the vacuum-bagging process, the interior hull surface can be smooth or quite rippled. Either way, the epoxy gives the boat a long-lasting smell similar to mouse droppings (we could still smell it on a five-year-old boat).

The popular Special Edition was described by the builders as a "luxury coastal cruiser." (If this was luxury, whatever happened to those World War II troop ships?) Although the Stiletto cost around $25,000, most sailors would eagerly opt for cruising on the $10,000 Catalina 22. The Special Edition's interior was completely covered—ceiling, overhead and sole—with Aqua Tuft marine carpeting. Owners say it is durable and does not mildew, but we feel that carpet belongs in houses, not in boats.

The Stiletto has the narrow hulls of a fast catamaran, which means that her berths are only 31 inches wide. The Special Edition has 14 feet of built-in berths forward of the companionway in each hull. For two people to sleep easily in a berth, they have to lie end-to-end. Crawling toward the bow to get to the forward berth is like crawling down a narrowing tunnel—it gave us claustrophobia. If a normal-sized couple really wanted a good night's sleep, they would have to bed down in separate hulls. There is stowage area under the berths, but access to it is just plain difficult.

The Special Edition has a self-contained head under one berth. Porta Potties and their ilk usually begin to reek before a weekend cruise is over. A pump-out head is not an option. The Special Edition also has a small galley built of "marble-finish" plastic laminate over plywood; we think that even the most "with it" cat sailor would consider it gaudy. The galley has a sink with a hand pump and a 2-gallon water tank. There is no permanently mounted stove; a portable stove is more practical for the weekend cruise.

A worthwhile option was the $695 mosquito-tight bridgedeck tent. The bridgedeck cushions that were standard on the Special Edition should make the tent, and hence the whole boat, somewhat livable. The Special Edition is also the only version of the Stiletto that has running and interior lights.

Perhaps the most distinctive feature of the Stiletto is her conical companionway hatches (canopies is what the builder called them). It's hard to be impartial about their appearance—you either like them or you don't. We don't. The canopies are formed of dark, bendy plastic. They open vertically like a pop-top hatch, and swing on flimsy aluminum tubes that are not well secured to their mounts.

Owners say the canopies are watertight, but the rubber gaskets in which they sit were rotting badly on the older boats we saw. For that matter, the rubber gaskets on the bridgedeck were rotting, too. Because the canopies rock forward as they "pop-up," it's hard to leave them open a crack like a conventional hatch, and there are no companionway boards. Trying to sleep in the Stiletto's hulls could be very stuffy on a rainy night.

CONCLUSIONS

There is probably no production hull built in the U.S. with a better strength to weight ratio that the Stiletto catamaran. Her Nomex honeycomb fabrication is truly impressive. But is it necessary? Just as some builders "overkill" with

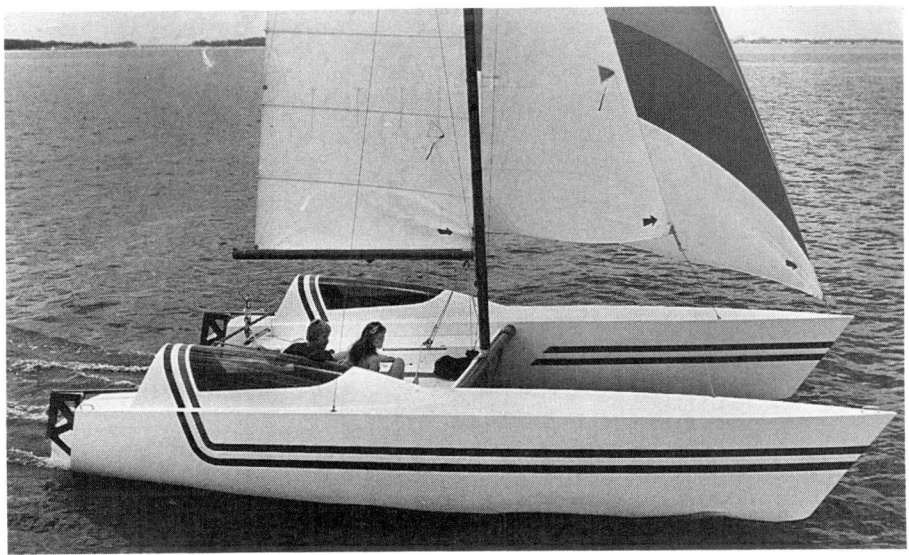

The Stiletto Catamaran

heavy solid laminates, we feel that Force Engineering overkilled in the other direction. Conventional coring probably could have created an adequately strong and light boat that would have provided just as much sailing fun for less money.

The next question is, "What do you do with her?" The Stiletto seems to appeal to the catamaran sailor hooked on high performance, but who wants a boat in which he can "go somewhere." Undoubtedly, the Stiletto is quick, but she won't get anywhere any faster than a smaller catamaran. She might be a little dryer, but she still lacks the creature comforts, such as comfortable seating and sleeping. When you get to where you're going, you will have very little comfort for $25,000 worth of boat. And when you get home, you have a considerable chore ahead of you if you plan to load her onto a trailer.

All the owners we talked to said they love the way the boat sails and have no complaints about her construction or about dealer service. Yet we still don't feel the Stiletto is practical. There are other, less expensive options for the multihull sailor who wants to weekend cruise. Any catamaran can be rigged with a tent on the trampoline/bridgedeck. Inflatable air mattresses stow easily and make fine temporary berths. And some catamarans, like the $5,000 P-Cat 2/18, have the dry stowage in their hulls to carry camping supplies. Small catamarans are ultimately safer, because they can be righted from a capsize, and they are infinitely easier to trailer.

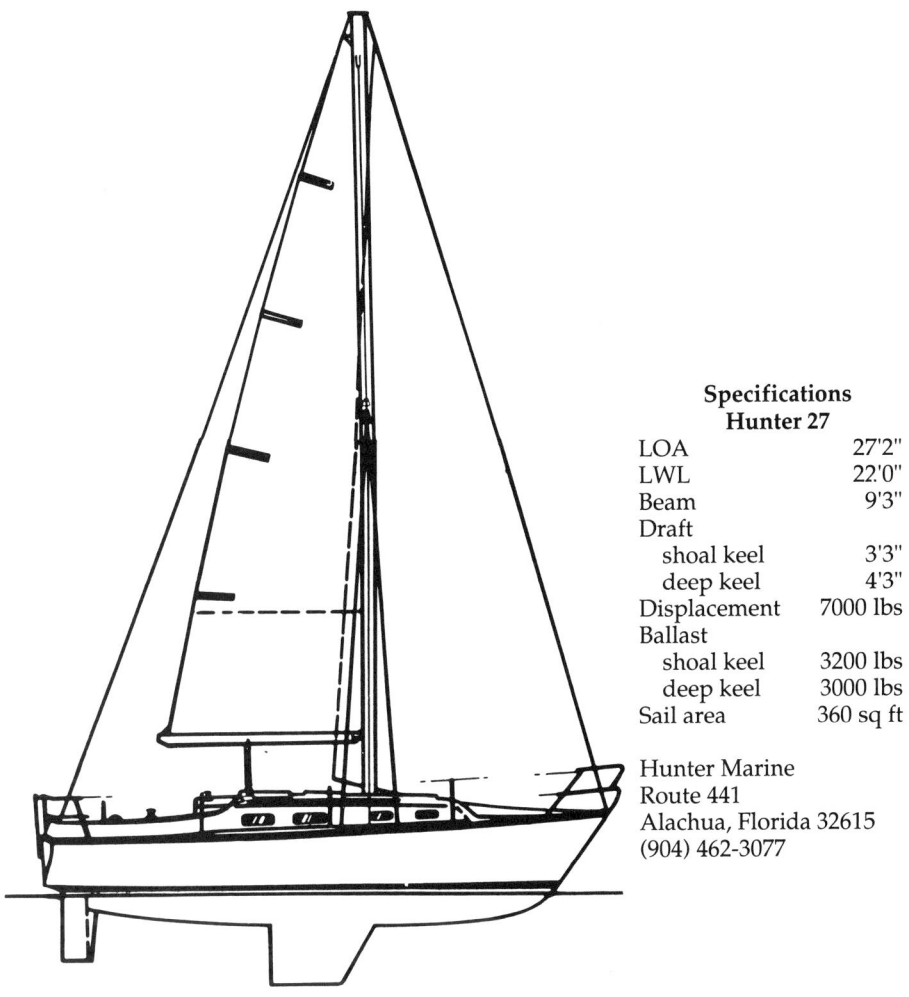

Specifications
Hunter 27

LOA	27'2"
LWL	22'0"
Beam	9'3"
Draft	
shoal keel	3'3"
deep keel	4'3"
Displacement	7000 lbs
Ballast	
shoal keel	3200 lbs
deep keel	3000 lbs
Sail area	360 sq ft

Hunter Marine
Route 441
Alachua, Florida 32615
(904) 462-3077

The Hunter 27:
A Popular Basic Boat

THE BOAT AND THE BUILDER

The Hunter 27 was dropped from the Hunter catalog in 1984 when Hunter Marine brought out a revamped line, including models of 23, 26.5, 28.5, 33.5, 37, 40, and 45 feet. Neither the 26.5 nor the 28.5 are close clones of the Hunter 27. Therefore, prospective buyers of Hunter 27s will have to shop the used-boat listings to still their cravings.

The Hunter 27 was a popular boat with first-time sailboat buyers, and with small-boat sailors purchasing their first auxiliary cruising boat. From the time the boat was introduced in 1975, until 1984, more than 2000 were sold.

Like other boats with a reasonably long production run, the Hunter 27 went through periodic changes. Wheel steering became standard. A split backstay was adopted to allow a stern boarding ladder, and to prevent the helmsman from hitting his head on a centerline backstay. All the ports become openable for ventilation. Later models came only in the diesel inboard version, rather than the inboard and outboard options of earlier years. The mainsheet lead was altered, and there have been other minor modifications—such as the switch to European-style pulpits and running lights.

Judging from the responses of the Hunter owners we contacted, *all* Hunters, including the 27, were bought for one reason: *price*. The Hunter 27 was just about the cheapest diesel-powered, 27-foot cruiser money could buy. The average price of the typical used Hunter 27 of any vintage is, for example, about $5000 to $6000 less than that of the typical Catalina 27 of the same year.

In their advertising literature, Hunter stresses that efficiency in construction, standardization of components, and low overhead keep their prices low. To some extent this is true, and it is neither new, nor something to be ashamed of. The much-venerated Herreshoff Manufacturing Company, known neither for cheap boats nor low quality, pioneered in component standardization and assembly-line construction.

By eliminating factory-installed options, every Hunter 27 was built the same. No going to the stockroom for an optional item; no time-consuming reading of each boat's specifications as it moved down the assembly line. There were trade-offs, however—the inability to customize a boat and a lack of flexibility in deck layout. The Hunter 27 buyer had to customize his boat at the dealer level, or do it himself. This, of course, makes dealers happy, as they often make as much on installation of options as they do on dealer mark-up and commissioning.

The Hunter 27 is a bit high-sided and sterile looking. The high freeboard and a high cabin trunk are almost necessary in a 27-foot boat that claims over six feet of headroom. The sterility comes from Hunter's bone white on bone white color scheme, and a paucity of external trim. Exterior teak is, of course, to the fiberglass boatbuilder what chrome is to Detroit. There are no hull or deck options.

CONSTRUCTION

The Hunter 27 is solid glass layup, with plywood reinforcement in high-stress areas such as winch mountings and locker tops. Gelcoat and finish quality of the hull molding are good. No roving print-through is evident, and the hull is quite fair—more than can be said for many more expensive boats.

The hull to deck joint of the Hunter 27 is quite simple and strong. The hull molding has an internal flange molded at right angles to the hull at deck level. This flange is heavily coated with adhesive bedding, the deck molding is laid over the flange, and the joint covered with a slotted aluminum toerail which is through-bolted with stainless steel bolts at six-inch intervals. This is an obvious and very satisfactory answer to the hull-to-deck question. The mating surfaces

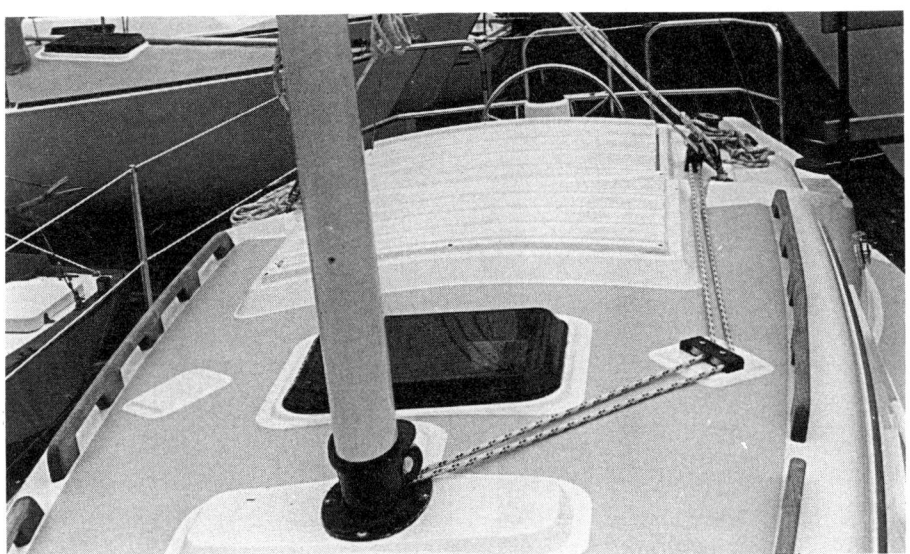

of the joint appear to match well, and the adhesive compound has squeezed out from the joint to where it can be inspected.

Across the transom, the joint is less satisfactory. The gelcoat and putty, with which the joint is faired at the stern, were sloppy on every boat we examined.

The keel of the Hunter 27 is a narrow, high-aspect lead fin weighing 3000 pounds. The shoal draft version has a much shallower lead fin weighing 3200 pounds. The additional weight of the shoal keel is to make up for the shift in the vertical center of gravity of the boat that would occur if a shoal keel of the same weight as the deep fin were to be used.

The keel-to-hull joint has caused problems in some Hunter 27s. The narrowness of the lead keel at the point of attachment to the hull results in considerable leverage on the hull when the boat heels. Several Hunter 27 owners who returned boatowner evaluations report oil-canning of the hull, leaking keelbolts, or vertical misalignment of the hull and keel. We have observed this vertical misalignment in the Hunter 25, but we have not seen it specifically in the 27.

The chainplates of the Hunter 27 consist of stainless steel U-bolts fastened through the anodized aluminum toerail. No backing plates are used with these. The chainplates are likely to carry any load to which they will normally be subjected. However, a simple U-bolt, no matter how heavy, is a poor choice for a primary chainplate unless the arc of the U-bolt is radiused to the diameter of the clevis pin which goes through it, and unless the strain on the bolt lines up with its vertical axis. U-bolt chainplates of the correct configuration are used in some European boats, notably the Nicholson and Bowman lines. Both of these lines of boats carry Lloyd's Bureau of Shipping classification certificates. We strongly suggest that Hunter 27 owners consider installing aluminum or stainless steel backing plates under their U-bolt chainplates, and check them periodically to be sure that the nuts are tight. With only two nuts on each shroud anchorage, this check is extremely important.

The rig is a modern, high-aspect-ratio masthead sloop. The mast is a deck-stepped, white Kenyon spar, supported by a wood compression column attached to the main bulkhead. We have seen no sign of compression stress in the Hunter 27 mast step.

Hunter uses gate valves on underwater through-hull fittings. We prefer seacocks. We also prefer some kind of shut-off valve on any through-hull remotely near the waterline. Few builders provide them. Hunter is no exception.

PERFORMANCE

Handling Under Sail

The Hunter 27 comes with a mainsail and 110 percent genoa. The total sail area with this configuration is 360 square feet, an average amount for a modern 7,000-pound boat. A larger genoa will be required for sailing in light-air areas.

Despite a ballast to displacement ratio of almost 43 percent, owners do not consider the Hunter a stiff boat under sail. They also consider the boat's performance under sail as only fair to good. There are several reasons for these mediocre sailing qualities.

The boat comes factory-equipped with sails. This means cheaper sails, for they are bought in quantity by the builder. It also means sails that won't be designed with specific local conditions in mind. Average sails make for average performance.

There is no provision for headsail sheeting angle adjustment. Without a genoa track, all headsails must sheet to the slotted toerail. On a wide 27-footer with this arrangement, the headsail slot will rarely be the proper width for good windward performance. With a small headsail, the lead will almost always be too far outboard. There is also no traveler for the mainsheet. This limits the creation of the proper angle of attack of the mainsail, and complicates draft control.

A relatively fat boat, such as the Hunter 27, rapidly acquires weather helm as she heels. This is due in part to the asymmetry of the boat's submerged sections. The judicious use of sail controls such as travelers, vangs, and flattening

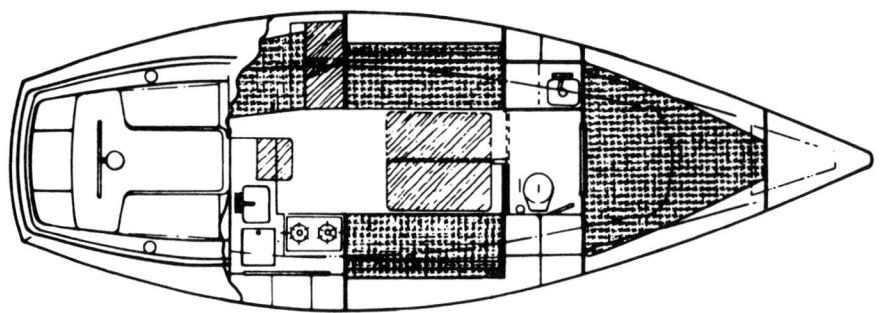

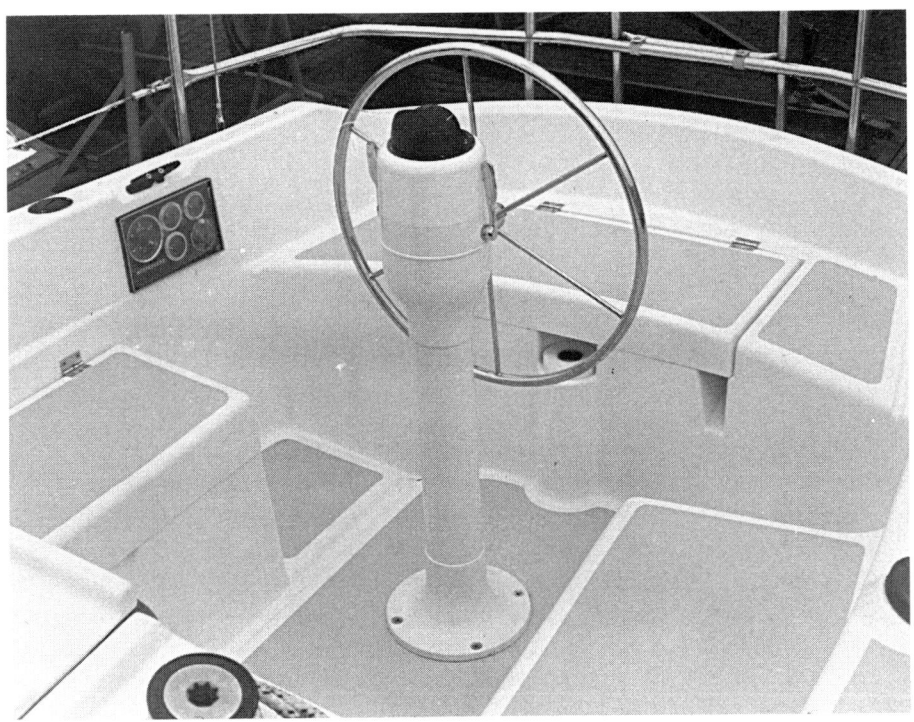

reefs greatly enhances the ability to keep the boat sailing on her feet, which will help reduce the weather helm. Hunter 27 owners complain that the boat suffers from extreme weather helm.

Chainplates set at the outboard edge of the deck also compromise windward performance. This arrangement makes it almost impossible to close the slot effectively with a large headsail.

If the Hunter 27 were equipped with well-made sails, inboard chainplates, inboard and outboard headsail tracks, a good vang, and a mainsheet traveler, we suspect that there would be a substantial improvement in the boat's windward ability.

There would also be a marked difference in price. Should you desire to make these changes, parts alone would probably run about $1500. Then the problems begin. How do you attach the chainplates? Will the deck take the vertical loading that will be on the track? Can the boom handle heavy vang loads? We are not talking about turning the Hunter 27 into a hot racer. We are only talking about improving the performance of the boat to a reasonable level for cruising.

Windward performance, then, is one of the trade-offs made for low price. Only the prospective purchaser, after considering how the boat is to be used, can decide how much that is worth.

Since the shoal-draft Hunter 27 is more heavily-ballasted than the deep-draft version, its stability is likely to be similar. However, the deep-draft, high-aspect-ratio fin is likely to be more efficient.

Handling Under Power

With only eight horsepower to push a 7000-pound, high-sided boat, don't expect spirited performance under power. In 1979, the powerplant of the Hunter 27 was changed from the eight-horse Renault diesel. The replacement Yanmar engines, though noisy and noted for their vibration, are also known for their reliability.

At lease one owner we talked to was, to put it mildly, disappointed with the Renault installation. Although the engine runs well, the attachment of the shifting mechanism to the transmission lever has the disconcerting habit of vibrating itself loose. When docking, the results of this shortcoming could be less than amusing to both the boatowner and his insurance company. Owners of Renault-powered Hunter 27s should definitely be aware of this potential problem.

Another owner reported leaking strut bolts and shaft wear due to improper shaft alignment. All engine installations should be realigned after the boat is launched for the first time. This should be a routine part of commissioning, but it rarely is.

Engine access is good, behind the removable companionway ladder. There is partial soundproofing in the engine enclosure, but not enough to shield the interior from a substantial amount of noise.

Fuel capacity is 12.5 gallons, in an aluminum tank located in the starboard cockpit locker. The tank is held in place by a stainless steel strap. There is no grounding jumper between the fuel fill and the tank. This is in violation of the standards for fuel tank installation of the American Boat and Yacht Council, which sets minimum standards used in the industry.

Owners consider the boat underpowered with either the Renault or Yanmar engines. They consider the boat's performance under power only fair to good.

LIVABILITY

Deck Layout

Because the Hunter 27 decks are relatively free of sail control hardware, there are relatively few toe-stubbers (even the grayest cloud has a silver lining).

Newer Hunter 27s have international-style running lights mounted on the bow and stern pulpits. These are far superior to the in-hull running lights on older Hunters, and better than those used on many more expensive boats. Newer boats also have a good-sized foredeck anchor well, incorporating a well-designed latch and a heavy stainless steel eye for the attachment of the bitter end of the anchor rode. The well has a large scupper which drains through the stem.

Although owners consider the cockpit of the Hunter 27 small, we find it comfortable for five, and certainly large enough for a 27-foot boat. Wheel steering has definitely made the cockpit seem roomier. With five people in the cockpit, the stern begins to squat. A larger cockpit would only encourage sailing with more people, causing the boat to squat even more.

The most recent models have Yacht Specialties pedestal steering. There is good provision for an emergency tiller, which is supplied with the boat. Access to the steering gear is excellent, through the lazarette locker. Unfortunately, because the steering gear, scupper hoses, and exhaust hose go through this locker, it cannot be used for storage. To do so would be to risk damage to vital parts of the ship's systems.

There is a large locker under the starboard cockpit seat. Unfortunately, because the fuel tank is located in this locker, nothing can really be stowed there without risking damage to the fuel system. Wet lines or sails stored in the locker would drip on the aluminum tank, inviting corrosion. Shelves installed in both these lockers would make them more useful. The shelves should not limit access to systems, however.

To raise the cockpit sill above the level of the lowest cockpit coaming, the lower dropboard must be left in place. This complicates access below when underway, but having the companionway blocked up to deck level is essentially for sailing in unsheltered waters or heavy weather. The cockpit bulkhead slopes forward. This means that a dodger must be installed if one wishes to ventilate the cabin in rain or heavy weather.

The high cockpit coamings provide good backrests for those sitting in the cockpit. They should also help keep the cockpit dry. These coamings have molded-in sheet winch islands. The owner wishing to upgrade to winches larger than the standard Lewmar 7s will discover that the islands are too small

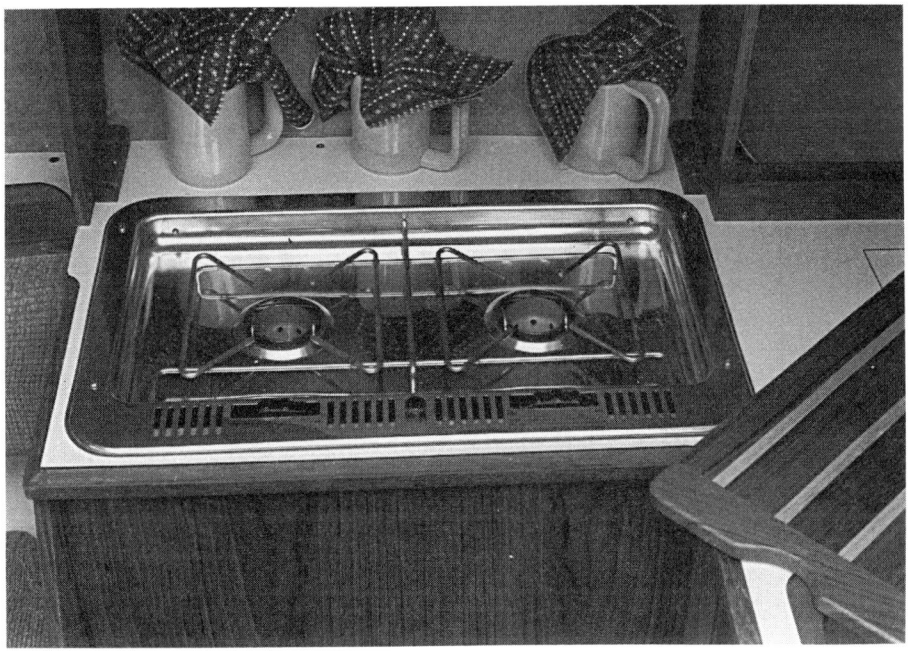

for a much larger winch. For the owner who wishes to use a large genoa, this could be a real problem. Despite these shortcomings, the T-shaped cockpit is reasonably comfortable, and is one of the boat's better design features.

Belowdecks

The Hunter 27 is a roomy boat. Headroom is just over six feet under the main hatch, and almost five feet, ten inches at the forward end of the main cabin.

The forepeak contains a double berth. Aft of this is a full-width head. Newer boats have a holding tank system; earlier boats usually have portable toilets.

The main cabin has settee berths port and starboard. These settees extend under the forward bulkhead. While this arrangement reduces seating area, it also allows more room for the galley and the quarterberth. This is a reasonable trade-off. To port, at the after end of the cabin, there is a quarterberth. To starboard is the galley, with sink, two-burner stove, and icebox.

Eight opening ports, two opening hatches, and the companionway, makes ventilation in newer Hunter 27 excellent at anchor in good weather. Older models have fewer opening ports. As with many boats, there is no provision for ventilation in heavy weather.

With a molded glass headliner, teak-finished bulkheads, solid teak trim, and teak cabin sole, the cabin has a finished appearance. There is good storage for a boat of this size for short-term cruising. Joinerwork is of fair stock boat quality. It is greatly improved over earlier Hunters, however.

CONCLUSIONS

At a sailaway price of $29,500, commissioned in southern New England, the Hunter was about the least expensive boat in its class—$4000 to $7000 cheaper than many boats of this size. The boat was also delivered with standard items that were optional on other boats; such as wheel steering, life jackets, anchor, and fire extinguishers.

However, it is not realistic to expect a boat that is 15 percent cheaper than another boat of the same size and type, to be of equivalent quality. There is just so much that efficiency, standardization, and bulk-buying can do toward reducing the price of a boat. Inevitably, the price of a boat is a function of the time, materials, and incidental costs that go into it. There is no magic way to reduce the cost of building a boat.

The Hunter 27 graphically demonstrates how costs can be reduced, however. Lots of time is saved in construction by hurrying finish work, by using staples instead of screws, by eliminating the option of factory-customizing the boat.

Hunter owners are the first to admit the influence low price has had on their buying decision. Many are happy with their boats; some are defensive about them; while others are really unhappy with them. For the relatively unsophisticated sailboat buyer, the new sailor or the powerboat convert, the Hunter 27 may have represented a good value. As a sailor's experience and expertise grows, however, we expect that he surely would be willing to *pay* more, in order to *get* more.

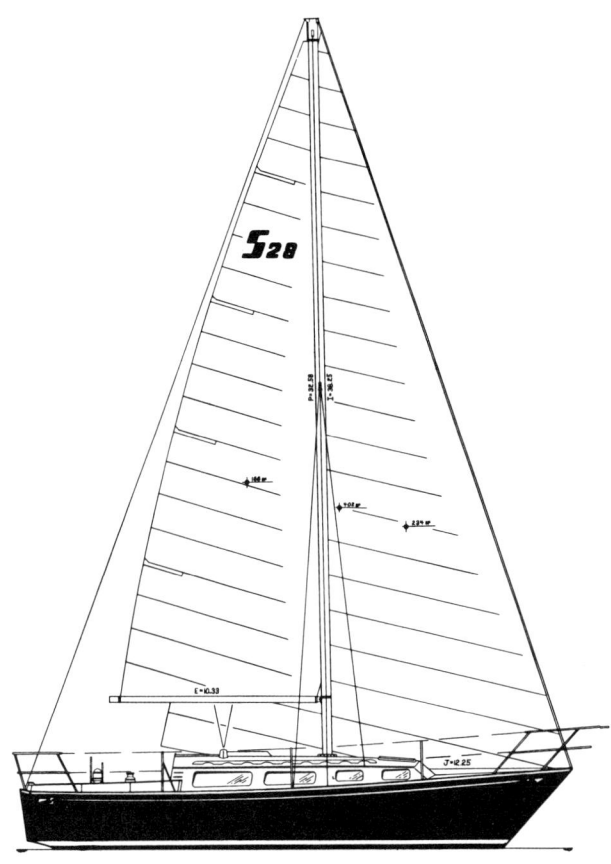

Specifications
Sabre 28

LOA	28'5"
LWL	22'10"
Beam	9'2"
Draft	
standard model	4'8"
shoal model	3'10"
Displacement	7900 lbs
Ballast	3100 lbs
Sail area	
cruiser	393 sq ft
standard	403 sq ft

Sabre Yachts
Hawthorne Road
South Casco,
Maine 04077
(207) 655-3831

The Sabre 28:
A Quality Cruiser-Racer

THE BOAT AND THE BUILDER

The Sabre 28 *was* the smallest boat in the line produced by Sabre Yachts of South Casco, Maine. Over 900 Sabre 28s were built between its introduction in 1972, and its termination in 1986. Although it was still available from 1984 until 1986, it was no longer a regular production line item, so only a few were built on special order. A used, 1985 Sabre 28 was bringing as much as about $53,000 in late 1987. Today, the Sabre 30 is the smallest boat in the Sabre fleet, along with the 34, 36, 38, and 42. The 1988 Sabre 30 will run about $63,000.

The Sabre 28 was the only model produced by the company until 1977, when the Sabre 34 entered production. In 1979, the gap between the Sabre 28 and the 34 was filled with introduction of the 30—a design very similar to that of her two sisters.

In 1982, the Sabre 38 was introduced, incorporating both standard and aft-cabin layouts, and shortly afterward, the 42 filled out the line. In a period when marginal sailboat builders have been biting the dust, Sabre has prospered and even expanded its line.

All boats in the Sabre line are of the modern cruiser/racer type, with fin keel and skeg-hung rudder.

With a 1981 base price of about $37,000, and an average delivered price (in southern New England) of about $40,000 without sails or electronics, the Sabre 28 was a relatively expensive 28-footer.

Despite a fairly high initial cost, the Sabre 28 proved to be a good investment for her owners. One, responding to *The Practical Sailor*'s boatowner's survey, reported that he paid $14,900 for his first boat in 1973. This same boat in 1981 was worth about $24,000. A Sabre 28 purchased in 1976 cost $22,000, and was worth about $29,000 in 1981. Of course, these prices reflect the inflation resulting from a dramatic petroleum price escalation, and don't imply that used Sabre sailboats will go on increasing in price forever. They do, however, hold their value.

Owners report that their primary motivation in purchasing a Sabre 28 was quality. Sabre is conscious of its image as a producer of high-quality boats. This fact attracts buyers willing to pay a little more than average—for a boat that is noticeably better than average.

As with all boats that have been in production for a period of time, the design of the Sabre 28 has undergone a gradual metamorphosis over the years. In particular, a number of changes were made in 1982, some of which are noted below. Therefore, the price of a used Sabre 28 may be a function of whether it has some of the more desirable features. For example, an older diesel-powered Sabre 28 brings about $2300 more than a comparable Atomic Four-equipped boat.

The Sabre 28 is conventionally modern in appearance. She has a modest concave sheer, straight raked stem, and short after overhang.

CONSTRUCTION

The hull of the Sabre 28 is a slightly heavier-than-average hand layup of mat and roving. Some roving print-through is evident but there are no visible hard spots in the hull. Gelcoat quality is excellent.

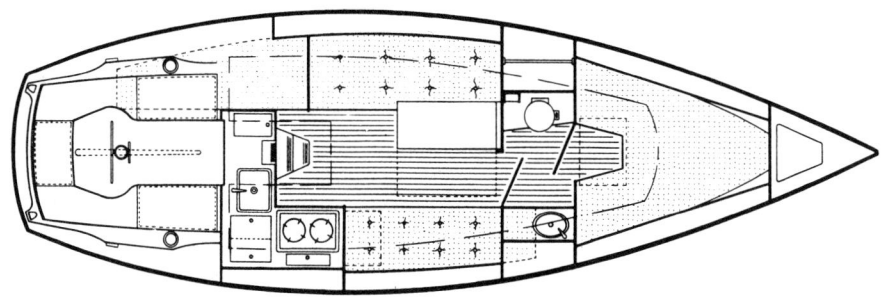

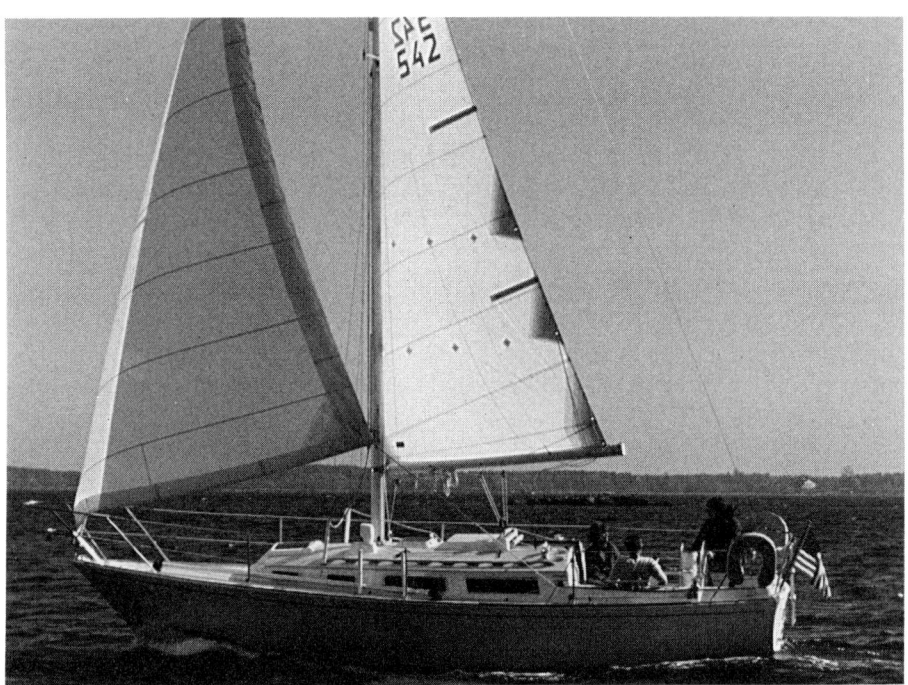

There were optional hull and deck colors beside the standard white on white. On an early Sabre 28 we examined, the red gelcoat had faded to a dull pink, and the boat was markedly past-due for painting. Of course, red hulls do fade more quickly than most colors.

The deck of the Sabre 28 is balsa cored for stiffness, with plywood inserts at such stress points as winch mountings. The hull to deck joint uses a fairly standard internal hull flange, and is butyl-bedded and through-bolted on six-inch centers with stainless steel bolts. These bolts also serve to attach a vinyl rubrail and a teak toerail. The hull to deck joint is also through-bolted across the transom.

All items of deck hardware, including stanchions, pulpits, and cleats, are through-bolted and backed with thick aluminum plates, which serve to distribute the load. The stemhead fitting is a well-finished aluminum casting.

Through-hull fittings are recessed flush with the hull surface. All underwater through-hull openings are fitted with bronze Spartan seacocks. Spartan seacocks have a short, lipped hose tailpiece rather than the more typical long straight tailpiece of other seacocks. This short tailpiece precludes double clamping of hoses. This single hose clamp on below-water fittings is fine as long as the hose clamps are kept tight. We recommend that they be checked at regular intervals.

In general, the construction details are among the best that we've seen on a production sailboat. All fillet bonding is absolutely neat. There are no rough

The Sabre 28

fiberglass areas anywhere. All exposed interior fiberglass surfaces, such as bilges and the inside of lockers, are gelcoated or painted.

Although tiller steering is standard, about 90% of the boats were delivered with Edson pedestal wheel steerers equipped with Ritchie compasses. The wheel steering option proved so popular that in 1976, the cockpit of the Sabre 28 was redesigned to accommodate the wheel without interfering with the seating arrangement. Access to the rudder stock for emergency steering is via a plastic plate in the cockpit sole. An emergency tiller is provided with wheel-steered boats.

The mast of the Sabre 28 is a straight, polyurethane-painted aluminum extrusion built by Rig-Rite. Internal halyards, internal clew outhaul, topping lift, and two-point jiffy reefing are standard; as is a transom-mounted, ball-bearing mainsheet traveler. The mast is deck-stepped in an aluminum casting. On newer boats, the mast step has been redesigned to incorporate attachment points for blocks, facilitating the leading of halyards aft to the cockpit. Halyard winches mounted on the cabin top were another popular option.

Mast compression is transferred to the hull structure by a teak compression column incorporated in the main bulkhead. Shroud chainplates are heavily through-bolted to the main bulkhead, which is solidly glassed to the hull.

Originally, the Sabre 28 was rigged with single upper and lower shrouds. In 1975, forward lower shrouds were added to reduce mast pumping under sail, and vibration at the mooring. Mast vibration in high winds, even at anchor, is a common problem with deck-stepped masts. Not all older Sabre 28's have been retrofitted with the additional set of lower shrouds. If the purchase of a pre-1975 model is contemplated, either ascertain if the forward lower shrouds have been installed, or contact Sabre for templates and parts to do the job yourself. It is a straightforward job, with the new chainplates bolting onto the cabin sides forward of the mast.

The ballast keel is an external lead casting, well-faired to the hull. Keel bolts are accessible in the bilge for periodic tightening. Construction of the Sabre 28 is strong, without being overly heavy. There is no evidence of careless work-manship anywhere on the boat.

PERFORMANCE

Handling Under Sail

With optional wheel steering, optional cockpit-led halyards, and optional self-tailing headsail sheet winches, the Sabre 28 can be easily be handled by one or two people. The mainsheet is within easy reach of the helmsman. Unfortunately, on older boats, the helmsman's head is also within easy reach of the mainsheet when jibing. The mainsheet was relocated to the cabin top in 1982.

With the chainplates set well inboard, the headsail sheeting base is quite narrow, particularly if the boat is equipped with the optional inboard genoa track, which supplements the standard toerail-mounted genoa track. The sheeting base is, for example, almost a foot narrower than the Hunter 27's. This allows the Sabre 28 to be reasonably closewinded. With her relatively small wetted surface and a big genoa, she will be fast in light air.

Unless the water in your cruising area is spread very thin, we suggest the standard keel version rather than the shoal keel. We suspect that the shoal keel presents a less efficient lateral plane for windward work.

Some attention will have to be paid to the size of the headsail used. Owners report that, although the Sabre 28 more than holds her own with other boats of her size and type, she is not a particularly stiff boat. Owners consider her performance well above average, although her PHRF rating suggests only average performance compared to similar cruiser-racers. Due to the off-center solid prop, the boat may be faster on one tack than the other, and owners who intend to race the Sabre 28 should experiment to see if this is the case.

Handling Under Power

Several different engines have been used in the Sabre 28. Until 1975, all were equipped with the Atomic Four gasoline engine. In 1975, a 10-horsepower Volvo diesel was offered as an option. In 1978, both these engines were dropped, and the Volvo MD7A diesel became standard. The MD7A is a two-cylinder engine rated at 13 horsepower. In 1981 it was replaced by the Westerbeke 13.

The propeller shaft on the right-hand-turning Atomic Four is offset to port. On the left-hand-turning Volvos, it is offset to starboard. On the earliest Sabre 28s the shaft was on centerline. This change in engines from right-hand to left-hand rotation means that replacement of engines in off-center located, Atomic Four-powered boats will be limited to either the Atomic Four gas engine, or some other right-hand-turning engine. Otherwise, there will be a considerable compromise in handling characteristics under power.

Owners report that engine access on earlier, Atomic Four-equipped models, is poor. On later Volvo-powered models, access for routine servicing is good. Some joinerwork disassembly is necessary for engine removal, but this has been anticipated by the builder. Routine service is via doors and panels. There is no oil sump under the engine. Access to the shaft stuffing box, required annually for repacking and adjustment, is poor.

Engine instruments—a full bank with no idiot lights—are mounted in the

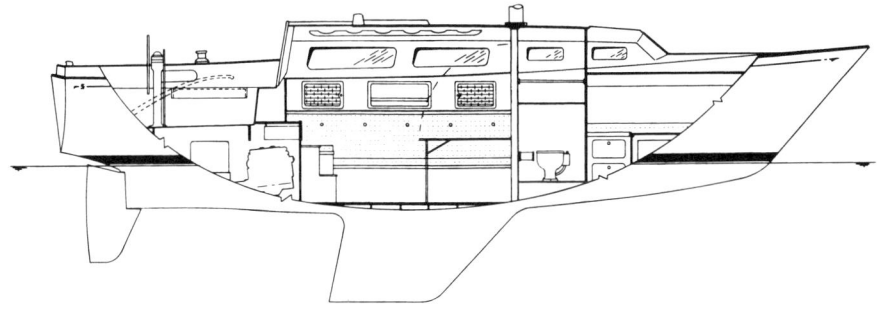

The Sabre 28
147

bridgedeck, with engine starting and stopping controls under the helmsman's seat. While this may seem awkward at first, it does protect the always-vulnerable ignition switch from water. This is an unusual, but certainly a reasonable arrangement.

Owners consider the boat's handling under power to be good. With her fin keel and spade rudder, she will turn in a tight circle. Owners report that any of the engines will drive the boat at or near hull speed under most conditions.

LIVABILITY

Deck Layout

In 1976, a foredeck anchor well was added to the Sabre 28. The well is large enough to hold adequate primary ground tackle for the boat. It has provision for securing the bitter end of the anchor rode, in boats built since 1982. We would add an eyebolt or a U-bolt to the well for this purpose if it is not already there.

The water tank vent is located in the anchor well. This is a rational location for an item whose position is commonly an afterthought. Frequently, tank vents are located in the topsides, just below the sheer. This can cause back-siphoning of salt water into fuel or freshwater tanks.

The Sabre 28 is one of the few boats we have seen that uses Skene bow chocks. Skene chocks effectively hold the anchor rode or mooring lines in the chocks, even if the boat sails around on her anchor. This is an important consideration in many modern boats, for the Sabre 28 (like many modern sloops of moderate displacement) probably sails as many miles around its anchor or mooring as are logged underway.

Heavy teak handrails, and a very effective molded-in nonskid surface, facilitate movement on deck in a seaway. The side decks are, of necessity, narrow, due to the wide cabin trunk.

The cockpit of the Sabre 28 is large and comfortable. It is as large a cockpit as we would consider safe for offshore sailing on a 28-foot boat. With wheel steering, the cockpit easily seats five.

The cockpit lockers deserve special comment. There are two molded-in recesses in the winch islands, handy for winch handles, sail stops, and other small items. There is a shallow lift-top locker under the port cockpit seat, a deeper locker under the helmsman's seat, and a deep locker under the starboard seat.

The deep starboard locker is bulkheaded off from the bilge, so sails, fenders, and lines will not migrate to the depths of the boat. This locker contains built-in holders for the companionway dropboards and emergency tiller, as well as a shelf arranged for line stowage. Although the lid of this locker is somewhat small for convenient removal of sails, it is one of the best designed cockpit lockers we've seen.

By comparison, the companionway is a bit of a disappointment. Although it is suitably narrow and has a good bridgedeck, the opening is sharply tapered, allowing removal of the drop boards by lifting them only about an inch. The drop boards themselves are 1/2-inch teak-faced plywood in early boats, solid teak in post-1982 models. The exposed edge grain of the plywood core will soon turn grey, unless the boards are well varnished. Eventually they may delaminate. We believe that plywood should not be used where it will be subject to weathering. Frankly, the plywood boards look a little cheap on a boat of this quality.

Newer boats have a translucent, smoked plexiglass companionway hatch top. Older boats have fiberglass hatches. The plexiglass hatch allows a good deal of light below. At night, when tied to the dock, it also allows people on the dock to stare into the main cabin. An often forgotten corollary to transparent hatches is that if they allow light below during the day, they allow it out at night. The glare of a white light belowdecks can wipe out the helmsman's night vision. Not a common problem, admittedly, but a real one nonetheless.

Belowdecks
The first impression of the Sabre 28 belowdecks is that she is roomy, neat and well-finished throughout. Headroom is six feet under the main hatch, and an honest five feet, eleven inches in the main cabin.

The forward cabin contains V-berths with a filler to form a double. The 30-gallon molded polyethylene water tank is located under the forward berths. There is a drawer and a bin under each berth. With the forward hatch open, it is possible to stand and dress comfortably with the berth filler removed.

The head is full-width and closed off from both the forward and main cabins by doors. The Sabre 28 comes with a standard 22-gallon holding tank. A Y-valve diverter was optional. One might consider replumbing the holding tank as a freshwater tank, to double water capacity. Then we would install either an overboard discharge sewage treatment system, or (if conscience allows) a direct discharge system.

Despite the teak bulkheads and trim, the main cabin is bright and attractive. There are substantial grab rails overhead. The port settee extends to form a double berth. With all berths filled, the Sabre 28 sleeps six. We would prefer an alternate four-berth interior arrangement providing a larger galley. Some older Sabre 28s are equipped with such a layout.

A bulkhead-mounted, fold-down cabin table seats four comfortably. It is secured in the folded position by a screw-type hatch dog—a good idea since a rattling table can drive one to distraction.

At the after end of the main cabin, the galley is located to starboard, with a quarterberth to port. Galley storage is good, with four drawers and several lockers. The galley sink is located just off the centerline, almost under the companionway. While this location is good for ensuring that the sink will drain on either tack, care must be taken when going below while heeled on the port tack to avoid stepping into the sink.

The galley stove is a recessed, two-burner Kenyon alcohol stove. Stoves of this type, which have integral fuel tanks with the fuel fill located between the burners, present a potential fire hazard if the fuel tank is refilled before the burners have cooled adequately.

On pre-1982 boats, the icebox is well insulated—with the exception of the top. Given the fact that Sabre has gone so far as to install an icebox pump to keep ice melt from smelling up the bilge, we were pleased to see them complete the otherwise good icebox in 1982 by insulating the top and lids.

Wiring and plumbing (in fact, all finishing details) are well designed and neatly finished. The location of the main electrical panel (next to the companionway where it is vulnerable to spray) is an exception to the generally well-thought-out installations.

Four opening ports are standard; an additional hatch over the main cabin is optional. We recommend this additional ventilation if the boat is to be used in a warm climate. The dorade box over the head is the only provision for foul-weather ventilation.

CONCLUSIONS

The Sabre 28 is an attractive, well-built, well-finished boat. Although her price is above average, construction and finish details are also well above average for a stock boat.

Sabre Yachts has an excellent reputation for service and personal attention. Owners repeatedly cite their personal dealings with Roger Hewson—Chief Designer, Chief Inspector, and Founder of the company—for superior service to owners. Dealers report excellent warranty support from the builder.

Despite her modern underbody, the Sabre 28 is a conservative design, conservatively built. She is neither an all-out racer, nor an all-out cruiser. She is a good compromise boat, strong enough to cruise with confidence and fast enough not to embarrass the performance-oriented sailor.

The Sabre 28 will probably not appeal to the hard-core traditionalist, nor to the flat-out modernist; she is good-looking in a modern way, without being so modern as to be trendy. Her appeal is as a well-thought-out coastal cruiser for the couple or a small family. The Sabre 28 may not be the ultimate swan, but on the other hand, she's light-years above the ugly duckling category.

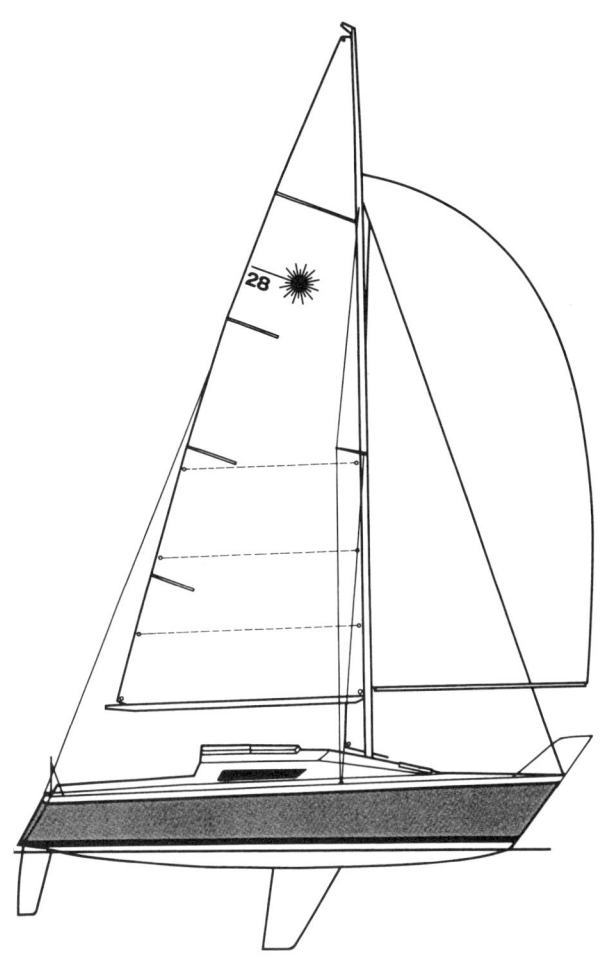

Specifications
Laser 28

LOA	28'5"
LWL	23'8"
Beam	9'6"
Draft	5'0"
Displacement	3950 lbs
Sail area	365 sq ft

Laser International
1250 Tessier Street
Hawkesbury, Ontario
Canada K6A 3C8
(613) 632-1181

The Laser 28:
An Offshore One-Design

THE BOAT AND THE BUILDER

Once in a great while, someone gets lucky in the boatbuilding business. Just occasionally, someone chances upon a great untapped market, and sells far more boats than anyone thought possible. Take, for example, the Hobie Cat, the J/24, the Windsurfer, and of course, the Laser. Rare as these success stories are, it's even rarer for a builder to strike two bonanzas in a row. Ian Bruce, sire of the Laser (and Performance Sailcraft of Canada) thinks he can do it.

Production of the Laser surpassed 100,000 units soon after introduction, but the Laser is a boat for the young in body, as well as heart; and bodies grow old. Of the more than 200,000 young people who have seriously sailed Lasers, a majority are now too old to "do it anymore." Many of these, Bruce hoped, would be ready for an affordable, family racer/cruiser, providing performance and durability, and built to the same strict one-design rules as the Laser. In reality, it would seem that Bruce was really betting on loyalty to the Laser logo.

To most of us, the Laser 28 is a new boat, a relatively untried and unproven design, that will have to be completely unique in both concept and performance to live up to its namesake. However, to the people who designed and now build her, she represents six years of hard preparatory work—at the previously unheard of development cost of $2.4 million. It's unlikely that any boat of her size has ever gone through such a lengthy and expensive development before introduction. In light of such a monumental investment, simple arithmetic would suggest that the Laser 28 will never return a profit.

For comparison, let's look at the J/30 and the Hobie 33. The J/30 was only one year in the works, at a cost of $200,000. After the first 80 boats were sold, this investment was recovered. Five years later, the total number of deliveries was over 500. To recoup the development costs of the Laser 28, 1250 boats will have to be sold.

Perhaps the Hobie 33 is an even better comparison. Like the Laser 28, it too was intended to capitalize on the success of a little sister—the Hobie Cat. The Hobie 33 was also designed with an eye toward the high performance that former small-boat sailors had learned to enjoy. Yet, after three years in production, less than 200 Hobie 33s were sold. Perhaps this was enough to recoup the $500,000 start-up costs, but alas, the builder was forced to admit that the Hobie 33 was a lost cause.

When you consider that the Laser 28's current builder, Laser International Holdings, is the end product of a series of developmental financing misadventures, you have to wonder about the ultimate future of such an ambitious project as the Laser 28.

The Laser 28 was conceived in 1978, when Performance Sailcraft was young and healthy under the leadership of Ian Bruce. After Bruce sold Performance, however, things began to become unhinged. Performance subsequently dropped the Laser project. To keep the project alive, a group of businessmen (including Ian Bruce and the boat's designer Bruce Farr) pooled their resources

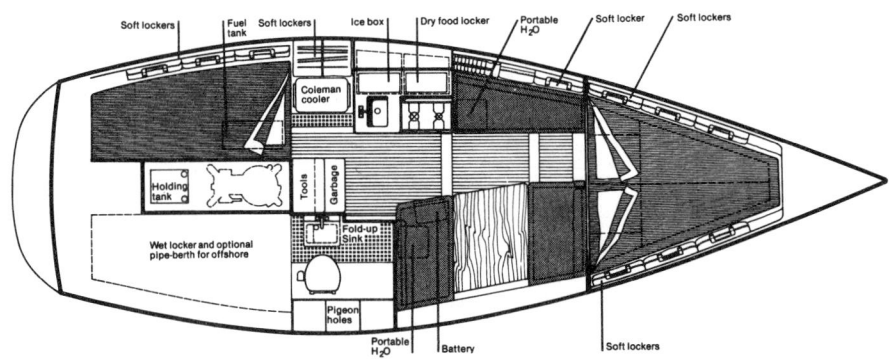

and began building prototypes in England. (An English licensee is producing Laser 28s in England today.) Originally, numerous interior, deck and rig configurations were tried, even including a flush deck model featuring a "pop-top" cabin.

Confident that they had their hands on a winner, the group decided on a method of construction that incorporated a two-piece "closed" injection mold. This method promises greater efficiency, and ultimately, a more affordable boat. But the capital investment in the specialized tooling is more than most boat builders would even consider. So the group secured financing for the more than $1 million still needed to actually begin producing the boats.

The Laser 28 is not designed to any rating rule. Marketing hopes hinged on her acceptance as an offshore one-design. When her little sister, the Laser, was designed in 1971, she was able to decimate competition because she clearly represented a performance breakthrough. The Laser 28 is faced with the same challenge. The idea of a mid-sized, offshore one-design is not new, and no one has, as yet, been able to make the concept work (except on a strictly regional basis, e.g. the Tartan Ten).

Production in North America was originally planned at two boats a week, with their prime market attraction a one-design racing potential. And how are things going as of this moment? New Year's Day 1988 celebrates the 245th boat in owner's hands. Peter Bjorn of Laser International Holdings reports that there are now 11 active one-design fleets along the east coast, with four in Canada and seven in the United States. Apparently, if anything can make the concept work, the Laser logo may do the trick. But how long will it take to reach that 1250-boat break-even point?

If the Laser 28 does survive and prosper, it will be because she tempts the prospective owner with a combination of qualities he won't find together in any other offshore one-designs: performance, durability, accommodations, trailerability, and low price. As of December, 1987, the sailaway price (f.o.b. Hawkesbury, Ontario) was $39,950. "But," Bjorn reminds, "that isn't a 'saila-way' price, it's a 'raceaway' price. Five sails, all gear ... you don't have to add *anything* to be competitive!"

CONSTRUCTION

The Laser 28 is built in a "closed" mold with a foam core encased in Kevlar skins. The closed mold process is not revolutionary, but it is a rarity in boatbuilding because of the tooling cost of the molds. In this process, the cloth and core are placed dry in a conventional female mold. Then a male mold is placed over the raw materials, inside the female mold, and the resin is injected. Except for spraying gelcoat, the procedure is "clean," and quicker than conventional layup methods. The inside, as well as the outside of the boat, is finished with gelcoat, so there is no need for a hull liner.

The resin used in the Laser 28 is an isophthalic polyester, formulated to flow through the closed mold without the need for thinners which would weaken the laminate. Isophthalic resins are less brittle and more resistant to water migration than the more commonly used orthophthalic polyester resins. This moisture resistance may help prevent gelcoat blistering, but the flexibility of the resin is essential when using a cloth with the strength of Kevlar. The flexibility of a resin should match the properties of the cloth used with it. Orthophthalic polyester, which is brittle, should be used with common fiberglass, as both will "fail" under approximately the same stress. An expensive, flexible epoxy resin is of dubious value when used with the conventional weak fiberglass, as the glass will break long before the resin cracks.

Along this same line, a flexible epoxy or vinylester resin would have been a better choice for the Kevlar cloth used in the Laser 28, but the cost would have been prohibitive. So, even though the isophthalic resin that they use might be considered less than ideal, we were impressed with its flexibility and the overall strength of the laminate.

For example, the stanchion bases on the first dozen boats (including one we evaluated) were much too small and had no backing plates. When any weight was put against the stanchions, the deck would flex alarmingly. On any other boat, we would expect to hear the laminate cracking with this amount of flex, but on the Laser 28 there was no discernible effect. The builder claims to have solved this flexing problem by increasing the size of the stanchion bases and inserting plywood "backing plates" within the core. These plywood inserts are used in the core wherever a fitting is mounted and no external backing plates are used. Fastenings for the hardware are flush mounted in the overhead. Reinforced plastic seacocks are used throughout.

The stanchion bases aren't the only item the builder had to beef up. The cockpit is not cored, and on the first dozen boats, it too flexed noticeably underfoot. More glass will be used to stiffen future decks, say the builders.

The Laser 28 is lightly built for a boat that boasts her interior accommodations. A great deal of weight is saved through the use of Kevlar (which is lighter and stronger than glass fiber) and through the lack of interior cabinetry and a hull liner. The foam used in her core is Italian-made Termanto, a close sister of Klegecell.

We don't like the Laser 28's hull to deck joint, an outward-turned flange protected only by a snap-on plastic rubrail. The flange is glued with a polyester slurry and fastened with an industrial stapler. The builder says there's more stainless steel in the staples than if #10 bolts were used at three inch intervals. Even so, we would worry about the stapler damaging the flange, and about the ability of the joint to withstand collisions. Leaks could develop should the rigid glue crack. We would prefer to see a flexible adhesive, such as 3M 5200, used in hull to deck joints.

According to the builder, the Laser 28 can be run hard aground at eight knots without damage to the hull. Many boats with a thin, externally mounted fin keel would suffer cracks in the hull behind the keel in such a grounding.

The keel and rig are carried by a molded internal floor structure which extends upward to form a ring frame around the mast support, and by hollow longitudinal stringers to support the keel and chainplates. This floor structure

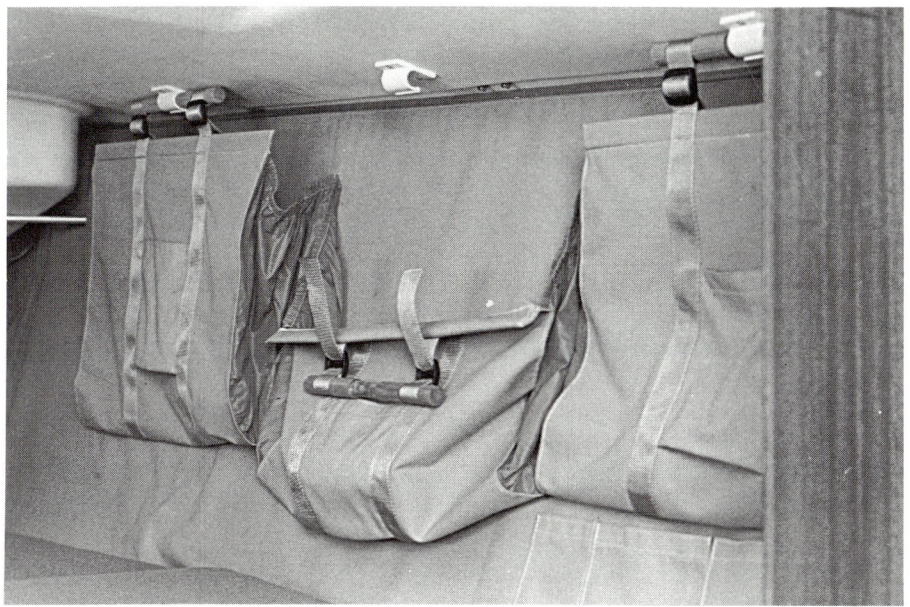

is built with unidirectional fiberglass, which provides good strength for its weight, and is glued to the hull on two-inch flanges. The flanges appear relatively accessible should repair be needed.

The chainplates are brackets attached to tie rods running from the deck to the stringers. The rods are threaded into a metal backing plate glassed into the stringer, and the stringer is glued to the hull in close proximity to the chainplate. This assembly appears strong, and even more important, is easily inspected.

The deck-stepped mast has a large compression post underneath, which sits on the ring frame. A hardwood block is set under the compression post inside the frame. No problems here.

PERFORMANCE

Handling Under Sail

The Laser 28's designer, Bruce Farr, is internationally recognized for his lightweight, performance-oriented boats. The choice of such a "big name" could be important if the boat is to achieve true international acceptance.

While there's no doubt that the Laser 28 will be faster than the average 28-footer, exactly how fast remains to be seen. Due to her lengthy development, she was a five-year-old design at introduction. She had trouble sailing to her initial PHRF ratings of 120-126 in moderate to heavy air. Reports are that she is at her best in light air. The builder expects the rating to settle in the 126-132 range (with genoa) after handicappers learn more about actual performance.

The boat comes equipped with an inventory of five sails. Like the original Laser, the Laser 28's class rules require that the manufacturer provide the sails.

The purpose is to make the boat a true one-design. However noble that purpose, it does present problems. First, sailmakers will not be attracted to racing the boat in order to promote their products. As much as we deride the presence of these "professionals" in our amateur sport, they are an invaluable promotional presence to a budding class. If the "rock stars" ignore the Laser 28, so too will many customers.

Owners who want to handicap race are also faced with a dilemma. Do they buy a second inventory of high-tech sails for PHRF racing? The Laser 28's sails were designed by Hans Fogh of North Sails. While they are modern by today's standards, they could be eclipsed in a few years by better construction techniques and superior materials.

"Freezing" a sail design and using a computer-driven cloth cutter may sound economical, but in our experience it does not result in more affordable sails for the boat owner. On the contrary, if you are forced to buy sails from a single source, he can set whatever price he wants. We have heard of markups of over 400 percent by some manufacturer-provided one-design sails.

The five sails included on the Laser 28 are: mainsail, tri-radial, spinnaker, working jib, a 108 percent "maxi" jib, and a choice of 153 percent genoa, storm jib, heavy air spinnaker, or cruising "lapper." The Laser 28 was intended to race as a one-design with only the 108 percent maxi jib. However, due to the predominance of light air in North America, the 153 percent genoa will be "legal" on this continent.

The sail inventory is all Dacron and nylon—no exotics—but a single full-length "compression" batten is used in the head of the mainsail, and two full-length battens are used in the maxi jib. These battens enlarge and stabilize the roach and make the sail shape more durable. The maxi jib carries 16 square feet of roach, yet its short foot makes it so easy to tack that you rarely need a winch handle. While full-length battens require that a sail be rolled instead of folded, there is ample space below to store "tube" sail bags for rolled-up sails.

The mainsail is loose footed with the clew attached to the boom with a sail slug. On a boat we sailed, the boom flexed considerably when the boom vang was tensioned hard, and the clew slug had deformed. The outhaul should be rigged with a track and car. The main comes equipped with two reefs, a third reef is optional. Like all lightweight boats, the Laser 28 will be sensitive to crew weight. Mindful of this, the one-design class rules limit crew weight to a maximum of 1000 pounds—about five or six bodies. We applaud crew weight limits. It makes for more balanced racing and eliminates the clutter of extra crew carried only as movable ballast.

The Laser 28 exhibits no bad handling qualities, save one. She turns quickly and is remarkably well behaved, especially on a tight spinnaker reach. However, the rudder is over-balanced. The rudder stock is placed 27 percent aft on the rudder blade to give the helm a neutral feel. But on the boat we sailed, the helm lacked that little bit of weather helm needed to steer the boat upwind. Downwind, the helm was so balanced that it would stay exactly where set—it

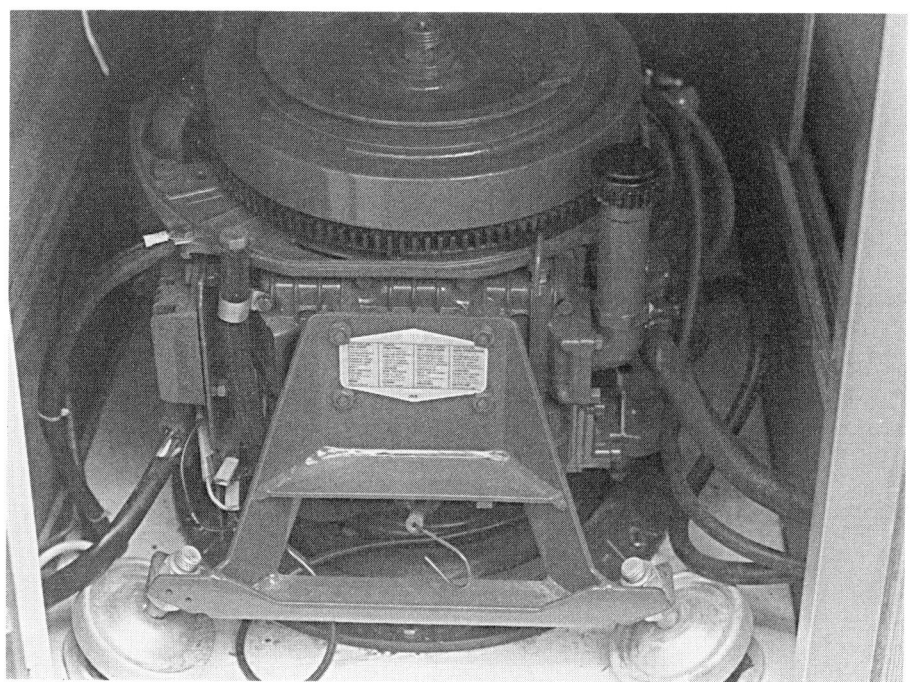

wouldn't return to center. This made it very difficult to steer, as the helmsman needs feedback from the rudder.

Handling Under Power
The Laser 28 was originally equipped with a Bukh 8.2 horsepower diesel saildrive with a folding propeller. A saildrive was chosen over a conventional inboard to keep the price of the boat down. Saildrives are much easier for the builder to install, as there is no need for space-robbing and time-consuming shaft installations.

The Bukh saildrive was installed in a shallow well under the cockpit. This well extended above the waterline, so the engine could be removed without hauling the boat. The engine mounts were hydraulically dampened. Access to the engine was excellent through side panels in the head and quarterberth, or by unfastening two toggle latches and sliding back the companionway step.

Saildrives developed a bad name for two reasons. First, studies done by the MHS (Measurement Handicap System) Technical Committee indicated that they cause more drag than a traditional shaft and strut. The Tartan Ten was originally equipped with a saildrive, but was later fitted with a conventional auxiliary to improve upwind performance.

The second problem with saildrives has been corrosion of the lower unit. Bukh claimed to have solved this problem by isolating the cooling water intake from the leg. While this would undoubtedly *retard* corrosion, it doesn't address the part of the problem caused by stray electricity from the alternator, other

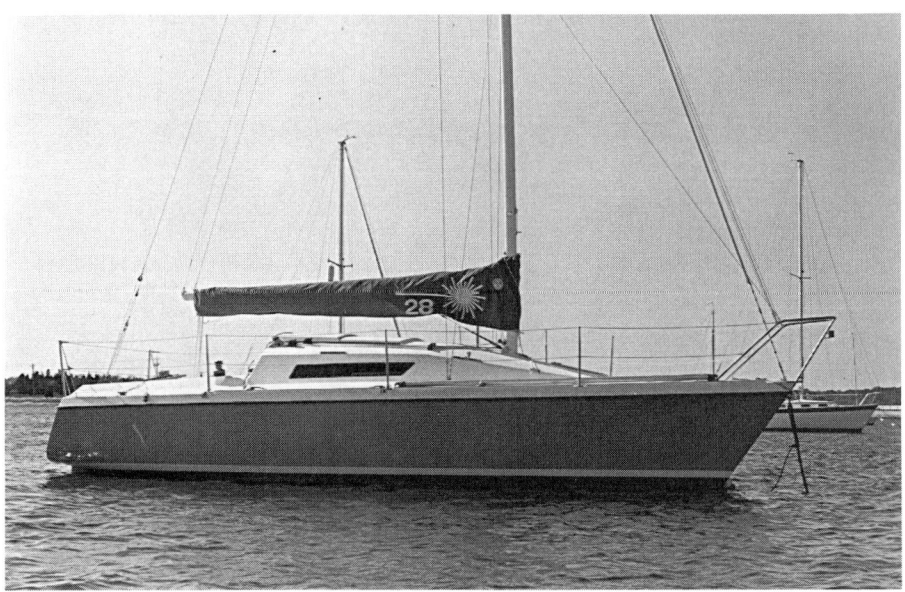

power sources in a crowded marina, or copper bottom paint. (It should be noted that saildrive corrosion is of concern only in salt water.)

Laser apparently came to agree, in time, with saildrive criticisms. Boats being delivered today are equipped with a Yanmar 10 horsepower diesel, a conventional shaft, and a Gori folding propeller.

LIVABILITY

Deck Layout

Like any sailboat with enhanced livability below, the Laser 28 has been forced to make concessions in deck and cockpit space to allow for a longer, higher cabin house. Despite these concessions, the deck layout of the Laser 28 is comfortable, and relatively easy to work on while racing.

The cockpit seats and seat backs are narrow, but angled for comfortable seating in port. The side decks slope upward from the rail to meet the seat backs, forming a slight coaming and providing more level seating for the crew members dangling their legs overboard while racing. The non-skid is excellent, a coarse molded-in sand texture (although we suspect that it won't wear as well as a finer textured non-skid.)

The cockpit lockers are very small but they are isolated from the interior, which makes the boat safer in the event of a capsize or severe knockdown. The starboard locker is barely large enough for two fenders; the port locker houses a propane tank.

The primary winches are two-speed Maxwell 22s, mounted on the coaming. While a position farther inboard would be more convenient, this would only be possible if the boat were flush-decked. Maxwell single-speed #14s are mounted on the cabin top, along with two banks of clutch stoppers. The

Maxwell 14s are all that's needed to handle the 108 percent maxi jib, and the stoppers are well suited for the task of leading the vang, cunningham, outhaul, reefing lines, and halyards back to the cockpit.

The Laser 28 makes prominent use of the cascade purchase principle in its rigging—a system we strongly recommend. For example, the backstay is made up of a 2:1, on a 2:1, on a 3:1 (for a total purchase of 12:1) without the friction typical of a tackle rigged on side-by-side sheaves. The backstay is led forward to each side of the cockpit. The vang is a 4:1 cascade and we would prefer more purchase. The mainsheet uses a doubled-ended cascade; one end is 3:1 coarse adjustment, led to a cam cleat which floats on the traveler car; the other end is a 6:1 fine-tune adjustment led to each side of the cockpit. The mainsheet system works like a charm, except that the fine-tune cleats are Easymatics. These don't work smoothly and the coarse adjustment can be difficult to cleat on a reach, from the windward side. (With a floating cleat, the angle changes as the sheet is eased.)

The spinnaker pole is stored on the boom in wire hoops—dinghy style. We see no clear advantage to this system on a boat with an excess of foredeck space. The pole controls are led to cam cleats on the mast.

"Twings" are used to pull the guy down and forward to a proper lead, allowing the boat to use a two-sheet (instead of a four-sheet) spinnaker system. The twings, along with barber haulers for the headsails, are mounted on an aluminum track which wraps around the foredeck. While a bit cumbersome in appearance, this box-shaped track makes an excellent toerail and improves footing. The twings and barber haulers are led back to cam cleats on the cockpit coaming.

The boat is rigged with a white painted, Canadian-made Espar mast. We would prefer anodizing. Although it is more expensive than paint, the finish is more durable. The mast is hinged at the deck with a sturdy-looking step, and this step incorporates the turning blocks for the halyards. It should be easy to rig when trailering. The Isomat gooseneck is fastened only with aluminum pop rivets, but side load is borne by a portion of the gooseneck that fits into the sail track.

The rig is fractional, with the shrouds swept aft—no running backstays are used. The spreaders and their brackets look solid, but the mast bends easily. Running backstays would probably improve her heavy air performance.

Belowdecks

The best way to describe the Laser 28's interior is "different." For a light-weight, less-than-beamy 28-footer without great interior volume, the cabin looks spacious indeed. A great deal of this "optical illusion" is due to the use of nylon storage bags in place of cabinetry. We would also consider this an asset in that the little woodwork provided is not of "yacht" quality.

As for the pouches lining the overhead, we counted over 60, ranging in size from minuscule, to as large as a duffel bag. They're removable for cleaning and available in a variety of colors.

There aren't many offshore one-designs with an interior that will please a woman. Most are stripped out, with no headroom or enclosed head. The Laser 28 is an exception. She has 5'10" headroom, a functional galley, and a spacious, enclosed head. The galley is located amidships, not tucked under the companionway. It is raised to normal counter height and has a deep sink with a double-action pump; a two-burner gimballed Primus propane stove; a fully insulated (though difficult to reach) icebox; and a slide-out cutting board. There is space for an additional Coleman-type cooler. The icebox drains overboard. The water supply is stored in portable plastic jugs under the settee and replacement jugs are inexpensive.

The Laser 28 has a quarterberth on only the port side. The head is on the starboard side, and while the head is partitioned off from the cabin, it is open aft to the transom—which makes it seem more spacious than it is. The starboard cockpit locker is formed in transparent plastic and floods the head with light when the locker hatch is open. A washbasin folds out over the toilet seat for shaving, and so forth. There are lockers and bins for toilet articles, and an optional hot and cold shower.

Looking aft from the head, there is ample space to store wet foul weather gear or rolled headsails. The V-berth is made of plywood-backed cushions sitting on aluminum bar. Easily removed for racing, they provide access to more storage space below the berth. Open stowage is plentiful and conventional closed lockers are scarce. Because closed lockers tend to devour and digest the seldom-used items we habitually leave on a boat, we like the Laser's approach.

The interior can comfortably accommodate a crew of three; two in the V-berth and one in the quarterberth. The quarterberth is wide enough to sleep two friendly souls in a pinch, and the dinette converts to a double berth as well. The V-berth cushions can be used to span the dinette and settee for more sitting room.

The dinette table also serves as a chart table. On the boat we sailed, the table was secured to a flimsy portion of the molded floor structure. The builder said that a backing plate is now used to solidify the table's attachment.

The combination of a vertical companionway that can slide four inches aft of the dropboards promises good ventilation in the rain. The forward hatch is custom-made by the builder. Unlike most off-the-shelf hatches where the hatch cover fits *over* its frame, the Laser 28's hatch cover fits *inside* its frame. This allows water to collect on top of the hatch. While a gasket in the frame *should* keep the hatch watertight for a few seasons, the conventional design would seem preferable.

CONCLUSIONS

If you buy a Laser 28 you can be sure of a few things—and unsure of a few others. You can be sure that you're getting a lot of boat for your money and you can be sure that you are getting about as much performance as possible out of a boat with this much interior.

You can be sure that the boat is built with modern materials and with highly engineered construction. You can't be as sure that the boat will be more durable than its fiberglass competition. The Laser 28 has not been proven yet. It's still a relatively new boat.

You can be sure that the boat can be trailered easily by a large automobile or mid-sized truck, and that a trailer is an affordable option. However, the boat is almost 9-1/2 feet wide (a foot and a half over the legal limit in the U.S.) so a special permit will be needed. In Europe, such a beam will make trailering impractical.

Finally, you can *hope* that the Laser 28 will make it as an international offshore one-design. Unfortunately, no one can be sure of this yet, and we're afraid that the odds might be against her. We hope we're wrong, however. The vitality of today's eleven functioning racing associations does lend encouragement to the hope.

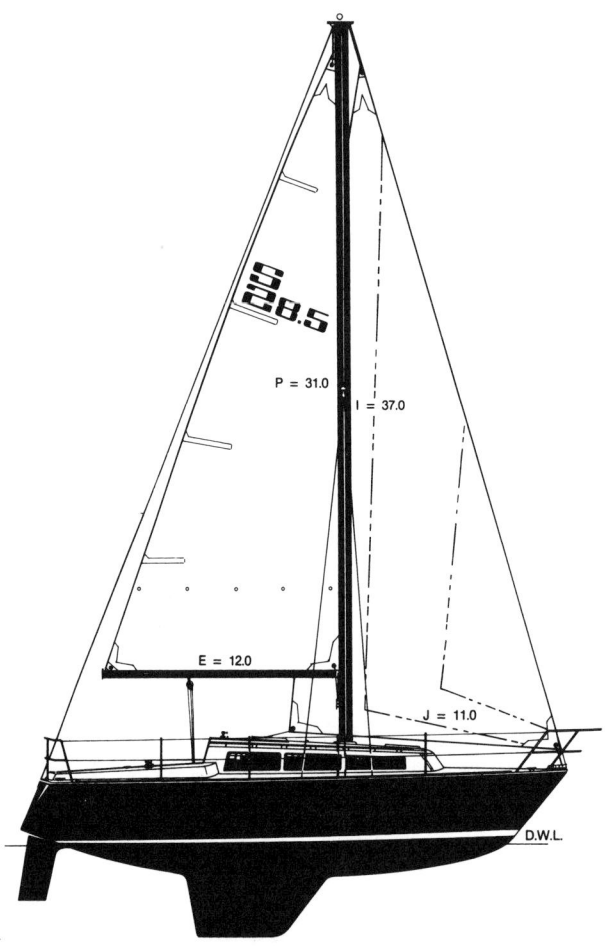

P = 31.0

I = 37.0

E = 12.0

J = 11.0

D.W.L.

Specifications
S2 8.5 Meter

LOA	28'0"
DWL	22'6"
Beam	9'6"
Draft	
deep keel	4'6"
shoal keel	3'11"
Displacement	7600 lbs
Ballast	3000 lbs
Sail area	400 sq ft

S2 Yachts Inc.
725 East 40th Street
Holland, Michigan 49423
(616) 392-7163

The S2 8.5 Meter:
Conventionally Modern

THE BOAT AND THE BUILDER

When Leon Slikkers founded S2 Yachts in 1973, much of the attention to detail that had characterized Slickcraft powerboats, Slikkers' earlier boatbuilding venture, traveled with him to the new boatbuilding company. Subsequently, S2 has produced a variety of modern cruising designs from the board of Arthur Edmonds, all characterized by longish fin keels, freestanding spade rudders, straight sheerlines, and a truly staggering variety of draft options and cockpit layouts.

S2 also entered the performance market with the Grand Slam series of small boats, and the newer 10.3 meter "offshore racer-cruiser." These higher performance boats were designed by Scott Graham and Eric Schlageter, well known for their MORC and smaller IOR designs. In addition the company produces a line of powerboats from 20 to 32 feet.

S2's nomenclature has always been confusing. Referring to their boats by their metric length (e.g. 8.0, 8.5, 9.2, 11.0) has probably caused a number of people to underestimate the size of the boats so designated. The 11.0, for example, is a 36-footer—not the 33-footer so often envisioned by those of us who are resistant to metric conversion.

The S2 8.5 is a 28-footer cast in the company's traditional mold. Her dimensions, sail area, displacement and general design characteristics put her right in the midst of such modern 28-footers as the Tanzer 8.5, the Newport 28, the O'Day 28, and the Pearson 28.

The boat's styling is conventionally modern, although the last one went down the ways in 1982. She has a fairly straight sheer, fairly high freeboard, and a low raked cabin trunk with dark tinted, flush ports.

S2 owners show considerable loyalty to their boats. The builder has a reputation for providing good warranty service. Surprisingly, owners report mixed results in their relationship with dealers. The two dealers that owners complained most about (one on the West Coast and one in Florida) have lost their S2 franchises. As one owner puts it, "If you have a problem, call S2 direct."

CONSTRUCTION

The hull of the S2 8.5 is a solid hand layup. Glasswork is excellent, and is noted by owners as one of the main considerations in buying the boat. Gelcoat quality is also excellent. Slight roving print-through is evident, but is not objectionable. Minor hard spots are visible in the topsides, probably caused by the attachment of interior furniture and bulkheads. The deck molding is cored with end grain balsa, giving a solid feel underfoot as well as providing reasonable insulating properties

S2's hull to deck joint is the basic type that we would like to see adopted throughout the industry. The hull molding has an inward-turning flange, onto which the deck molding is dropped. The joint is bedded in flexible sealant, and through-bolted at six inch intervals by bolts passing through the full-length slotted aluminum toerail. The joint is also through-bolted across the stern.

All deck hardware is properly through-bolted, although pulpits, cleats, and winches merely use nuts and washers on the underside of the deck, rather than the aluminum or stainless steel backing plates we prefer.

Another feature of the hull to deck joint is a heavy, semi-rigid vinyl rubrail at the sheerline—quite aptly termed a "crash rubrail" by S2. This will go a long way toward absorbing the shocks of those inevitable encounters with docks and pilings. Although this rail is black when the boat is new, it had dulled to a chalky gray on the older S2s we examined.

The builder advertises "bronze seacocks on all through-hull fittings." These are not traditional tapered plug seacocks, but are ball valves mounted directly to through-hull fittings. A proper seacock—whether it uses a ball valve or a tapered plug—has a heavy flange to allow through-bolting to the hull. This is

The S2 8.5 Meter

an important safety feature. Should a valve seize, it may become necessary to apply a great deal of leverage to the handle in order to open or close the valve. The deeply threaded through-hull stem can easily break under these conditions, and more than one boat has been lost in this manner.

We also suggest that seacocks be installed on the cockpit drain and the bilge pump outlet—both of which may be under water while the boat is sailing. Light air performance would benefit by the fairing in of the through-hull fittings, particularly the head intake and discharge, both of which are far enough forward to have a significant effect on water flow past the hull.

Ballast is a 3,000-pound lead casting, epoxied inside a hollow keel shell. We prefer an external lead casting bolted to the hull for its shock-absorbing qualities and ease of repair.

Much of the boat's interior structure is plywood, glassed to the hull. Fillet bonding is neat and workmanlike with no rough edges to be found.

The chainplates are conventional stainless steel flat bar, bolted to bulkheads and plywood knees in the main cabin. These are properly backed with stainless steel pads. Due to the fact that the hull is lined throughout with a carpet-like synthetic material, it is not possible to examine the bonding of the chainplate knees to the hull. The stemhead fitting is a stainless steel weldment, through-bolted to the deck and hull, and reinforced inside the hull with a formed stainless steel gusset, to prevent deflection of the deck from the pull of the headstay. We'd like to see a metal backup pad behind this fitting, rather than the washers that are used.

General construction is thoughtful and well executed, with excellent glasswork, a strong and simple hull to deck joint, and reasonably well installed hardware and fittings.

PERFORMANCE

Handing Under Power
Although some early models of the 8.5 used a 7-horsepower BMW diesel, the 1982 version employs an 8-horsepower Yanmar. The new generation of small Yanmars are quite impressive, light in weight and far smoother than the company's engines of a few years ago.

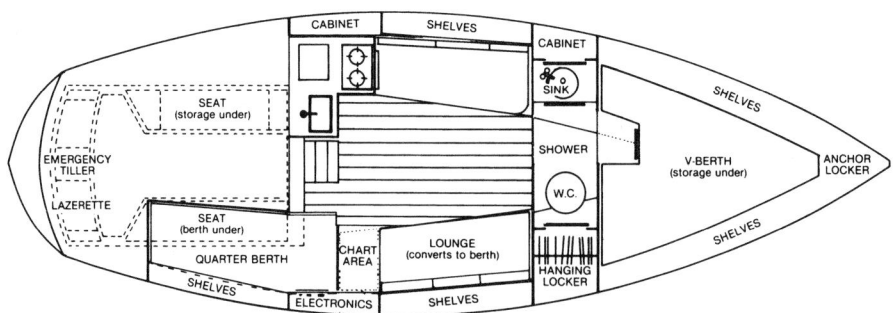

Because of the high freeboard and considerable windage of the 8.5, the standard engine provides minimum power for the boat. Recognizing this, the company offered a 15-horsepower, two-cylinder Yanmar as an option. For another 75 pounds (and $1150) we would certainly choose this model if the ability to navigate under power was a prime consideration.

The extra fuel consumption of the larger engine will scarcely be noticed. The 18-gallon aluminum fuel tank will probably give a range of over 250 miles—more than adequate for a 28-foot cruising boat.

The fuel tank is located under the cockpit and is securely mounted and properly grounded. There is an easily reached fuel shut-off between the engine and tank. Unfortunately, the fuel fill is located in the cockpit sole. Spilled diesel oil turns even the best fiberglass nonskid into an ice skating rink.

Engine access is via a large removable panel on the inboard surface of the quarterberth. This panel lacks any kind of handhold for convenient removal, which could work to discourage regular inspection of the engine oil level. The top companionway step also removes for access, but it's a long reach to the dipstick. There is no oil pan under the engine. It will be necessary to be very careful when changing oil to keep the bilge clean.

With the quarterberth panel removed, access for routine service is excellent. The quarterberth has remarkable headroom, so that the mechanic will not feel like a trapped spelunker after a half hour of work. Engine removal will require some joinerwork disassembly.

Handling Under Sail

The S2 8.5 is no slug under sail. Her PHRF rating of 174 to 180 compares favorably with other boats of similar size and type. The Sabre 28, for example, has a rating of 198, the Pearson 28 about 195, and the O'Day 28 about 198.

Part of this is no doubt due to the fact that the standard sails on the boat come from the North loft. While North's OEM sails may not be the vertical cut Mylar-Kevlar wonders that adorn custom boats, they're a good bit better than most.

S2 uses Hall spars. The simple masthead rig is extremely clean, with airfoil spreaders and internal tangs. The boom features an internal outhaul and provision for two internal reefing lines, with cam cleats at the forward end of the boom.

The deck-stepped mast is mounted in a stainless steel deck plate incorporating plenty of holes for the attachment of blocks. Halyards and cunningham lead aft along the cabin house top to a pair of Lewmar #8 winches. Lewmar #16s are optional, but hardly necessary.

The main is controlled by a six-part Harken tackle mounted on the end of the boom, and a Kenyon traveler mounted on the aft cockpit coaming. This will work fine with the tiller-steered version of the boat. With wheel steering, the mainsheet is likely to be a nuisance to the helmsman.

Because of the end-of-boom sheeting, a boom vang will be essential for full mainsail control. Ironically, the boat's drawings show almost midboom sheet-

The S2 8.5 Meter

ing, with the traveler mounted on the bridgedeck at the forward end of the cockpit. This is probably a better arrangement, although it heavily loads the center of the boom and requires more sheeting force.

Despite the fact that the shrouds are set well in from the rail, the boat lacks inboard headsail tracks. Rather, you are limited to snatch blocks shackled to the toerail track. A six-foot piece of track set inboard of the rail would be a useful addition.

Standard headsail sheet winches are two-speed Lewmar #30s. Options include both larger winches and self-tailers, both of which are worth considering for either racing or cruising. The cockpit coamings are wide enough for mounting larger primaries and secondaries.

The high-quality rig and sails add to the price of the S2, but they are well worth the cost.

LIVABILITY

Deck Layout

The deck layout of the 8.5 is clean and functional, with no toe-stubbers to catch you unaware. There are two foredeck mooring cleats, but no bow chocks. The necessity to lead an anchor rode well off the boat's centerline, coupled with high freeboard forward, is likely to result in a boat which sails around on her anchor or mooring. The 8.5 has a pair of wide stainless steel chafing strips at the bow which will effectively protect the deck from the chafe of the anchor line.

The 8.5's foredeck anchor well is one of the best we've seen. It is shallow—just deep enough to hold an anchor and adequate rode. There are double scuppers, which offer less likelihood of clogging. The lid is held on by full-length piano hinge, and there is a positive latch. The shallow locker, well above the waterline, means that water is less likely to enter through the scuppers, which can be a real problem with a deep anchor well. When the bow pitches into waves, a deep anchor well can fill with water, and if the scuppers clog with debris, you can find yourself sailing around with several hundred pounds of extra weight in the worst possible location. There is no provision for securing the bitter end of the anchor rode, but a big galvanized eyebolt installed in the well by the owner will solve that problem.

The running lights leave something to be desired. Their location at deck level just aft of the stem makes them vulnerable to damage when handling ground tackle. We much prefer an international style bicolor mounted on the pulpit, another two feet off the water; easier to see, and out of the way. Wiring for the running lights is exposed in the anchor well, and should be secured out of the way.

A recessed teak handrail runs the full length of the cabin trunk, serving the dual function of heavy weather handhold and cabin trim piece. Its shape makes it far easier to oil or varnish than the conventional round handrail, although the wide, flat section seems somewhat awkward after years of grabbing round rails.

The 8.5's cockpit is the maximum size we'd want to see on a boat of this size. The T-shape is designed to accommodate the optional wheel steerer, yielding a somewhat odd layout for the tiller-steered version. A bench seat spans the aft end of the cockpit. Although this makes good seating in port, we doubt that you'd want anyone sitting there under sail; too much weight in the end of the boat. It does make a natural helmsman's seat for wheel steering. Engine controls and instrument panel are also located at the aft end of the cockpit, basically inaccessible to the tiller-steering helmsman.

There are two lifting lids in the aft cockpit bench, giving access to a cavernous space under the cockpit. To be useful, dacron bags should be fitted to the inside of these lockers for handy stowage for spare sheets and blocks.

There are comfortable contoured seats along each side of the cockpit. The large cockpit will accommodate up to six for sailing, and eight for in-port partying, although the seats are both too narrow and too short for sleeping. There is a huge locker under the port seat. Although plywood pen boards somewhat separate this locker from the engine space under the cockpit, it would be far too easy for deeply piled junk to get knocked over the board and into the engine. This locker should be partitioned into smaller spaces unless it is to be used exclusively as a sail locker. The battery boxes, fitted at the forward end of the locker, could benefit from plywood or fiberglass lids to keep battery acid off gear which might find its way onto the batteries. The box is designed to take two batteries (one battery is standard) stored in plastic containers. A single lid covering the whole box would be more efficient.

The forward end of the cockpit is protected by a narrow bridgedeck. However, the cockpit coamings extend a full foot above the level of the bridgedeck. To block the companionway to the level of the top of the coamings will require leaving two of the three drop boards in place when sailing.

Although there is moderate taper to the sides of the companionway, making it easier to remove the drop boards, it is still necessary to lift each board above five inches before it can be removed. This is far safer than many tapered companionways, where the boards practically fall out if touched. As on many boats, the aft cabin bulkhead slopes forward, rendering it impossible to leave the drop boards out for ventilation when it rains.

The companionway slide is one of the best we've seen. It's a contoured piece of Acrylic fitted with a convenient grabrail. It slides easily in extruded aluminum channels, and is fitted with a fiberglass seahood.

Belowdecks

Owners consistently praise the interior design and finishing of S2 sailboats. From looking at the 8.5, it's easy to see why. There are no exposed interior fiberglass surfaces except the head floor-pan molding. The hull and cabin overhead are lined with a carpet-like synthetic fabric. While this will undoubtedly cut down on the condensation, but we wonder how this fabric will hold up over time. Inevitably, the hull liner and even the overhead will get wet. In freshwater areas, this is no problem. The water will eventually evaporate. In salt water, however, wet fabric never seems to dry. Salt draws moisture like a magnet draws steel. Although the fabric-covered interior is attractive, Formica, wood, or even gelcoated surfaces are probably more practical in the long run on boats used in salt water.

The interior layout is fairly conventional, with V-berths forward, and a full-width head just aft of these. The head can be closed off from both the forward cabin and the main cabin with solid doors—a real luxury. There is a large hanging locker in the head, and reasonable storage space for toilet articles.

The word for the main cabin is "wide," with the settees pushed as far outboard as they can go. Decor is a little rich in teak for our taste, but it is one of the better coordinated interiors we've seen. S2 has a good interior decorator.

A fold-down dining table seats four. When folded against the bulkhead it is held in place by a single latch, which makes us nervous.

Neither settee is full length. The foot of the port settee runs under the galley counter, making it long enough for sleeping, although your feet may feel a little claustrophobic in the tiny footwell. The starboard settee is of an unusual configuration. The aftermost 12 inches of the settee fold up to form an armrest, leaving a gap between the end of the settee and the quarterberth. Inexplicably, this gap is referred to on the accommodation plan as a "charting area," although there is no chart table.

Over this hypothetical charting area, is the best electrical panel we've seen on a 28-foot boat. The panel has a locking battery switch, battery test meter, and a panel with room for 14 breakers, although only half this number are used on the standard boat.

Most quarterberths tend to induce claustrophobia. That of the 8.5 is more likely to magnify any tendency toward agoraphobia. At last, there is a quarterberth that won't cause a concussion when you sit bolt upright in the middle of the night when your neighbor drags down on you in the anchorage.

The standard cabin sole is carpet-covered fiberglass. For another $325, teak and holly was available for the traditionalist. Unfortunately, there is no access to the bilge in the main cabin—none! This is inexcusable, and could be dangerous. A few hours with a sabre saw could solve this problem.

The galley is workable and accessible, with no awkward posturing necessary to do the dishes. The sink deserves high marks. It is a full nine inches deep, is large enough to take a frying pan, and is mounted close to the centerline. In contrast, the icebox gets a low score. It is larger than normal for a boat of this size, but it drains to the bilge, has a poorly insulated top, and a tiny, uninsulated hatch without even a suggestion of a gasket.

Because of limited counter space, the two-burner Kenyon alcohol stove is mounted athwartships, rather than fore and aft. This means that the stove cannot be gimballed, and that it necessary to reach across the inboard burner to use the outboard one. Given the fact that countertop gimballed stoves are usually dangerous, the lack of gimballing doesn't bother us much. What does concern us is that if you want to upgrade the stove to something more functional, the limited space will stretch your ingenuity.

A fold-down table at the end of the galley counter gives additional counter space, but it must be left up in order to use the port settee for sleeping.

Roominess, excellent execution, and good color coordination are trademarks of the interiors of all S2s, and taken as a whole, the 8.5 fits well into this enviable tradition.

CONCLUSIONS

With a base price of $37,200 and a typical sailaway price of about $40,000, the S2 8.5 Meter was not a cheap boat. With a full-blown list of options, including such items as hot water, larger engine, spinnaker, genoa and wheel steering, the price could easily exceed $45,000.

The option list for this boat was the most extensive we've seen on a 28-footer—including a wide range of both performance and comfort packages. For the person who wants to personalize a 28-footer, and doesn't mind spending the money, the options list is intriguing. We quickly ran the price of an 8.5 over $50,000 by drooling over the options list.

With money becoming tighter, dock space tougher to find, and boatowners generally downscaling their size expectations, we're likely to see more lavishly equipped, well finished small boats. The cost of these smaller boats, however, can be a little staggering.

The S2 8.5 is a good boat for cruising the Great Lakes or any coast in comfort and a certain amount of style. Her appearance may be a little modern for traditionalists, with her straight sheer and European-style cabin windows.

Pricey? Yes, but when you look at the things that go into the boat—the rig, good sails, and a comfortable, well finished interior—the price may seem a little less painful. You still pay for what you get.

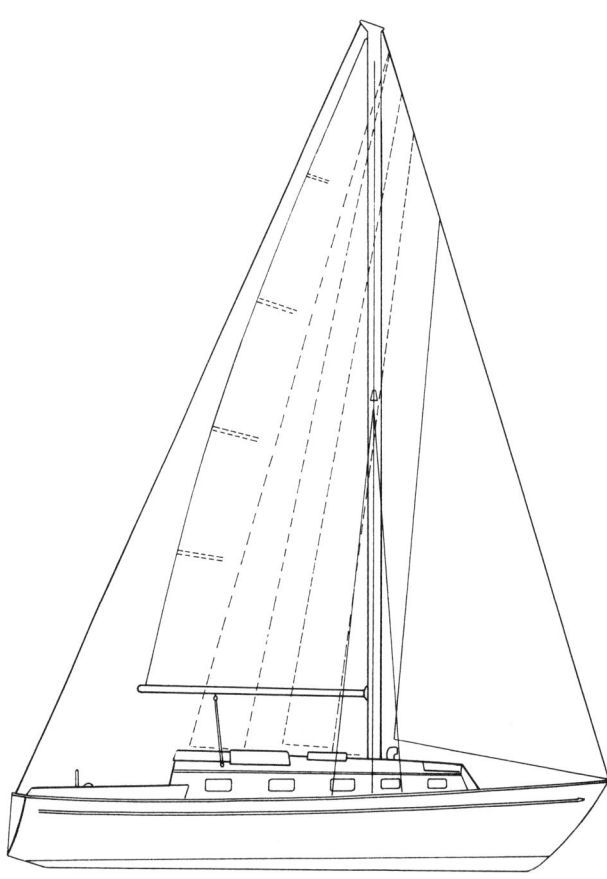

Specifications
Bristol 29.9

LOA	29'11"
LWL	24'0"
Beam	10'2"
Draft	
standard	4'4"
centerboard up	3'6"
centerboard down	7'6"
Displacement	8650 lbs
Ballast	3600 lbs
Sail area	391 sq ft

Bristol Yachts
Franklin Street
Bristol,
Rhode Island 02809
(401) 253-5200

The Bristol 29.9:
Solid, Comfortable, and "Low-Tech"

THE BOAT AND THE BUILDER

A Bristol yacht has always been characterized by a conventional sheer, capped by a high, cambered cabin house. The 29.9 has all these features, along with a freeboard of less than attractive height, and a slightly pinched stern. The phrase "bulky looking" has been used by more than one 29.9 owner.

The Bristol line has traditionally exhibited a conservative approach to design that emphasized increased displacement, labor intensive interiors, and less than sprightly performance. The 29.9 is no exception. She is of moderate displacement, has a long, shallow keel, and a cruising rig. Perhaps surprisingly, the builder and designer conceived her as a potential participant in IOR and MORC racing/cruising events. She was not a racing success, however, and was quickly relegated to the role of cruiser and daysailer.

Since her introduction in 1977, over 200 Bristol 29.9s have been built. Construction continued until 1985, when production facilities (and hopefully, prospective buyer's attentions) were shifted to the newer Bristol 31.1.

Bristol Yachts is located in Bristol, Rhode Island. Despite their occasional allusions to "Bristol fashion," this term has its origin in Bristol, England—not Rhode Island. The heritage of Bristol Yachts barely spans the era of fiberglass. General Manager Clint Pearson helped introduce fiberglass sailboat auxiliaries to the public as co-founder of Pearson Yachts in the late 1950s. After selling out to Grumman Allied Industries, Pearson founded Bristol Yachts. While a financial crisis brought the company to the brink of bankruptcy in the 1970s, it has since regained its health and stands today as one of the dwindling number of "survivors" of the big mid-'80s sailboat depression.

Bristol 29.9 owners who returned *The Practical Sailor's* Boatowner Questionnaires are generally happy with their boats. Only one filed a warranty claim with the builder and felt he was not treated satisfactorily. He recommended inspection of the boat before accepting delivery. Of the owners who purchased their boats from dealers, a majority said they were not treated satisfactorily by the dealers. One even called a major Bristol dealer "unpleasant and hostile."

CONSTRUCTION

The construction of the 29.9 was conventional and sturdy. We consider it above average for a production cruiser and would not hesitate to use this boat for coastal cruising. The hull is a heavy layup of solid fiberglass and the deck is cored with balsa. The counter is stiffened by a stringer. The topsides derive stiffness from the interior furniture (for example, the V-berth is positioned relatively high to more effectively lend stiffness to the flat surfaces of the forward topsides).

The 29.9 is not typical of production sailboats in that the interior is built in pieces and glassed into place (except the head/shower and the overhead). Most production boats use a one-piece molded interior liner which, because it is attached to the hull in fewer places, offers less stiffness. Liners also have the bad habit of working loose during the later years of a boat's life, and are far more difficult to refasten than a pieced-in interior.

The hull-to-deck joint is done in a fashion we recommend. It has an inward-directed, horizontal hull flange, overlapped by the deck, which is through-bolted at close intervals. In fact, on the 29.9, the bolts are installed even closer than necessary.

Originally, this joint was sealed with butyl tape, a clay-like substance which provides good waterproofing but no chemical bond. We have no reports of this joint leaking, but on later models, Bristol used 3M 5200 outside the butyl to provide a clean, glued joint. (3M 5200 is a strong, semi-rigid adhesive.) On the older boat we inspected, the butyl had not been trimmed where it had oozed from the joint inside the cabin lockers. Also, the hull flange had been cut away to allow a stanchion backing plate to be positioned flush against the deck. It would be better practice to shim one side of the backing plate to provide flush positioning against the hull flange.

The 29.9 has an internal keel which is set into the boat with fiberglass mat, and then glassed over to seal the ballast from the interior of the boat. It is difficult to prevent voids between the hull shell and the internal ballast. In the event of a hard grounding, water could enter the shell and repairs would be more difficult than with external ballast.

Bristol offered both keel and centerboard versions of the 29.9. Although the centerboard was a $3400 option, the BUC Used Boat Price Guide shows that it adds no value to the boat. The centerboard version draws only 10 inches less with the board up, so any advantage to the gunkholer would be minimal. The centerboard version also lacks the sump of the keeled version, so water is prone to slosh up under the quarter berth. The board is hoisted by a wire pennant on a worm-driven reel winch, and works well. This is advantageous because owners will want to hoist the board when moored, to keep it from slatting in the trunk.

The rudder is supported by a skeg and driven by an Edson wheel-steering system. There is a propeller aperture in the skeg. Access to the steering cable (or to fit an emergency tiller) is through a hatch under the lazarette.

Seacocks are used on all through-hull fittings, but until 1984, a gate valve was used on the engine coolant intake. Hoses are double clamped and seacocks are bedded with 3M 5200.

The spar is a non-tapered, non-bending, anodized section—very simple, safe and "low-tech." It is keel-stepped, with fore and aft lowers. Until the early '80s, the spreaders were simple tubes fitted into small brackets, which also served to anchor the lower shrouds. Now, the 29.9 is rigged with more modern tapered spreaders and a cleaner shroud anchorage. The halyards are still externally led, which simplifies maintenance but dramatically increases windage.

The chainplates are gunwale-mounted and are bolted to small knees tucked under the hull to deck joint, a method which should remain secure, given the strength of the hull-deck joint. This method is more seaworthy than mounting the chainplates inboard and attaching them to knees glassed to unsupported hull panels. The price of having outboard shrouds is, of course, loss of upwind ability.

PERFORMANCE

Handling Under Sail

Although the 29.9 was designed with racing in mind, her actual performance has been hampered by her underbody and her rig. A shallow, low-aspect keel, outboard shrouds, and an undercanvassed sailplan do nothing to enhance performance in light to moderate winds. The 29.9 is available with an optional "tall rig" which adds 2-1/2 feet to the mast height—but few boats have been ordered with this option. The performance of the standard rig seems to suit the cruising mode of most 29.9 owners.

The centerboard option has seen greater acceptance than the tall rig (with about 25 percent of the boats so equipped), but we don't recommend this alternative. It reduces the draft only slightly when raised, and appears to

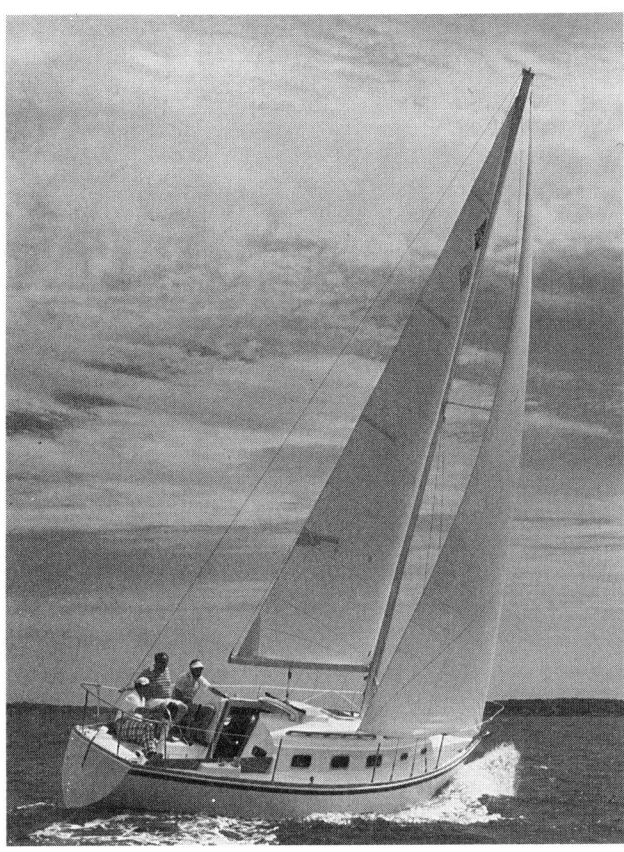

unbalance the boat when down. Many owners of the centerboard model complain about the boat's balance. She has "extreme weather helm, no matter how the board is positioned," said one owner. No owners of the standard keel version complained about balance. In fact, comments like "we sail unattended when the wind is forward of the beam" were common responses to our questionnaire.

The rig of the Bristol 29.9 is immovable in the fore and aft direction as the step and the mast partner are fixed. There is no space for partner blocks and the mast steps through a tightly fitted hole molded into the head's floor pan. Therefore, you can't change the rake to balance the helm.

In general, responding owners were satisfied with the 29.9's stability and said the boat's overall speed was better than average for a boat of her size. The PHRF rating questions their evaluation, however. The 29.9's ratings range from 180 to 216 (depending on the handicapper) and average 193. At this rating, she is just about 10 seconds per mile slower than a Catalina 30; 13 slower than a Hunter 30; 16 slower than a Pearson 30; 18 slower than a Sabre 30; and 20 slower than a Tartan 30.

Handling Under Power

The standard engine in the 29.9 was a Universal 11 horsepower diesel, with a 16 HP Universal available as an option. Earlier, a Yanmar 12 HP diesel was standard, with a 15 HP Yanmar optional. In both cases, the prospective owner was wise to choose the larger engine. When a builder offers such an engine cption, it usually means that the smaller engine is of marginal utility.

Owners report that both the Yanmars and Universals are reliable, and that power, especially with the larger options, is adequate. One owner says his 16

HP Universal pushes his boat at 6-1/2 knots. Maneuverability is rated good as the propeller is located close to the rudder.

Most owners cite marginal engine accessibility. To check the oil in either the Yanmar or the Universal installations, a panel must be removed inside the cockpit locker, which means emptying this locker of all contents. There is no sound insulation around the engine.

The aluminum fuel tank has a capacity of 18 gallons, which is more than adequate. On models built before 1981, the fuel tank was of steel, and one owner reports replacing his due to rust. On the boat we checked, the straps securing the tank were not padded to prevent chafe. The fuel fill is in the cockpit floor, which can make the floor slippery in the event of spillage or overflow during fueling. There is no oil pan under the engine and owners of older boats commonly mention problems with engine mounts and shaft mis-alignment.

LIVABILITY

Deck Layout

The cockpit of the Bristol 29.9 is small but uncluttered. Except for the sheets, there are no lines to tangle underfoot. The halyards cleat on the mast but the standard mast is equipped with only one halyard winch. Most owners add at least one extra. There is no mainsail reefing system. The traveler is short and is mounted forward of the companionway. To compensate for the poor purchase of a traveler so mounted, the mainsheet is led forward to the mast, and then aft to a winch on the cabin house.

The cockpit is wide—a bit too wide for many people to comfortably brace their feet against the leeward seat—yet not long enough to seat more than four in comfort. The seat backs are straight and the coaming is of wood trim—attractive in appearance but uncomfortable when sitting on the rail while sailing to weather.

The Edson steering is equipped with a 22-inch wheel to allow free movement fore and aft through the cockpit, but one owner reported easier steering after installing a larger wheel. Despite the high cabin house, visibility from the cockpit is adequate.

Teak trim is standard on the 29.9. On our test boat, the scuppers in the teak toerail were too few and too small. Because the cockpit coaming doesn't extend

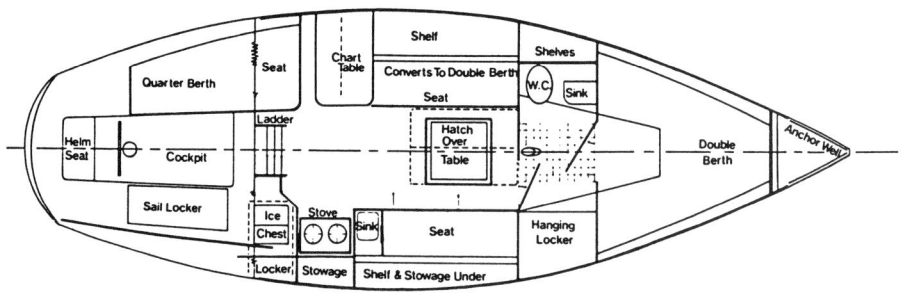

to the stern, water on deck tends to work its way into the cockpit before the scuppers can drain it overboard.

The companionway sill is lower than the cockpit seats, so the lower drop board should be kept in place when sailing in rough weather. The taper of the companionway is gradual, so there is little tendency for the boards to float out should the cockpit be pooped. There is no coaming molded into the deck to accept a dodger, which implies that a dodger will be less than completely effective in keeping water out of the cockpit.

The non-skid on the deck is of a woven pattern and less effective than the pyramid or random patterns found on some boats. Single lifelines were standard, double were optional, but only necessary if sailing with children.

The 29.9 is equipped with black-painted Bomar hatches. On the six-year-old boat we examined, this paint was flaking off. Until 1982, the forward running lights were deck-mounted Perkos. Peters and Bey stanchion-mounted lights, more visible and watertight, replace these on later models. The standard primary winches are Lewmar 30s which, though marginal for racing, should be adequate for cruising and daysailing.

There is a locker for ground tackle in the foredeck. It is shallow enough to hold little water when beating into a sea, but on the boat we inspected the drain was not canted enough to completely drain the locker.

Belowdecks

The Bristol 29.9 has a well built and reasonably livable interior. The piece-by-piece attachment of the interior components results in better bonding and reinforcement of the hull, and also makes interior modifications easier. Pre-1982 models had interiors of quality Philippine mahogany (lauan) marine plywood. On subsequent models, teak veneer plywood was utilized. The cabin sole is of teak and holly. A worthwhile option was a wood ceiling for the quarterberth and V-berth.

The arrangement of the interior is conventional, with berths for six. Of course, sleeping six on a boat of this size can involve heroic forbearance. The quarterberth is tucked almost completely under the cockpit to make room for a

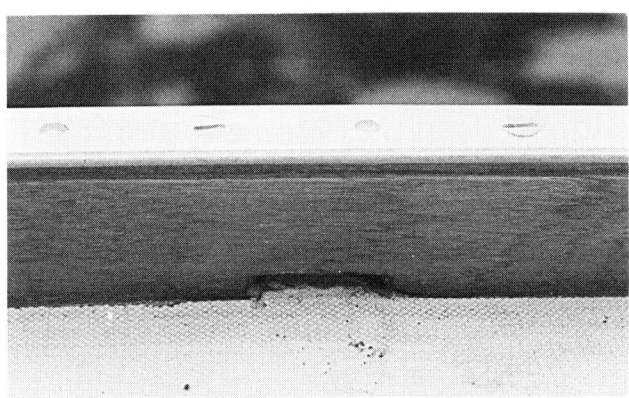

good sized navigation table forward. The high freeboard aft is no doubt a result of seeking some clearance above this berth.

Throughout the cabin, headroom is six feet or more, which is greater than necessary for most people, especially on a thirty-footer. The galley is convenient, with a deep sink. Hot, pressured water is an option. Small storage bins are numerous throughout the boat, and all bins and shelves have doors to prevent spillage of contents as the boat heels.

"We could use more ventilation on rainy days," is a common complaint by owners. On one boat we examined there was excessive mildew in the bilge. The companionway is angled forward so dropboards must be left in to exclude rain. While the boat has a good sea hood to keep water from the companionway hatch, the mast boot is only a cloth gasket. Owners report difficulty in sealing the mast. One owner reports having the builder install optional dorade vents, but complained that they were positioned to snag the jib sheets when tacking. The storage lockers in the cabin are poorly ventilated.

The head, shower, and wet locker lie between the main cabin and the V-berth. Although there is a hatch above the V-berth, this area inevitably takes on the odors of the head, so opening ports in the V-berth area were a desirable option. The icebox drains into the bilge but the shower pumps overboard.

The 29.9 carries a whopping 63 gallons of water in fiberglass tanks in the cabin and under the V-berth. The weight of this much water can affect the boat's trim. The vent for the water tank is in the topsides, which makes it possible for saltwater to find its way into the tank.

Exposed wiring in the cockpit locker, and a fuse panel on the starboard bulkhead (just inside the companionway), could prove vulnerable to water intrusion. Later models use circuit breakers. An interior headliner hides the wiring running forward from the fuse panel, making it inaccessible for repair.

Perhaps the most commendable interior item is the cabin table. It is both rugged and rigidly attached to the main bulkhead with a screw-down hatch dog. It doesn't rattle when folded, and like the galley, is surfaced with plastic laminate. The interior joinerwork isn't as extensive as on some of the boats coming out of Taiwan, but more workmanlike—simple, sturdy, and well done.

CONCLUSIONS

While Bristol sold more than two hundred 29.9s since the boat's introduction, you can't call this model an unqualified success. Perhaps it's her appearance. She wasn't as modern looking as many of her contemporaries, but at the same time her high, boxy profile wasn't "classic" enough to appeal to many traditionalists. She isn't a true offshore cruiser, yet her underbody and rig are too conservative to make her a spirited daysailer.

For the most part, owners generally like their 29.9s. The complaint of most merit is that the centerboard version doesn't balance well upwind, but most comments are positive. For example, "She inspires confidence and will carry a lot of sail comfortably." Or, "She's sturdy, and makes good use of the space."

Bristol Yachts isn't a large boatbuilder. They built the 29.9 only on order, and with the pieced-in interior, were willing to customize. Prospective buyers of used Bristol 29.9s can therefore expect to find a number of variations from standard on the boats they'll inspect, and probably some nice owner-installed modifications as well.

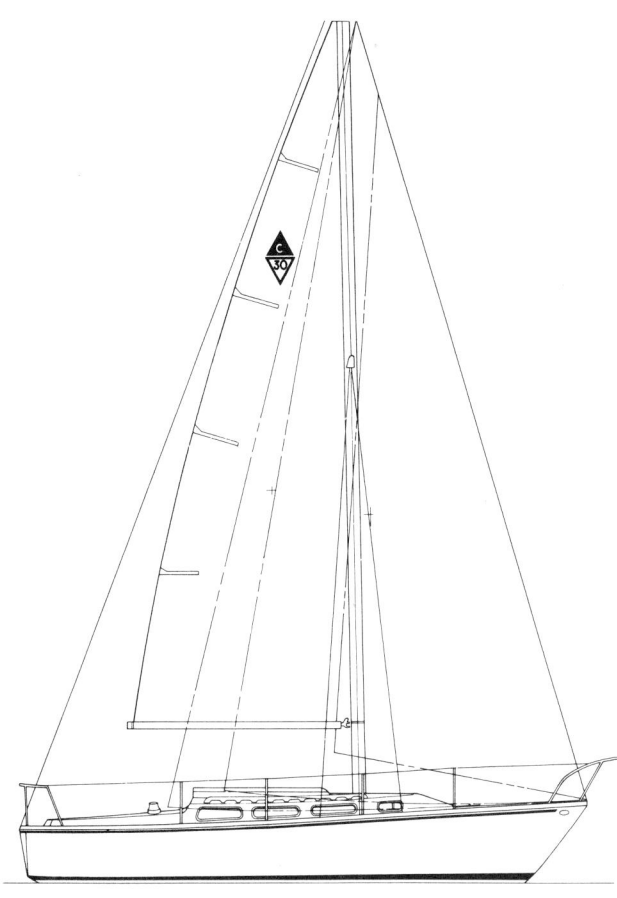

Specifications
Catalina 30

LOA	29'11"
LWL	25'0"
Beam	10'10"
Draft	
standard	5'3"
shoal	4'4"
Displacement	10200 lbs
Ballast	4200 lbs
Sail area	444 sq ft

Catalina Yachts
21200 Victory Blvd.
Woodland Hills,
California 91367

The Catalina 30:
More Boat for Less Money

THE BOAT AND THE BUILDER

Catalina Yachts is one of the world's largest manufacturers of fiberglass cruising and racing sailboats over 21 feet. The company has two plants, one in Largo, Florida, and the other in southern California. Between the two, they turn out several thousand sailboats a year. The Catalina 22 is probably the most popular small trailerable cruiser ever built.

Since the Catalina 30 went into production in 1975, output has been at a steady rate of about 470 boats per year. Dealers report that they could easily sell more, if they could only get their hands on them. One New England dealer reported that he requested 18 Catalina 30s one year, but because of demand for the boat from other dealers, received only nine. These nine were sold before they were even delivered.

The success of the Catalina is even more remarkable when you consider that the company does no advertising. You won't find a single Catalina ad in any national magazine. The company depends on its extensive dealer network—about 150 dealers nationwide—and on word of mouth recommendations from satisfied owners.

Most boat manufacturers spend between five and ten percent of gross revenues on advertising. Catalina may well be saving several thousand dollars per Catalina 30. However you look at this, it comes down to a lower price per boat.

The entire Catalina line is extremely popular with new boat dealers, who are required by Catalina to represent other lines as well. Usually, the Catalina line is priced about five percent lower than a comparably equipped boat of the same size and type from some another manufacturer. For example, the typical out-the-door price for a Newport 30 is consistently about $2000 more than for a Catalina 30. These two boats are almost identical in layout, design, and appearance. The customer who resists the higher price of the Newport 30 might logically be directed to the Catalina 30.

Catalina owners frequently trade up through the line. Some dealers make it a policy of offering the customer full trade-in value for a smaller Catalina, traded up for a larger one, within the first two years after purchase. A remarkable number of owners do just this.

The Catalina 30 is a typical modern design of fairly light displacement. The boat has a swept-back, moderately high-aspect-ratio fin keel of the type made popular by IOR racing boats in the early 1970s. The high-aspect-ratio spade rudder is faired into the underbody with a small skeg.

On a waterline length of 25 feet, the Catalina 30's displacement of 10,200 pounds is slightly above average for modern cruiser-racers. By way of comparison, the Newport 30 displaces 8000 pounds; the Cal 31, 9200 pounds; and the O'Day 30, 11,000 pounds.

The boat is conventionally modern in appearance. She is moderately high-sided, with a fairly straight sheer and short ends. The cabin trunk tapers slightly in profile, and is slightly sheered to compliment the sheerline of the hull. Coupled with the tapered cabin windows—a Catalina trademark—this yields a reasonably attractive appearance compared to many modern boats.

CONSTRUCTION

The hull of the Catalina is a hand layup of solid fiberglass. In areas of high stress, such as the tops of the cockpit coamings where winches are mounted, the laminate is reinforced with plywood inserts.

The external lead keel is bolted to the hull with stainless steel bolts. On most Catalinas inspected, there was a slight cracking at the joint between the hull and ballast, which is typical of boats with narrow external ballast keels. The surface of the keel is roughly faired with polyester putty at the factory. This must be sanded fair by the owner or commissioning yard, or light air performance will suffer. The bottom of the hull must also be heavily sanded before paint is applied or there will be a problem with paint adhesion.

The hull to deck joint is simple. The deck molding is wider than the hull molding. At the outboard edge of the deck, the molding forms a downward-facing, right-angle flange. This is slipped over the hull molding, and the joint filled with what appears to be fiberglass slurry. The joint is finished with a soft plastic rubrail held by an aluminum extrusion. The aluminum extrusion is held in place by stainless steel self-tapping screws, which reinforce the chemical bond. An integral solid wood sheer clamp, laminated into the hull, further strengthens the joint.

There was some play in the rudder stock of every Catalina 30 we examined. This is similar to the problem found in the Pearson 30. It is more likely to be a minor annoyance than a serious problem.

Lifeline stanchions are more closely spaced than on almost any production boat we have seen. Double lifelines are standard, as are double bow and stern rails. Stanchions are through-bolted, but with washers rather than the backing plates we prefer. Some owners report problems with leaking stanchions. This is easily corrected, as the stanchion fastenings are readily accessible from inside the boat.

The rig is a simple masthead sloop, with a straight section aluminum spar, double lower shrouds, and (on older models), wooden spreaders. The mast is stepped on deck, supported by a wooden compression column belowdecks. All the boats we examined showed local deflection of the top of the cabin trunk in the way of the mast step. This varied from as little as 1/16-inch to over 1/4-inch. There was no evidence of stress in the form of cracks around any of the steps, however.

It is difficult to assess the method of attachment of the chainplates and bulkheads to the hull. The interior of the hull is completely lined, showing no raw fiberglass—nice to look at but preventing examination of the internal structure of the hull. Lower shroud chainplate attachments have been beefed

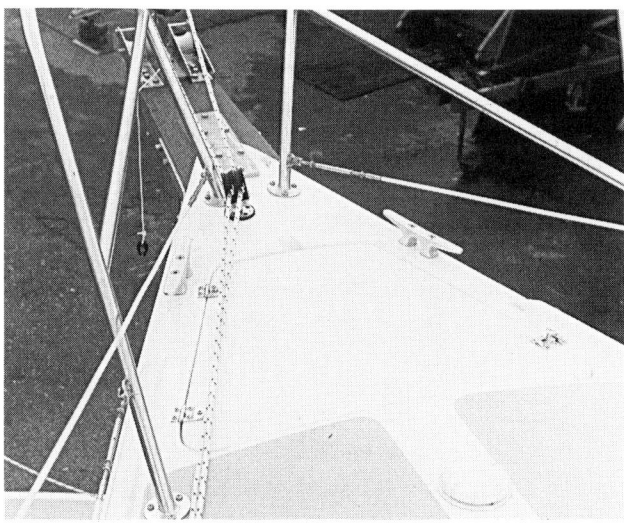

up since the first hulls were produced. Owners warn that when considering the purchase of a used Catalina 30, be sure that the chainplates have the new reinforcements installed.

A shoal draft model, drawing 11 inches less than the standard model, is popular in some areas where the water is spread thin, such as Florida and the

The Catalina 30

Chesapeake. A taller rig is also offered, and might be recommended in traditionally light air areas, such as Long Island Sound.

PERFORMANCE

Handling Under Sail

With the standard rig, the Catalina 30 will be slightly undercanvassed in areas with predominantly light weather conditions. In areas with normally heavier conditions, such as San Francisco, the standard rig should yield good performance. The working sail area with the standard rig is 445 square feet. For comparison, the Pearson 30, with the same sail area, weighs 1900 pounds less than the Catalina 30. To get good performance in light air, the boat will either have to be ordered with the taller rig, or very large headsails must be carried. If headsails larger than a 150 percent genoa are carried with the normal rig, turning blocks will have to be added aft in order to get a proper lead to the headsail sheet winches.

The Catalina 30 is a very stiff boat. The combination of a high ballast to displacement ratio, extraordinary beam, a deep fin keel, and a fairly small sail plan produces a boat that stands on her feet well. Owners consider the boat to be just about as fast as other boats of the same size and type. PHRF ratings suggest that the tall rig boat is substantially faster than the boat with the standard rig. With the tall rig, and well-cut racing sails, the boat should be competitive with other cruiser-racers that are actively raced, such as the Pearson 30, the O'Day 30, and the Ericson 30-2.

Sails are available from the factory. At a total of less than $2000 for a main, 110-percent lapper, and a 150-percent genoa they are cheaper than one is likely to find from a local racing sailmaker, or one of the big national names. If the boat is to be used only for daysailing and cruising, the factory-supplied sails are likely to be adequate. If, however, you are concerned with performance, it is always advisable to have sails made either by a national sailmaker with a local loft, or by a local racing sailmaker. The sailmaker who is familiar with local weather conditions, and who probably races himself, is most likely to provide a faster suit of sails than those provided as a factory option.

The Catalina 30 does not have any particularly disturbing or exciting charac-

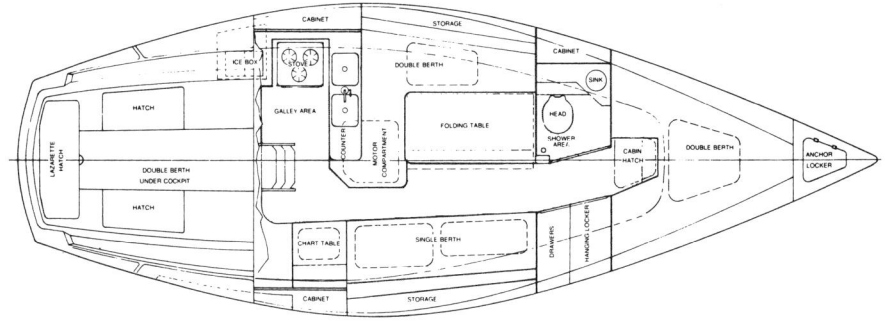

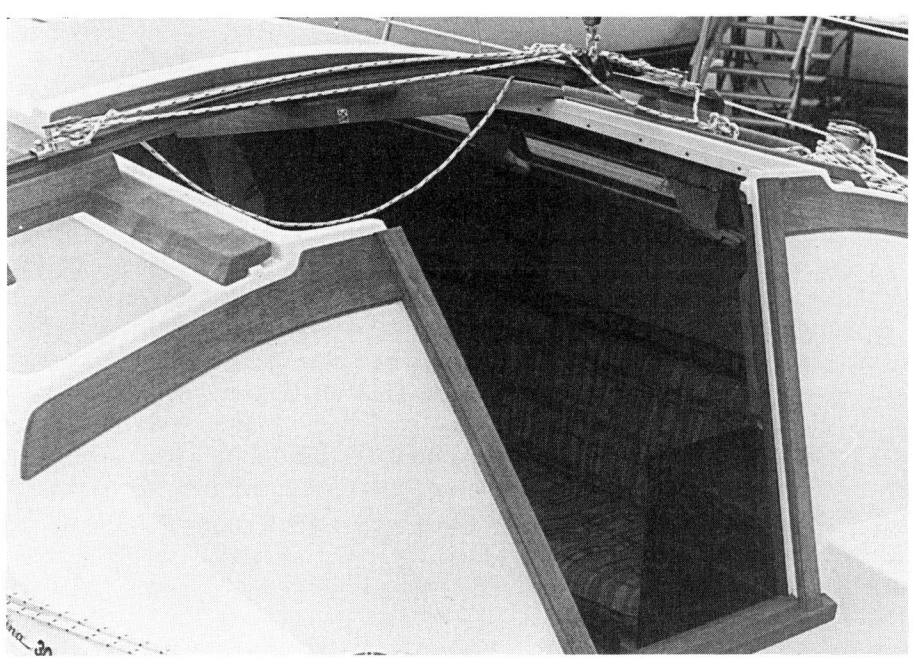

teristics under sail. Like many wide modern boats, the Catalina 30 rapidly develops weather helm when heeled. The boat should be sailed on her feet. Because she is quite stiff, headsail changes will not be as frequent as with a boat such as the Pearson 30.

Handling Under Power
For many years, the standard engine in the Catalina 30 was the workhorse Atomic 4 gasoline engine. For several years, an 11-horsepower Universal diesel was an option. Now that the Atomic 4 has been discontinued, a Universal diesel is the standard inboard powerplant, and the boat is fitted with engines as large the three-cylinder Model 25 Universal diesel.

The big Universal diesel is by far the best engine for a boat that weighs over 10,000 pounds, since it should be able to push it to hull speed. The Atomic 4 could do that with ease.

Although the engine has flexible mountings and a flexible shaft coupling, some owners report there is substantial vibration under power with the small diesel engine. This is felt most acutely in the cabin, because of the midships location of the engine. The engine box has no soundproofing. The main cabin is very noisy under power. Long periods of powering would be rather uncomfortable for the crew belowdecks.

With a fin keel and spade rudder, the boat is quite maneuverable under power, both ahead and astern. With the wheel steerer—one of the most popular options—very little steering effort is required.

LIVABILITY

Deck Layout

The deck layout of the Catalina 30 is typical of small cruiser-racers. There is a small foredeck anchor well. Access to the hull-mounted running lights is via this well. The running lights are protected from damage inside the well by molded fiberglass covers. We are not fond of running lights mounted in the topsides, which almost invariably short out. Other manufacturers who mount the lights in the hull could take a lesson from Catalina, however. Neither C&C nor Cal protects their running lights on the inside of the anchor well.

Despite the wide cabin trunk, it is reasonably easy to maneuver on deck. The shrouds are placed far enough inboard to allow going outside them on the way to the foredeck. There are also well-mounted teak grabrails on the cabin top.

The cockpit is large and comfortable. With wheel steering, it easily accommodates the helmsman and four companions. There is a large sail locker under the port cockpit seat, and a smaller locker under the starboard seat. There is also a fair-sized lazarette locker. The sail locker is properly separated from the under-cockpit area.

The cockpit is large by offshore standards. There are only two fairly small cockpit drains, whose sizes are greatly reduced by strainers. Despite the fact that the companionway has a fairly high raised sill, at least two of the three companionway drop boards would have to be in place to raise the sill to the level of the main deck.

The strong vertical taper of the companionway allows the drop boards to be removed by lifting them only about one and a half inches. In a bad knockdown in severe weather, the boards could fly out, or float out, much easier than if the companionway sides were more parallel. The sliding companionway hatch is unnecessarily large. This is useful when sitting in a marina in a hot climate, but is a disadvantage at sea.

Because the main cabin bulkhead slopes forward, the drop boards cannot be left out of the companionway for ventilation when it rains. For this reason, boats used in raining climates frequently have cockpit dodgers. There is no provision for ventilation below in rain or heavy weather.

There is a permanently mounted manual bilge pump, operable from the cockpit. Although other manufacturers would do well to include such a pump as standard equipment, not many do.

Belowdecks

The interior of the Catalina 30 is roomy, and quite well laid out. The forward cabin has large, tapered V-berths which form a large double when the filler is added. A molded hatch, which forms part of the front of the cabin trunk, will provide good ventilation in port, but may be a leaker in heavy weather.

The head is quite comfortable. The optional shower drains directly to the bilge. Marine toilet installations are all optional. There is good storage space for clothes in a hanging locker and drawers opposite the head.

Interior bulkheads are teak-faced plywood. The hull is completely lined with fiberglass hull liners, yielding a very finished appearance. The main cabin is large and comfortable for a 30-foot boat. There is an L-shaped settee to port, and a straight settee to starboard. The cabin table folds up against the forward bulkhead when not in use.

The engine is mounted under the settee and part of the galley counter. It's a tight fit. Access for service is excellent through traps in the settee. The location of the engine in the lowest part of the bilge does make it vulnerable to bilge water, however.

Under the cockpit to starboard, there is a large double quarterberth. Unfortunately, the occupant of the inboard half of the berth had better be thin and non-claustrophobic. Headroom over this area is a little over one foot. It makes an excellent single, however.

A large, U-shaped galley is to port. A gimballed alcohol stove with oven is standard, as are double sinks. On older boats, the icebox is uninsulated, except for the side facing the stove, and drains directly into the bilge. Storage space is in the galley is plentiful (although not as much as it might first appear) as the lockers under the sink are filled with hoses for the engine and water tanks. Batteries are well-mounted under the small chart table opposite the galley.

The general appearance of the interior is one of spaciousness and good design. This initial impression breaks down somewhat on careful examination of details. Interior finish is of average, production boat quality.

CONCLUSIONS

According to Frank Butler, President and Chief Designer of Catalina, the company's sole goal is to provide "as much boat for the money as we can." The Catalina 30 is definitely priced among the lowest of the 30-foot cruiser-racers. This boat is similar in price to the Hunter 30. For their displacement, these are two of the least expensive 30-footers made. It is not reasonable to compare these boats with more expensive 30-footers like the Ericson 30+ or the Cal 31. The Catalina 30 is a lot of boat for the money. What you get for the price is solid and well executed. The refinements and extras you don't pay for, however, you won't find on the Catalina 30

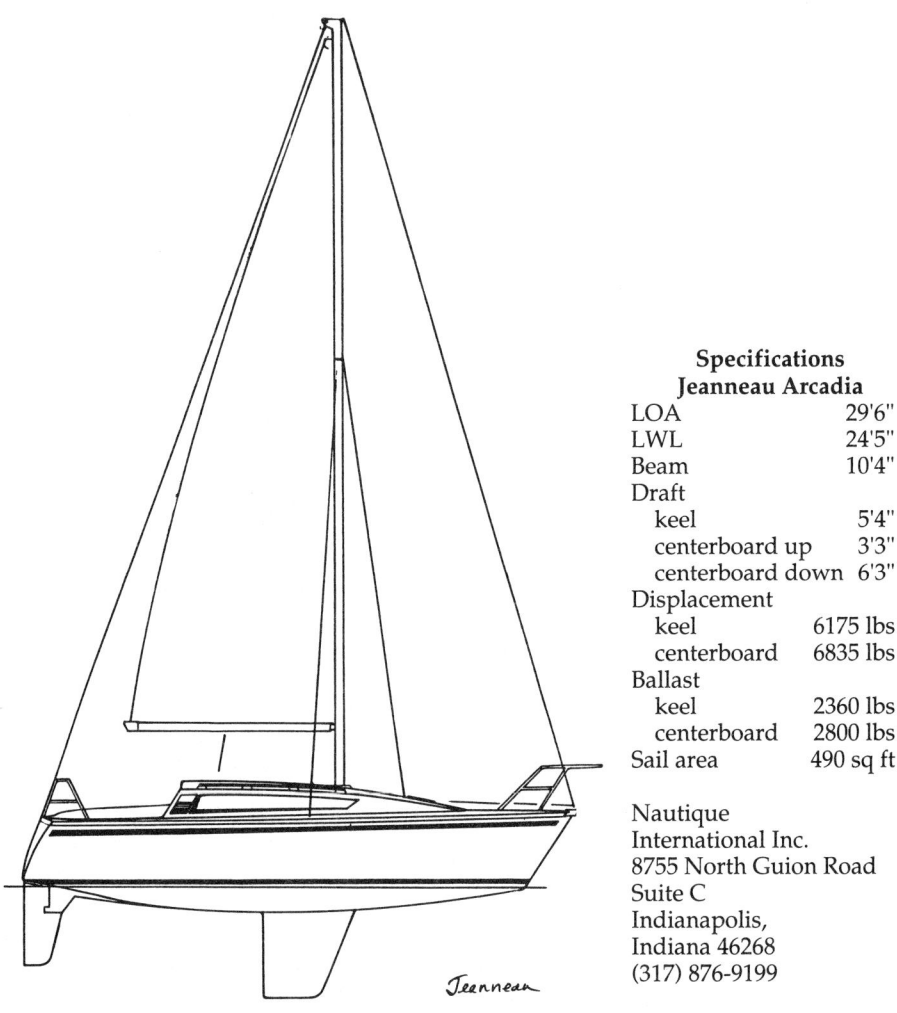

Specifications
Jeanneau Arcadia

LOA		29'6"
LWL		24'5"
Beam		10'4"
Draft		
	keel	5'4"
	centerboard up	3'3"
	centerboard down	6'3"
Displacement		
	keel	6175 lbs
	centerboard	6835 lbs
Ballast		
	keel	2360 lbs
	centerboard	2800 lbs
Sail area		490 sq ft

Nautique
International Inc.
8755 North Guion Road
Suite C
Indianapolis,
Indiana 46268
(317) 876-9199

The Jeanneau Arcadia:
Style, in the European Tradition

THE BOAT AND THE BUILDER

Constructions Nautiques Jeanneau advertised itself as Europe's largest boatbuilder, and often boasted of its production capacity. "We have a new Sunrise 34 coming off the lines every three and a half hours." At the same time, the company referred to the 1300 production workers in its 600,000 square foot factory in different terms. "In a quiet country town on the west coast of France, French craftsmen—not ruled by timeclocks—produce boats of exceptional value."

This mixture of the old and the new, of reality and hype, seems to character-

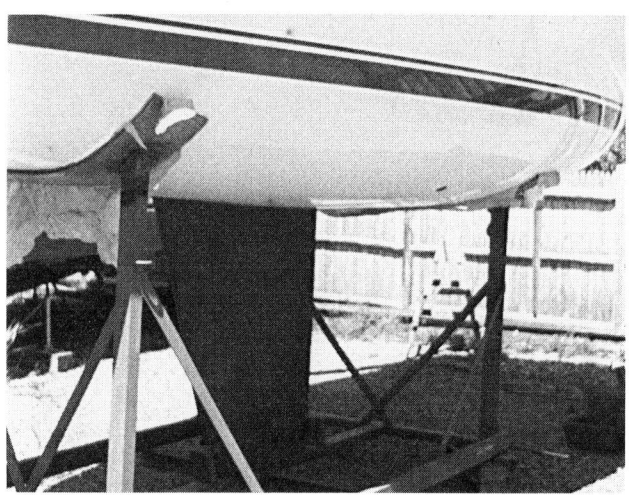

ize the Jeanneau Company and its boats ... bit of old-fashioned attention to detail, a bit of high-tech, high volume production ... a bit of conventional engineering, a bit of "to hell with tradition, let's make this boat different."

To most Americans, Jeanneau boats seem to have appeared suddenly, but the company has been around since 1956. In addition to previously favorable currency rates (which made the boats attractive to Americans), aggressive entry into the American market resulted when Lear Siegler bought Jeanneau and the other Bangor Punta boat companies (Cal, O'Day, and Ranger), in 1983.

"Only" ten models of Jeanneau sailboats have been imported into the U.S.—just a fraction of the bewildering array of models, model names, and variations in the total Jeanneau line. We could get no exact figures on the number of models currently in production, but from brochures and advertisements, we estimate Jeanneau has about 25—not counting variations such as "owner" or "chartering" interior options.

Like most of the Jeanneaus, the Arcadia (pronounced "Are-caw-dee-yah") is not a common boat in America. About 40 have been imported. Again like most of the Jeanneaus, total production is incredible. The factory popped out 600 completed boats in the Arcadia's first two years. The only American company that could claim such numbers in a 30-footer is Catalina, and they produce a minuscule number of models when compared to Jeanneau.

A unique element in Jeanneau's organization is the diversity of designers—almost all "big names"—at least in Europe, and almost all with Grand Prix racing credentials. Guy Dumas, Doug Peterson, Phillippe Briand, Jacques Fauroux and the Joubert/Nivelt team are examples.

The designer of the Arcadia is Tony Castro; a new name to Americans, perhaps, but an established designer in Europe. Of Portuguese descent, Castro began his work with Ron Holland in Ireland, then set up his own shop in 1981 and achieved success designing IOR racing machines. Now a British citizen, he has two other designs in production at Jeanneau, and a third (an IOR half-tonner) scheduled for production.

The design of the Arcadia is not IOR. We would call it "moderate modern." It is of relatively light displacement; with a shallow, beamy hull; a high aspect-ratio keel; and a separate spade rudder.

The Jeanneau Arcadia
185

Her appearance is "European." The flat sheer, a doghouse that slopes forward into the foredeck, long black windows (you can't call them "ports"), and blunt ends make up that "European" look which is decidedly—almost blatantly—non-traditional. "Thoroughly modern" is a term that appears several times in Jeanneau's advertising copy.

CONSTRUCTION

In contrast to the boat's image, the construction of the Arcadia is anything but high-tech. The hull is standard hand-laid fiberglass mat and roving. The deck is also hand-laid fiberglass with balsa core in spots. The balsa-core "spots" seemed to be less extensive than normal (we couldn't examine much of the deck molding because of the interior liner), but the deck was stiff underfoot. The deck hardware we could examine was through-bolted with large washers, but there were no backing plates.

The hull to deck joint typifies the construction of the boat. The joint appears to be a standard inward-turning flange on the hull, on which the deck molding rests. Quarter-inch stainless bolts are set through an aluminum toerail, the deck, aı.d the hull flange.

Pretty normal so far, but Jeanneau finishes off the joint on the inside by laying a thick layer of fiberglass over everything—from the deck, over the seam, covering the bolts, and onto the hull. It looks strong, and appears to be a good way to finish the hull to deck joint on a fast-moving production line. If the joint is damaged, however, it will be tough to examine thoroughly and hard to repair. The joint should never leak, but if it does, tracking down the source will be nearly impossible. Generally, the rest of the glass work and gelcoat look good; the two hulls we examined were smooth and fair.

The boat's strength and stiffness probably come from Jeanneau's practice of bonding everything to everything. Not only are the athwartship bulkheads bonded to the hull and deck with fiberglass tape, but cabinet fronts are bonded to bulkheads too. Cabinet sides are bonded to the fronts and to bulkheads. The head door frame, for example, is bonded to the engine box frame, which is bonded to the hull and to the cockpit, and on and on. The whole interior is obviously prefabricated in typical production line fashion, but we've never

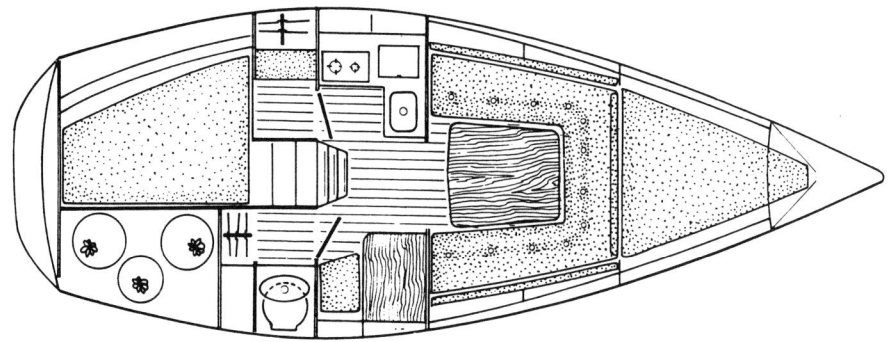

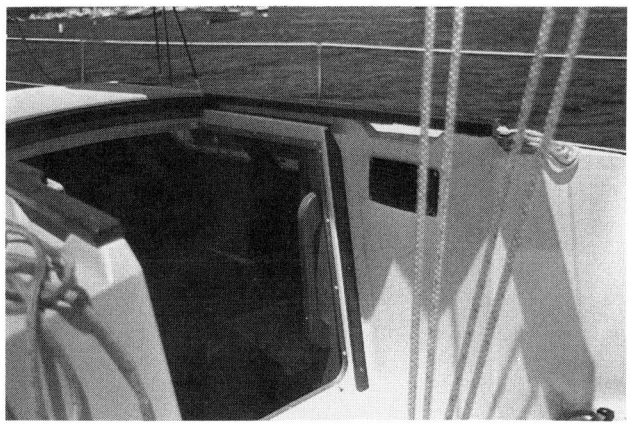

seen a production boat in which the interior parts were so thoroughly fiberglassed to each other and to the hull. This is a good "low-tech" method of acquiring stiffness without skeletal framing or coring of the hull.

Like many of the Jeanneaus, the Arcadia comes with either a centerboard or an external keel—about 70% being keel models. The keel is unusual in two respects. First, rather than lead, it is iron, coated with fiberglass to prevent corrosion. Next, the keel bolts are not vertical in the normal fashion. Instead they are set in pairs, angled from the sides of the keel inward. Inside the hull, were the bolts long enough, they would converge and touch. Once the keel is attached, a heavy layer of fiberglass is laid in the bilge to fully cover the bolts. As with the hull to deck joint, this looks strong and leakproof, but again we would be concerned about the difficulty of repairs, or finding leaks following a hard grounding. The keel we examined was fair and well finished. We did not inspect a centerboard model.

The spade rudder is supported by a small skeg, and well finished except for a rough trailing edge. Tiller steering is standard on the Arcadia but both boats we examined had the optional Plastimo wheel steering with a "European-size" wheel of about 24 inches diameter. Most Americans like a larger wheel. Unfortunately, a larger one could not be fitted without major modifications to the cockpit seats.

The rig generally looks to be standard issue—a masthead-rigged sloop with upper and aft-lower shrouds, and a "baby stay" forward. The boat we examined had double spreaders, but the company literature and photos show a single-spreader rig. Partly because of language problems and shipping time, and partly because of the speed with which these boats are produced (a dozen boats can come off the line before the marketing department learns of a change), we can't say which rig is normal.

The company advertises an optional (tall) "lake rig," but the importer says this is designed only for European inland lakes and would be unsuitable for coastal, Great Lakes, or offshore sailing. None have been imported into the United States.

The upper shroud chainplates are anchored to a transverse overhead frame which begins as a settee bulkhead on the hull, and then extends up over the cabin and down to the hull on the opposite side, with a compression post in the middle of the cabin under the mast. This frame is bonded to the hull and deck

The Jeanneau Arcadia
187

and should provide adequate strength and mast support. The lower shroud chainplates are anchored to a similar frame, bonded to the hull and side decks.

We asked the dealer who showed us the Arcadia to pick out one thing that made the Jeanneau different from the three American brands he also handled. "They are dry," he said. "I don't know how they do it, but they just don't leak, either from the top of the deck downward or from the bottom of the hull upward." From a dealer who has sponged out a lot of bilges before bringing customers on board, those are words of praise.

PERFORMANCE

Handling Under Power

The two Arcadias that we looked at had two-cylinder diesels—one a Yanmar, the other a Volvo (production line changes, again). Sales literature lists an outboard version (thankfully no such monster is likely to be imported), and a version with either a one- or two-cylinder Yanmar. For a boat of more than 6000 pounds, we would consider the one-lunger very marginal, and recommend the two-cylinder along with the optional folding prop.

The engine installation is well done (stringers and beds bonded to everything in sight) with soundproofing on the compartment walls, a waterlift muffler, and a seven-gallon fuel tank. There is good accessibility to the engine through the aft cabin and through the removable companionway steps, except that the dipstick on the Yanmar is hard to reach.

Two details impressed us: The engine compartment has a small electric bilge pump as standard equipment in a sump below the prop shaft's packing gland—one place that is likely to receive water. And, in the front of the companionway step that opens into the engine compartment, there's a 2-inch hole with a plastic cover, the function of which baffled not only us, but also the person who first demonstrated the boat. Finally, the dealer explained its purpose. In the event of an engine room fire, pull the plastic cover, insert the working end of a fire extinguisher, and discharge it. This is eminently more practical than pulling off the companionway steps and feeding more oxygen to the flames (and an idea that should be considered on any boat).

Under power with the folding prop, the boat handled satisfactorily, backing where we wanted and with adequate power in forward and reverse. Visibility from behind the wheel is decent, but there is no comfortable place to sit aft, and the wheel is too small to reach from the sidedeck. The engine had no more vibration than you'd expect from a two-cylinder diesel, and was bit quieter than on many boats, probably because of the insulation in the engine compartment.

Handling Under Sail

We were able to sail the Arcadia for only about an hour. Unfortunately, we had too few responses from readers of *The Practical Sailor* to make any valid judgements about the Arcadia's performance under a variety of conditions. (Most of our owner's responses were based on a single season's sailing or less).

In our limited experience, however, we found that she went to weather, reached, and ran very much like other contemporary racer-cruisers. She pounded a bit in a short chop, as you might expect with her shallow hull design, but we saw no other bad habits. (Her sails are from a small French loft, "Ton," and are adequate. Racers will want better.)

Her PHRF rating of 150 suggests that overall performance under sail is about midway between older racer-cruisers (like the Pearson 30 or Tartan 30) and the newer, hotter racer-cruisers (like the Santana 30/30 or the S2 9.1). We were hoping—considering that she's a Tony Castro design—that she might be a rocketship. She's not. She is a fast cruiser and an owner will be able to race her under PHRF.

LIVABILITY

Deck Layout

With inboard shrouds, wide decks, and a sloping cabin top, the Arcadia is easy to move about on, and to work under sail. We noted only two problems. First, the foredeck becomes very narrow, an impediment to easy headsail and anchor handling that is common on all "modern" designs. Second, the cockpit was uncomfortable—the seats a little too narrow, the backs too vertical, and the footwell a trifle too deep. We also had trouble reaching the small wheel from either the windward or leeward sidedecks, where one would normally sit while racing.

Deck fittings are generally of good quality and size, with everything necessary for racing (except spinnaker and gear) as standard equipment. We did feel that the designer could have placed a higher priority on crew positions, how-

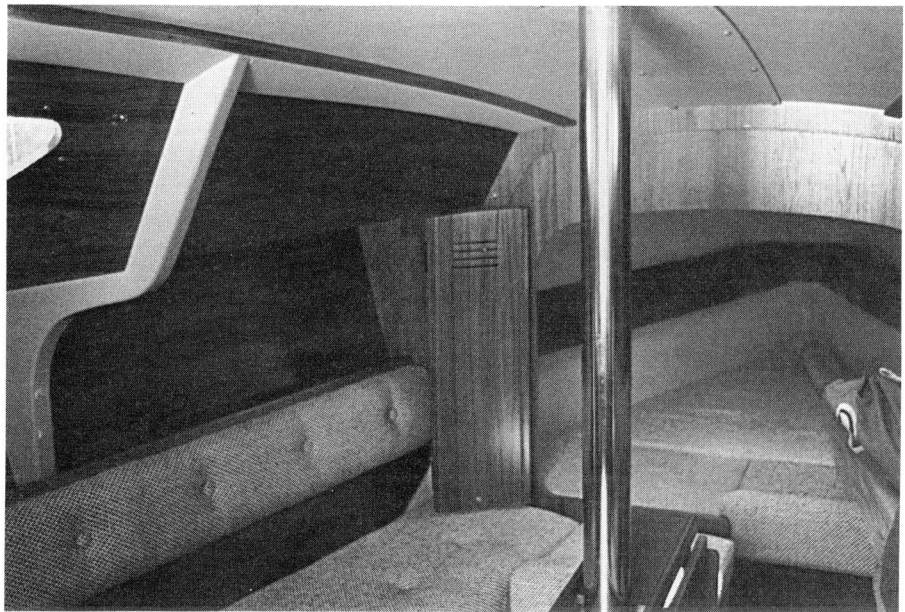

The Jeanneau Arcadia

ever; what should be done at the mast, what from the cockpit, and so forth. Most owners will probably rearrange things after a season's experience.

The non-skid is average, but there are nice details on the deck, such as the twin bow rollers for anchor handling, the sturdy latch on the anchor locker, and the large mooring cleats. There is a space at the back of the cockpit for life raft stowage and for propane bottles. A stowage bracket is built into the stern pulpit for horseshoe buoy stowage, and the stern pulpit opens up into a folding stainless steel boarding ladder.

Belowdecks

It is "downstairs" that Jeanneau really spits in the eye of tradition, not just in the Arcadia, but in most of their models. Most obvious is the layout, with the Arcadia's head and owner's double-berth cabin packed into the rear third of the boat, partly under the cockpit. Both head and owner's cabin are a little cramped, but for a smallish 30-footer, it's still a surprisingly innovative use of the space. The rest of the cabin is wide open. A small galley and navigation table are opposite each other, then settee berths on either side of a fold-up centerline table, then a crawl-in forward berth.

We noted three drawbacks. First, the forward V-berth is too short for adults. Second, anyone over 5'8" or so cannot sit upright on the settee berths without banging the overhead. Third, the standing headroom at the aft end of the cabin disappears as you walk forward under the sloping deck house.

This last item we find hard to understand as headroom is a marketing plus, and the only possible justification for the sloping deck is obeisance to "style." There *is* a marginal amount of weight saving, which could be important for all-out racers, but hardly valuable in this model. Oddly, the same headroom problem exists in the 34-foot Jeanneau Sunrise we inspected.

The interior of the Arcadia is all "woody." There is teak-faced plywood all over. We thought the veneer work was good for a production boat, especially where the veneer is used to cover plywood edges (for example, in the window cutouts). The wood has a light coating of varnish, even inside the lockers and drawers. The overhead has a soft vinyl covering that looks somewhat better than bare fiberglass. The hardware inside the boat, like hinges and latches, is noticeably superior to that found on most American production boats. A strange detail is the manual bilge pump, the handle of which sticks out at the side of the chart table, into the middle of the cabin.

Oddly, the boats we inspected were not "Americanized." Most owners might want shore power, but this is not a company option; it must be installed by the owner. The galley stove comes with a hookup for butane—not propane—and must be converted. And many Americans looking at a 30-footer might expect a shower, but this would be difficult to install on the Arcadia.

CONCLUSIONS

Overall, the Jeanneau Arcadia surprised us. We were expecting a boat comparable in quality to mid-line American production boats. We found the Jeanneau to be somewhat better in construction and in many details. Being fond of tradition, we have problems with the style of most of the Jeanneaus, including the Arcadia, but ultimately, style is a tenuous criticism of a boat—unless it is certifiably ugly.

A large part of the appeal of the Arcadia (and many other European boats), was dependent on the relationship of the American dollar to European currencies. The franc was Jeanneau's strongest selling point in America—until the dollar began to drop.

Unfortunately, as the dollar began to plummet and the franc to soar, this artificial advantage evaporated. Then came the big jump in interest rates, with the soft sailboat market following—and importation of Jeanneau boats ceased.

You can't buy an Arcadia on the new-boat market today, but they offer many interesting features for the perceptive used-boat purchaser. And who knows, as economic forces back and fill, Arcadias may show up again, "reborn," as a result of the next international economic cycle.

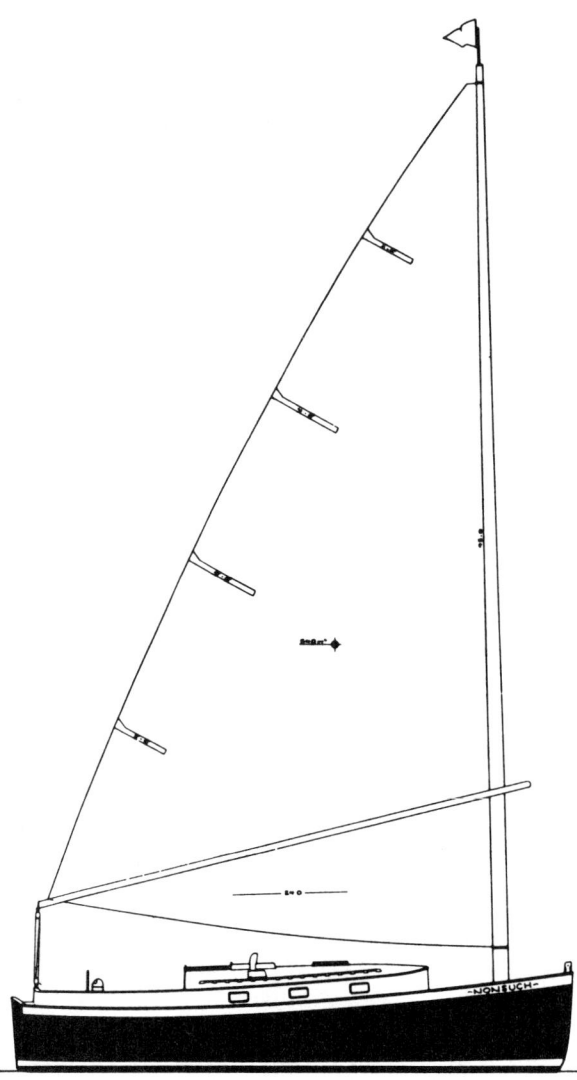

Specifications
Nonsuch 30

LOA	30'4"
DWL	28'9"
Beam	11'10"
Draft	5'0"
Displacement	10500 lbs
Ballast	4500 lbs
Sail area	540 sq ft

Hinterhoeller Yachts Ltd.
8 Keefer Road
St. Catherines, Ontario
Canada L2M 7N9

The Nonsuch 30:
An Odd Eye-Opener

THE BOAT AND THE BUILDER

The Nonsuch 30 at her introduction in 1979, was an oddity. Her fin-keel, spade-rudder, and unstayed wishbone cat rig was strange. Now, with more than 400 built plus having two smaller (22 and 26 feet) and one larger (36 feet) sisters, the Nonsuch 30 and the whole Nonsuch concept is no longer weird. Indeed, in conjunction with the similarly successful Freedom Yachts (with similar unstayed wishbone rigs), the idea of simple, easily handled cruising

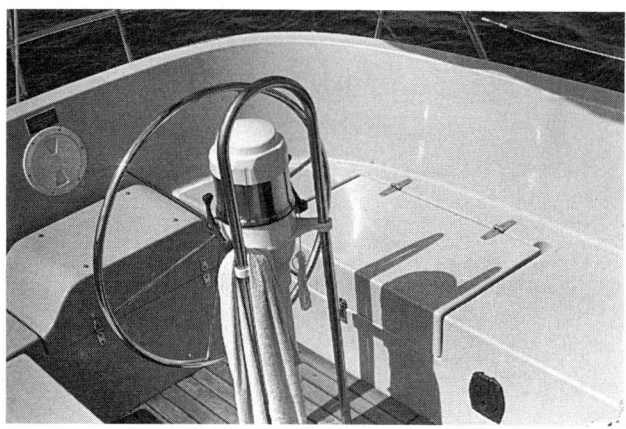
Nonsuch cockpit is deep, plain and spacious.

boats has arrived. They are boats that deserve a close look by anyone who has qualms about large genoa jibs and masts held up by wires.

The Nonsuch 30 is built in Canada, whose main boat-building export has been C&C sailboats. Come to think of it, all her construction details look very much like those of C&C boats. This isn't unusual, since George Hinterhoeller, the original builder of the Nonsuch, was formerly the president of C&C, and one of the founders of the three-company merger that finally created C&C Yachts.

When Hinterhoeller left C&C to recreate Hinterhoeller Yachts Ltd., he took with him those characteristics that have given C&C a reputation for quality: good attention to finish detail, and high-quality balsa-cored hull construction.

The Nonsuch 30 is the concept of retired ocean racer Gordon Fisher, the design of Mark Ellis, and the creation of Hinterhoeller. Hinterhoeller is one of the few production boatbuilders with the legitimate title Master Boatbuilder, earned the hard way through apprenticeship in Europe.

The original Nonsuch 30 layout, used in the first 215 boats, was dubbed the "Classic." In 1983, the 30 was upgraded with a new interior and the new version was called the "Ultra." So successful was the Ultra that, despite the continued availability of the Classic, there has been almost no demand for the original layout. Still, with more than 200 boats of each version already on the market, this look at the boat will deal with both.

CONSTRUCTION

George Hinterhoeller's reputation as a builder is not unearned. His balsa-cored hulls are known for being light and strong. It is probably not an exaggeration to say that he knows as much about cored construction as any boatbuilder around.

Both hull and deck of the Nonsuch 30 are balsa-cored. The hull and deck are joined by a through-bolted, butyl-bedded joint, capped with an aluminum toerail. The butyl tape used for this purpose has no real structural properties but does create a good watertight seal. A sealant such as 3M 5200 provides equivalent sealant properties with greater structural properties, and we prefer its use in hull to deck joints. It is hard to quibble with the Nonsuch's strongly through-bolted joint, however.

The external lead keel is bolted on with stainless steel bolts. These pass through floors of unidirectional roving, transferring keel loading from the garboard section to a greater area of the hull.

The cockpit seats and coamings contain a surprisingly large number of sharply radiused turns. Gelcoat cracks are likely to develop here earlier than anywhere else in the hull.

The freestanding mast requires modification of the normal construction methods. While no chainplates are required, substantial bulkheading is required in the area of the mast to absorb the considerable forces generated by the unstayed mast. The forward six feet of the hull is strongly bulkheaded for this purpose, and no sign of undue strain could be detected.

Because there is no rigging to hold the mast in the boat should she capsize, alternative means must be found. This is accomplished by lagging a cast aluminum, hexagonally shaped female mast step to the hull. The butt of the mast is fitted with a hexagonal male counterpart which is strongly joined to the mast step by stainless steel set screws. The mast is further connected to the hull by a deck-level pin which passes through the mast and the cast aluminum deck collar.

Deck hardware is properly backed for load distribution and, in all, construction is generally to standards well above average for the industry.

PERFORMANCE

Handling under Sail

First of all, let's face it, there *are* some limitations on performance. The 30 does little better than chug to windward in sloppy conditions. The full hull shape forward needed to support the weight of a spar stepped but a couple of feet abaft the stemhead and the lesser efficiency of a cat rig over a jib-headed rig, do little to provide power through slop.

The Nonsuch 30 is one of the most boring boats we have ever sailed. (Tacking requires no yelling, releasing of sheets, cranking, tailing, or trimming.) Yet, tacking the 30, while a somnambulent exercise of merely moving the wheel a half turn, does result in the bow falling off and slow acceleration on the new

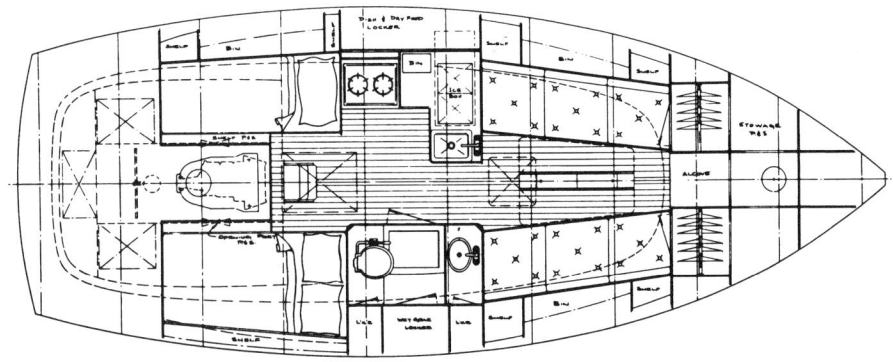

tack (briefly easing the main sheet and/or increasing mainsail draft seems to help). Similarly, sailors who enjoy the feel of a fine-performing sloop charging to windward will find the catboat asking to be driven, well balanced as she is. There is no letting the 30 "find her head" and "settle into a groove" as one might on a proper performing sloop.

This doesn't mean that she is necessarily easy to sail well. Getting the most out of the boat upwind definitely requires some practice. The aluminum mast is quite flexible, allowing the top of the mast to fall off as the wind increases. The sail's draft will shift, changing its efficiency. In about 10 knots of breeze, the top of the mast falls to leeward about a foot. This can be a little disconcerting to those used to a fairly rigid stayed mast.

Optimum performance for the 30 is directly related to the care and attention one lavishes on mainsail trim and shape control. For the average afternoon sailor this may make little if any difference, but there are a lot of us who remain uneasy unless a boat is sailing close to her best. In short, the 30 may be lazy to sail, but that is only because there is less of the hard work; there remains plenty of opportunity for fussy tweaking.

Sail shape is controlled by the "choker," a line which controls the fore and aft trim of the wishbone and functions as a clew outhaul. Tensioning the choker pulls the wishbone aft, flattening the sail. The sail is slab-reefed much the same as a conventional mainsail.

The Nonsuch mainsail is 540 square feet, with a hoist of 45 feet and a foot of 24 feet. By way of comparison the mainsail of the Irwin 52 is 525 square feet, and the Cal 31's is 210 square feet. The sail does not handle like a sail of 540 square feet, fortunately. The wishbone is rigged with permanent lazy jacks which hold the sail as it is dropped. Furling merely involves tying ties around the neatly cradled sail for the sake of aesthetics. Dousing the main or reefing is easily accomplished by one person, as all sail controls lead back to the cockpit.

The Nonsuch does not suffer from "catboat disease"—the tendency to develop monstrous weather helm as the breeze pipes up. She is remarkably well-mannered, with a surprisingly light helm. Downwind she holds course with the wheel brake off and hands off the wheel. Performance was almost as good upwind at moderate angles of heel.

She is a stiff boat. The flexible mast allows a substantial amount of air to be spilled from the main as the wind pipes up, removing much heeling force. We found that the boat goes better upwind with a reef in the main even at moderate angles of heel once the upper mast begins to fall off. Getting sail off the more flexible upper part of the mast allows better draft control as the wind increases.

The Nonsuch 30 is no Cape Cod catboat under the water. She has a moderate aspect-ratio fin keel, low wetted surface, and a freestanding semi-balanced spade rudder. These characteristics greatly add to her performance.

With all sail controls led back to the cockpit, she is a natural candidate for singlehanding. We strongly recommend self-tailing winches for all functions if shorthanded sailing is contemplated.

The Nonsuch 30
195

The Nonsuch 30 is not the boat for the hard-core Grand Prix racer. Her entire sail inventory consists of that one big sail, with perhaps a single downwind sail. You will not become the bosom buddy of any racing sailmaker by owning a Nonsuch. Then again, no sailmaker will ever have a second mortgage on your boat, either.

Handling Under Power

The Nonsuch 30 was originally equipped with a 23-horsepower Volvo MD 11C diesel with saildrive. This virtually eliminated engine installation and alignment problems for the builder, saving both time and money. These units have an integral cast zinc anode to protect the vulnerable aluminum lower unit from galvanic corrosion. A special Volvo-supplied zinc is required—not an item that you can pick up in any boatyard. About hull number 125, this installation was changed to a more conventional engine and shaft arrangement, utilizing a 27-horsepower Westerbeke diesel.

Either engine will drive the boat to hull speed. We prefer the conventional engine installation, which is understood and can be worked on by most boatyards. It is less vulnerable to corrosion, and runs quietly and smoothly.

Because of her high freeboard, the Nonsuch 30 will be susceptible to cross-winds when docking. With most of her windage forward, her bow has a tendency to blow downwind. A good hand on the throttle and gearshift will be a real plus in tight docking situations.

Incidentally, mocking the oft heard complaints about the adventure of sailboats backing down under power is the ability of the Nonsuch to do exactly that. We got ours up to five knots in reverse—and without slewing off before she got moving. It may not be something the harbor-master or the steering system appreciates but it is an impressive exhibition.

LIVABILITY

Deck Layout

Because the Nonsuch 30 has no standing rigging, her sidedecks are devoid of obstacles. Because she has no headsails there are no sheeting angles to be concerned with.

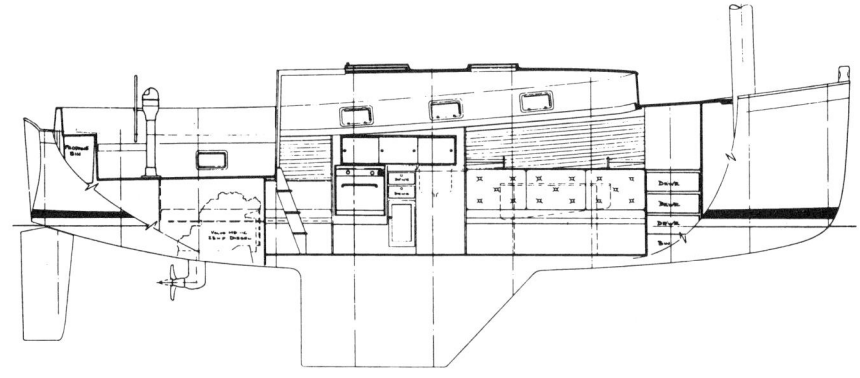

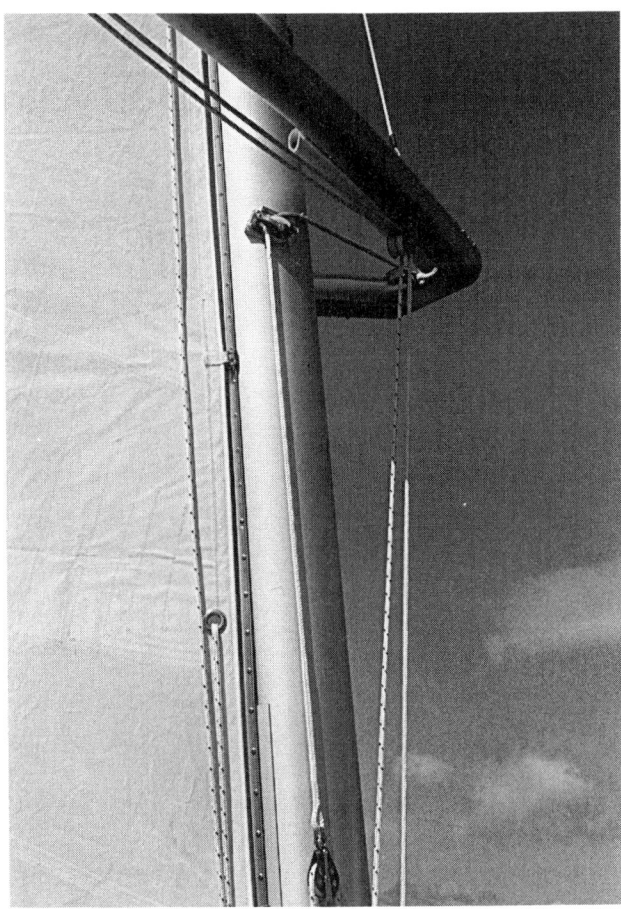

For cruising, the optional bowsprit/anchor roller with a hawsepipe to the otherwise unusable forepeak is highly desirable. Otherwise, anchor and rode must be stored in one of the cockpit lockers and dragged forward every time one wishes to anchor. We also recommend the installation of a bow pulpit. With no shrouds to hold when forward there is a great feeling of vulnerability on the bow. These things may make the Nonsuch 30 "uncatboat-like" in appearance, but they will add considerably to the safety and convenience when sailing and anchoring.

The wishbone boom flattens or "chokes" the mainsail by being moved aft closer to the mast by means of tackle running to the cockpit.

The cockpit is the most spacious we have found on a boat under 35 feet. The visibility forward is better than any sloop with a genoa set, albeit not as unobstructed under power (with the mainsail "furled") as conventional 30-footers with their mainsails piled on a boom well above the line of sight forward.

The large cockpit creates other problems. First, you should never raft up with other boats at anchor. A friendly crowd of eight could easily fit in the cockpit.

There are more serious problems associated with the cockpit design. The standard cockpit is not suited to offshore use. There is no bridgedeck. The companionway goes almost to the level of the cockpit sole—about three feet below the level of the lowest point in the cockpit coamings. Coupled with the huge cockpit volume, this creates a situation that cannot in any good conscience be called an offshore configuration. If this boat is to be called an offshore sailboat, we think there should be an optional cockpit arrangement—a large bridgedeck which could incorporate life raft storage, two more large cockpit drains, and perhaps a raised cockpit sole to further reduce the cockpit's volume.

There are three cockpit lockers: deep port and starboard lockers, and a lazarette set up to hold two 10-pound propane gas bottles.

When tacking or jibing it is easy for the helmsman to get caught by the mainsheet as the boom comes over. A better lead would be welcome here, perhaps having the mainsheet system incorporated into the stern rail.

Belowdecks

The interior volume of the Nonsuch 30 is an eye opener even to those used to the modern trend toward maximum interior volume on minimum overall length. To anyone used to the interior space of an older boat, the interior of the Nonsuch 30 is absolutely stunning.

The waterline and beam of the Nonsuch 30 are about the same as that of a modern 36-foot cruiser-racer, and that beam is carried quite a bit further forward. Coupled with high topsides and a highly-crowned deckhouse, this yields a boat with tremendous interior volume for her overall length.

The layout of the original 30, the "Classic," was as unusual in its day as it was practical. There is no forward cabin in the conventional sense. This isn't a real drawback. The forward cabin on the typical 30-footer is only useful for sleeping or sail stowage, and frequently has berths which are far too narrow at the forward end.

The forwardmost six feet of the boat is given over to two huge hanging lockers and a great deal of storage space. This space has been created by the three transverse and two fore and aft bulkheads that stiffen the hull in the way of the mast.

The rest of the boat is essentially one large cabin. The saloon occupies the forward third of the interior. There are shelves and bins outboard of the two long settees that face each other across the cabin, with a dropleaf table on centerline. Varnished pine ceiling behind the settees is a welcome note in an otherwise dark teak interior.

The galley is amidships to port. The cook is out of the traffic flow yet located in the center of activity if there are people both below and topsides. The galley has a gimballed propane stove with oven, a well-insulated icebox with (hurrah!) an insulated, gasketed lid, and a deep sink nearly on centerline which will easily drain on either tack. The icebox melt water is pumped into the galley sink.

The head is opposite the galley. Because of the pronounced deckhouse camber, headroom there decreases rapidly as you move outboard.

There are quarterberths port and starboard aft of the galley and head. The standard berth starboard is a double, with a single to port. An option provides doubles on both sides, although filling all the berths on the boat requires an open mind and no highly-developed sense of privacy.

The impression of spaciousness created in the original layout is even greater in the "Ultra." With its saloon aft, double berth in the forward cabin, amidships galley, and head serving to isolate the forward cabin, the new layout represents a significant improvement. Gone are the two coffin-like quarterberths and the need to go all the way to the forward cabin for comfortable sitting. In their place with the new layout is a spacious main cabin, better suited to socializing.

Ventilation of the interior is excellent, with seven opening ports, two hatches, and two dorade boxes. The propane heater vents overboard through its own exhaust stack.

CONCLUSIONS

Perhaps it is an exaggeration to say that this 30-footer is comparable in price, speed, and space to a more conventional 35-footer, but the Nonsuch is more boat than her modest LOA would suggest. She is indeed easier to handle and has more versatile accommodations than most production boats up to five feet longer. Moreover, her rig, while once "innovative," if not "weird," now has gained the acceptance it deserves.

The Nonsuch 30 is not a traditionalist's catboat. She lacks the sweeping sheer, low freeboard, gaff rig, and barn-door rudder of the Cape Cod catboat. However, she also lacks the traditional catboat's weather helm, poor windward performance, and man-killing mainsail.

At the same time the Nonsuch is well-built, simple, and comfortable. She makes an excellent coastal cruiser for a couple or a small family, with space and a modicum of privacy. She also seems an ideal boat for an older couple who desire to minimize the heavy work of sailing—the winching, the furling, and the lugging of sailbags.

At $84,000 reasonably well equipped, there is nothing cheap about the Nonsuch 30. That is a price that comes close to a comparably equipped 34- or 35-footer of modest quality, and doesn't even take into account the $5,000 or so of additional sails included in the price for the conventionally rigged counterpart. Still, there is a mitigating circumstance; the Nonsuch may be 30 feet overall, but length has always been a deceptive indicator of size, let alone quality, roominess, or even performance. In short, if you want bragging rights on the basis of length, not price, there are a lot of boats you might consider before the Nonsuch.

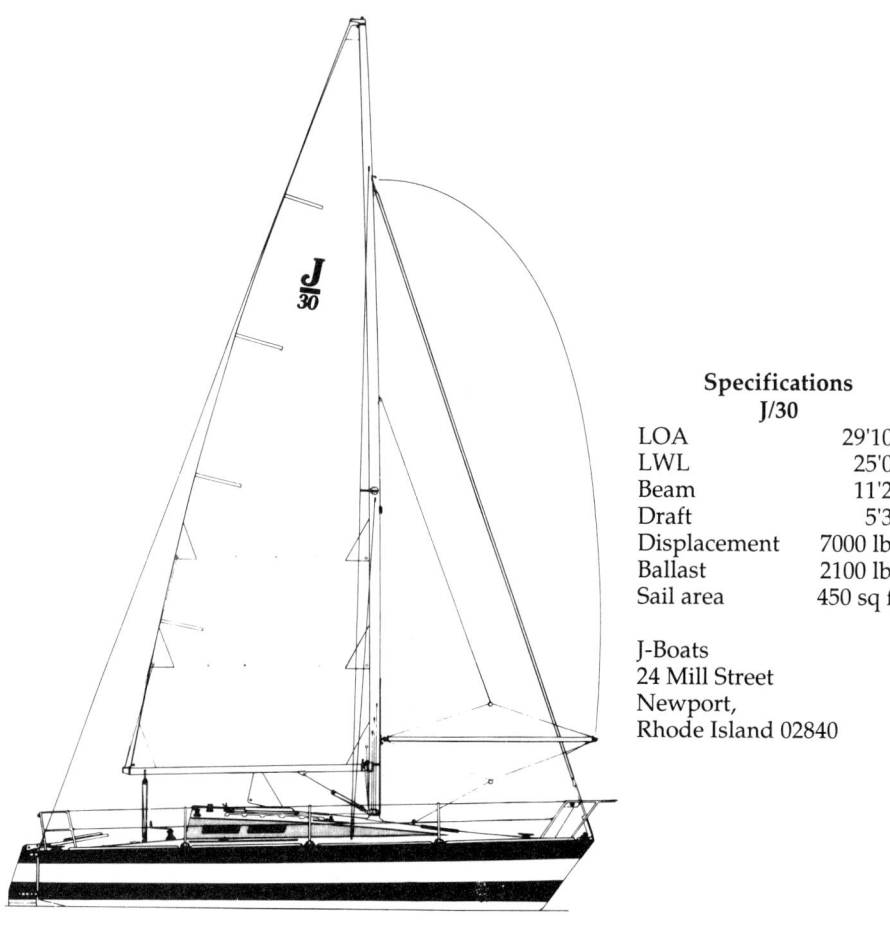

The J/30:
A True Racer/Cruiser

THE BOAT AND THE BUILDER

No one has blanketed the market with such a line of so basically similar boats for so long as has J-boats. Starting with the J/24 in the mid-1970s, J-Boats in the next 10 years put nine models on the market, all of them aimed at performance on either the one-design or PHRF race course, most of them on both. Even the J/40 introduced in 1985, the J/28 the following year, and the J/37 new in 1987, with their primary emphasis on cruising, come with the promise of better than average performance.

J-Boats in that 10 years thus became the foremost name in producing performance sailing craft, helped in no small measure by formation of class associations, maintenance of strict one-design standards, and considerable promotion of the idea of performance as the primary desirable characteristic of its boats. Moreover, no major builder has managed so ably to control the after-market for its products as has J-Boats. An informative newsletter, an instructional program (J-World), and a network of knowledgeable dealers and sailmakers have also done much to contribute to the J-Boat success story.

Despite the primary intention that its racing boats should lead the way on the race course, J-Boats has had its share of racing setbacks. Only in the hands of top-notch sailors has any J-Boat except the 24 done well in Grand Prix-style racing. PHRF handicappers have tended to take J-Boats at their advertising word and rate the boats as fast. Worse still (for the beginning sailor) is that highly experienced sailors have been attracted to J-Boats and sail them well. As a result, J-Boats tend to be difficult to sail as fast as they are rated. Nevertheless, no production boats have had the overall success in PHRF racing as has the extensive line of J-Boats.

The J/30, the second J-Boat after the super-successful J/24, was introduced in 1979. The J/30 was designed to let the type of sailor who had outgrown the J/24 (or whose family had outgrown her) step up to a similarly smart-performing boat, but with full cruising accommodations and a bigger boat "feel." The one-design racing capability of the J/24 is retained in the J/30, but the 30 offers her owners the chance of competing in at least semi-serious overnight handicap events. In short, unlike the racy 24 with her spartan accommodations, the J/30 is intended to be the best of both worlds: a comfortable family cruiser and racer at a more modest cost than most of her competition.

By the end of 1986 about 600 J/30s had been built. Moreover, in 1984 J-Boats modified the cockpit and interior layout, changes intended to make the J/30 a more pleasant boat to cruise, yet the changes were done in such a way as to retain the one-design capabilities of the class.

CONSTRUCTION

The hull of the J/30 is cored with end-grain balsa. After the balsa core is glassed to the outer hull skin, the two-part mold is bolted together, and the centerline joint heavily glassed over. The layup is then finished the same as any one-piece molded hull.

Exterior finish quality of the molding is good, with little evidence of gelcoat blistering or roving print-through. The hull to deck joint is made by laying the deck molding over the internal flange of the hull molding. This joint is heavily bedded in 3M 5200 and through-bolted on eight-inch centers with quarter-inch stainless steel bolts. The joint is covered on the outside by the teak toerail, which is cut away around the lifeline stanchion bases to provide deck scuppers. The toerail is through-bolted, further backing up the hull to deck joint. This joint can be visually inspected on the inside of the boat throughout most of its length.

The outboard high-aspect-ratio rudder is strongly attached to the boat with stainless steel pintles and gudgeons. The bolts which attach these to the rudder should be periodically tightened.

The J/30

The tillerhead is also a strong stainless steel fabrication. A stainless steel tiller extension on the ash tiller allows the helmsman to sit on the weather rail with the rest of the crew. The steering system is simple, strong, and cheap. It should give little or no trouble if the fastenings are checked periodically.

Many J/24s had a disconcerting structural shortcoming; the main bulkhead tended to come adrift. Since the main bulkhead provides almost all of the transverse rigidity of the J/30, quite a bit more thought has gone into it. The main bulkhead of the J/30 is a fairly sophisticated combination of cored and solid construction—solid where the chainplates attach, cored elsewhere.

This bulkhead is glassed to the hull along its outer perimeter and butt-jointed with 3M 5200 to the deck molding. A recess in the deck molding to receive the bulkhead would be better than a simple butt joint. There is no evidence of this bulkhead's moving, panting, or creaking, as the boat works to windward. In fact, the inside of the boat is remarkably quiet going to weather.

Two large fiberglass moldings form the floor pans and the basic furniture structure.

Water tanks are cast polyethylene. Although these have glassed-in retainers, we would want to reinforce them before going offshore for any period of time. Large storage bins under the berths and settees have polyethylene liners, a practical solution to keeping anything dry in these areas. The boat also has a good-sized bilge sump, an absolute necessity in a boat with flat bilges.

The J/30 has a bendy, fractional rig with swept-back spreaders and single lowers aft of the mast. Both uppers and lowers share a single stainless steel chainplate. Playing with the rig adjustments is an integral part of making the J/30 go fast. Despite the apparent fragility of the rig, it has shown little tendency to crumble.

PERFORMANCE

Handling Under Sail

The original idea behind the J/30 was to provide a racing-cruising boat capable of sailing competitively against more sophisticated and more expensive boats. The 30, despite her then light displacement and innovative fractional rig, did not succeed. Her IOR rating (about 25.8) proved more than she could handle,

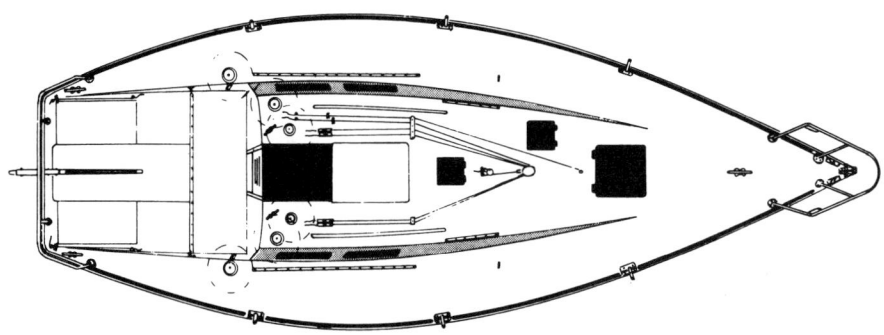

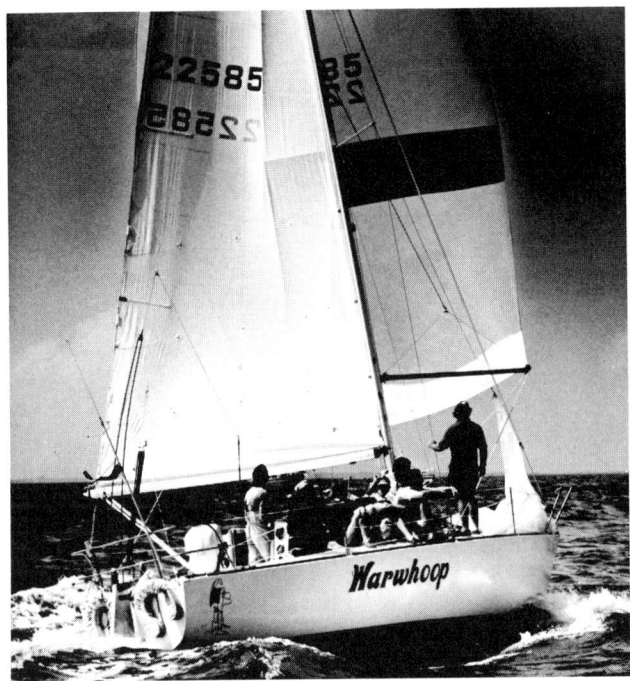

and even PHRF tended to give her a rating (130-145) she could sail to only in a breeze. The best J/30 racing became one-design fleets. Recognizing the limitations on the 30 for racing, J-Boats in 1983 introduced its J/29, a boat with minimal accommodations, 1000 pounds lighter and $10,000 cheaper than the J/30. J-Boats then upgraded the 30 for cruising.

As a handicap racing boat, the J/30 has distinct liabilities. She is sluggish in light winds, especially in a chop. At the same time, for optimum performance in her most favored conditions (a breeze), she needs weight on the windward rail—four or five lumps of live ballast. For club or family racing this is a demanding requirement, yet she does not sail to her rating without it. Her fractional rig makes depowering the mainsail easy and the headsail is small, but the boat is initially tender and a heel angle in excess of 15 degrees hurts windward performance.

This tenderness is her most critical liability for family cruising. Few sailors find sitting on the rail to be the way to cruise. Thus, while the liveliness and basic weatherliness of the 30 is a virtue, it does carry a price.

The J/30 is a delight for the sailor who loves to tweak rig and sails for maximum performance without spending a fortune. The boat is the ideal choice for the racing sailor with Two-Ton aspirations and a Half-Ton pocketbook. The J/30 one-design class specifications limit sails to mainsail, three jibs, and one spinnaker when racing. There are minimum specified cloth weights for all sails.

Wisely, the Johnstones have not insisted on a single sailmaker for one-design racing. Sailmakers have become the gurus of the modern racing sailor, and like charismatic religious or political leaders, each racing sailmaker has his own band of faithful followers. Specifying a single sailmaker is the sure kiss of death for a boat intended to be mass-marketed throughout the country.

With 18 to 22 knots of wind over the deck, the J/30 will do up to six knots to windward in a slight chop using the 105-percent genoa and a single-reefed mainsail. In puffy conditions, the mainsheet traveler should be played constantly to keep the boat on her feet. This is typical of fractionally rigged boats with their relatively large mainsails. As with all modern, low-wetted-surface boats, the J/30 goes fastest when sailed almost upright, and a great deal of sailing effort should be directed to keeping her in that upright trim.

With light displacement for her waterline, the J/30 should be sailed around waves rather than into them. It is important to keep the boat from bobbing in a chop.

When reaching under spinnaker, the boat is far more stable than the typical IOR boat, which has a pronounced tendency to round up when overpowered by the spinnaker. This lack of broaching tendency is the characteristic that makes the J/30 sail well above her rating off the wind in heavy air. Under these conditions, the typical IOR boat spends a substantial part of her sailing time dragging her rudder through the water sideways in an attempt to keep the boat on her feet and pointed in the right direction. The J/30 has a straight, relatively flat run aft, with the rudder well aft of the normal waterline. This produces a boat which surfs easily and quickly while maintaining fairly straightforward steering characteristics.

Sailing any fractional rig is substantially different from sailing the masthead rig. The mainsail is far more important in the fractional rig, both because of its size and the fact that the leading edge of the main is the highest sail on the boat. For this reason, J-Boats recommends that the full main be carried whenever possible, to keep the upper part of the sail in clear air.

Handling Under Power
The J/30 comes with a two-cylinder, raw-water cooled 15-horsepower Yanmar diesel. Fresh water cooling is an option. This is more than adequate power for a 7,000-pound boat. The Yanmar engines have a reputation for a fairly high level of vibration and noise. The one in the J/30 is no exception. Owners, however, report excellent handling under power.

The engine of the J/30 is unlikely to accumulate many hours. The boat sails so well that there is little excuse to use the engine except to charge batteries and for motoring in a flat calm. With the optional shower, the engine may acquire a few more hours heating water for a post-race cleanup—a luxury on a 30-foot racing boat.

LIVABILITY

Deck Layout
Under the strict one-design class rules, the deck layout of the J/30 is tightly controlled. Since the deck layout is the product of much careful thought by the Johnstones, it is unlikely that anyone would want to alter it substantially.

As with most modern boats, less thought goes into the arrangement for mooring and anchoring than in the arrangement for sailing. The J/30 does have two bow chocks, but their location well back from the stem accentuates the boat's tendency to sail around on the mooring or anchor. The class rules allow for the changing of the mooring cleats and chocks. Sailors who plan to cruise the boat much are likely to take advantage of this allowance.

There is an excellent self-draining anchor well in the starboard deck abreast the mast. This is designed to hold a Danforth 22-S or 20-H, either of which is more than adequate for the boat, depending on the type of holding ground. The anchor rope is carried in the forepeak locker, feeding onto the deck via a hawsepipe. A second anchor can easily be carried in one of the cockpit lockers, which are too small for sails anyway.

It is easy to move around the deck of the J/30, even when the boat is heeled. The deck features excellent molded-in nonskid.

The original cockpit is not particularly comfortable. There are minimal cockpit coamings. The helmsman and crew sit on extensions of the sidedecks in the fashion of racing boats where crew efficiency and keeping weight to windward are more important than crew comfort. Water running aft on the sidedecks runs over the vestigial coaming and except for the dubious support of the lifelines, even if padded, there is no back support. This cockpit configuration did nothing to encourage use of the J/30 for cruising.

In 1984, the cockpit was redesigned to make it more of a "sit in," rather than a "sit on" type. Since that same modification did away with the port quarterberth, the 30 also acquired a much-needed cockpit seat locker. While an improvement for cruising, the cockpit retains the athwartships traveler, and the relatively awkward winch locations of the original.

A word of caution: the cockpit of the J/30 and her outboard rudder plus the racing heritage of the design virtually preclude installation of wheel steering. While wheel steering on a lively boat of this size and weight is hardly the norm, for cruising, wheel steering is one way to make a cockpit at least seem more spacious, by eliminating the space needed to accommodate the swing of the tiller.

Belowdecks

The interior of the J/30 is light, roomy, and well thought-out. The general appearance is high-tech traditional, with varnished white cedar ceiling, laminated ash trim, and an optional teak and holly cabin sole.

When the J/30 underwent modification in 1984, the interior layout as well as the cockpit was redesigned. The original interior had six berths, the argument being that for racing, the off-watch should all be sleeping to windward. The result was a pair of matched quarterberths, a configuration that raised hob with the size and convenience of the galley. Cooking, for instance, meant having to reach across a sink to operate the stove.

With the redesign, the galley moved aft, replacing one quarterberth and more than doubling its size, not to say its efficiency and safety. The result is a simple, practical layout for a 30-footer, capable of comfortably sleeping a crew of three or four.

Overall, the main cabin of the J/30 is quite remarkable for a 30-footer whose primary purpose is performance. The interior is wide, comfortable and attractive. While a chart table may be an arguable use of space on a boat as small as 30 feet, in the J/30 it is a useful, if not a necessary, amenity.

Headroom is a good six feet at the after end of the main cabin, tapering to about five-feet, six inches at the forward end of the cabin.

The forward cabin features a large V-berth with molded storage alcoves over and watertight bins under. A privacy curtain can separate the forward cabin from the head.

The head compartment is surprisingly comfortable. Both the mast and grabrail offer good handholds and bracing points. It is most comfortable to use the sink while sitting on the toilet seat, a practical solution in a small boat.

Ventilation is provided in all three interior areas by three plastic-framed opening hatches. There is no provision for ventilation in heavy weather.

While the J/30 is no luxury cruiser, the interior is quite habitable, and intelligently finished. Joinerwork and finish are of good production boat quality. We would strongly recommend the optional cabin table, a well mounted and fiddled dropleaf unit with storage bins in the center section. The table will seat six for dinner in reasonable comfort.

At the same time, buyers considering the J/30 for cruising should be prepared to accept the compromises that give the boat performance. It is no easy job to make a boat fast and comfortable, no easy job to have a layout that can accommodate a racing crew of six for an overnight race as well as a family for two weeks of cruising. For all the spaciousness of the basic interior, storage is at a premium and so too is privacy.

CONCLUSIONS

The boat buyer looking at the J/30 has to have performance as his highest priority, whether that performance is lively daysailing and cruising or some level of competition—or most likely, some combination of both. The J/30 makes little sense for an owner not interested in keeping sails well trimmed and working to get the last quarter-knot of boat speed the conditions and his boat can produce. This is a boat for a small, active family whose idea of a good car is a sports car rather than a station wagon. The J/30 may be no harder to sail than any other 30-footer, but she fairly pleads with her crew to busy themselves making her go.

While attractive and functional, the accommodations of the J/30 are subordinate to performance. At the same time, there aren't many 30-footers on the market that can boast as much performance and belowdecks comfort as is found on the J/30.

Throughout its production run, the J/30 has represented a good value for her price. When she was introduced, the base price was $35,000 plus electronics and class sails, a figure 20 percent under good quality production boats with less performance. By 1985, the price had risen to over $50,000 equipped, still a tab substantially under such similar-sized boats as the Sabre 30 with comparable accommodations and notably less performance.

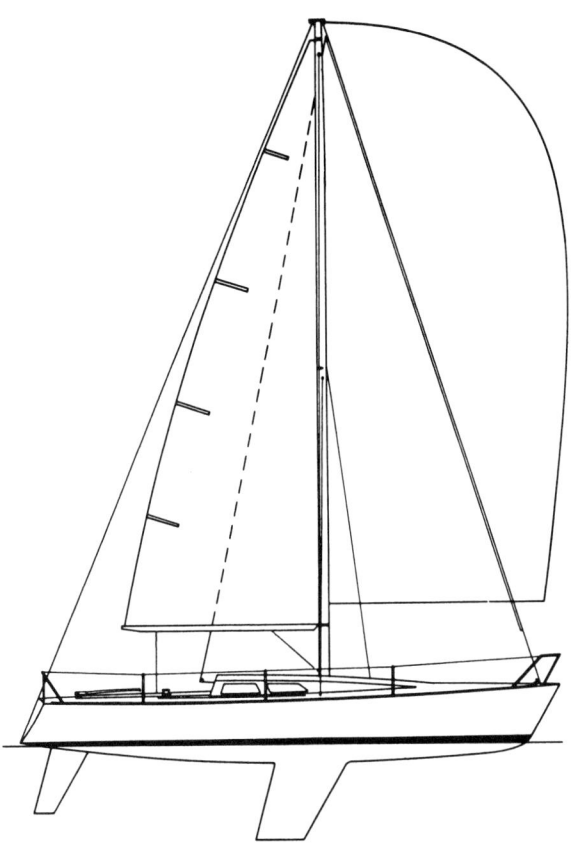

The Olson 30:
Ultra Light, Ultra Fast

THE BOAT AND THE BUILDER

The Olson 30 is one of a breed of sailboats born in Santa Cruz, California called the *ULDB*, an acronym for *ultra light displacement boat*. ULDBs basically are big dinghies—long on the waterline, short on the interior amenities, narrow in the beam, and very light in both displacement and pricetag. ULDBs attract a different kind of sailor—the type for whom performance means everything.

For some yachting traditionalists, the arrival of the ULDB has been a hard pill to swallow. Part of this is simple resentment of a ULDB's ability to sail boat-for-boat with a racer-cruiser up to ten or twenty feet longer (and a whole lot more expensive). Part of it is the realization that to sail a ULDB might mean having to learn a whole new set of sailing skills. Part of it is a reaction to the near-manic enthusiasts of Santa Cruz, where nearly 100 ULDBs race for pure fun—without the help of race committees, protest committees, or handicaps (in Santa Cruz, IOR is a dirty word). And part of the traditionalists' resentment is their gut feeling that ULDBs aren't real yachts.

In 1970, Californian George Olson tried an experiment and created the first ULDB. He thought, if he took a boat with the same displacement and sail area as a Cal 20, but made it longer and narrower, it might go faster. The boat he built was called *Grendel* and it did go faster than a Cal 20, much faster than anyone had expected. The plug for *Grendel* was later widened by Santa Cruz boatbuilder Ron Moore, and used to make the mold for the Moore 24, a now popular ULDB one-design.

In the meantime, George Olson teamed up with another Santa Cruz builder by the name of Bill Lee. Together they designed and built the Santa Cruz 27. Olson also helped Lee build his 1977 TransPac winner, *Merlin*, a 67-foot, 20,000-pound monster of a ULDB. (She has subsequently been legislated out of the TransPac race.) Then Olson and several other Lee employees started their own boatbuilding firm in Santa Cruz—Pacific Boats.

The first project for Pacific Boats was the Olson 30, which was put into production in 1978. Over 200 of these 3600-pound ULDBs were sold, and the builder claims they have gathered in sufficient numbers to support one-design racing in Seattle, the Great Lakes, Annapolis, Texas, and Long Island Sound, as well as several spots in California. Pacific Boats was a small firm that built only the Olson 30 and the Olson 40, both to quality standards.

CONSTRUCTION

Some people wonder how the ULDB can be built so light and still be seaworthy offshore. The answer lies in the fact that a light boat is subjected to much lighter loads than a heavy boat when pounding through a sea (there is tremendous saving in weight with a stripped-out interior). And perhaps more importantly, ULDB builders have construction standards that are well above average for production sailboats. The ULDB builders say that their close proximity to each other in Santa Cruz, combined with their open sharing of technology, has enabled them to achieve these high standards.

The Olson 30 is no exception. The hull and deck are fiberglass, vacuum-bagged over a balsa core. The process of vacuum-bagging insures maximum saturation of the laminate and core with a minimum of resin, making the hull

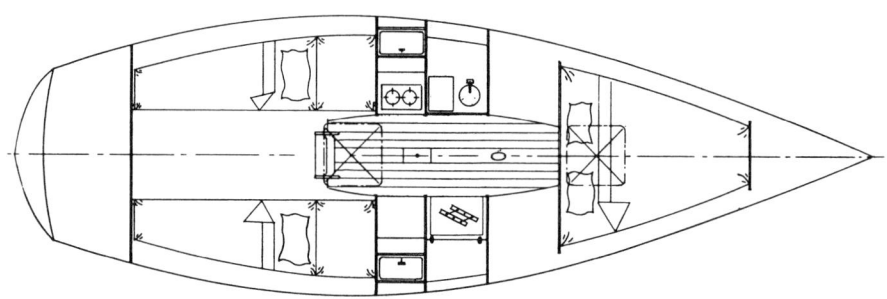

light and stiff. The builder claims that they have so refined the construction of the Olson 30 that each finished hull weighs within 10 pounds of the standard. The deck of the Olson does not have plywood inserts in place of the balsa where winches are mounted, instead relying on external backing plates for strength.

The hull to deck joint is an inward turned, overlapping flange, glued with a rigid compound called Reid's adhesive, and mechanically fastened with closely spaced bolts through a slotted aluminum toerail. This provides a strong, protected joint, seaworthy-enough for sailing offshore. The aluminum toerail provides a convenient location for outboard sheet leads, but is painful for those sitting on the rail.

The Olson 30's 1800-pound keel is deep (5' 1" draft) and less than five inches thick. Narrow, bolted-on keels need extra athwartship support. The Olson 30 accomplishes this with nine 5/8-inch bolts, and one one-inch bolt (to which the lifting eye is attached). The lead keel is faired with polyester putty and then completely wrapped with fiberglass to seal the putty from the marine environment. Too many builders neglect sealing autobody putty-faired keels, and too many boat owners then find the putty peeling off at a later date. The Olson's finished keel is painted, and, on the boats we've seen, remarkably fair.

The keel-stepped, single-spreader, tapered mast is cleanly rigged with 5/32-inch Navtec rod rigging and internal tangs. The mast section is large enough for peace of mind in heavy air. The halyards exit the mast at well-spaced intervals, to avoid creating a weak spot. The chainplates are securely attached to half-bulkheads of 1-inch plywood. In addition, a tie-rod attaches the deck to the mast, tensioned by a turnbuckle. While this arrangement should provide adequate strength, we would prefer both a tie-rod and a full bulkhead that spans the width of the cabin to absorb the compressive loads that rig tension puts on the deck.

The rudder's construction is labor-intensive but strong. Urethane foam is hand shaped to templates, then glued to a two-inch diameter solid fiberglass rudder post. The builder prefers fiberglass because it has more "memory" than aluminum or steel. Stainless steel straps are wrapped around the rudder and mechanically fastened to the post. Then the whole rudder assembly is faired, fiberglassed, and painted.

PERFORMANCE

Handling Under Sail

For those of you who agonize over whether your PHRF rating is fair, consider the ratings of ULDBs. The Santa Cruz 50 rates 0; *that's right, zero.* The 67-foot *Merlin* has rated as low as *minus* 60. The Olson 30 rates anywhere from 90 to 114, depending on the local handicapper. Olson 30 owners tell us that the boat will sail to a PHRF rating of 96, but she will almost never sail to her astronomical IOR rating of 32 (the IOR heavily penalizes ULDBs).

ULDBs are fast. They are apt to be on the tender side, and sail with a quick, "jerky" motion through waves. Instead of punching through waves, they ride over them. You may get to where you are going fast, but with the motion of the boat and the spartan interior you won't get there in comfort. Olson 30 owners tell us that they do far less cruising and far more racing than they had expected to do when they bought the boat. They say it's more fun to race because the boat is so lively.

Like most ULDBs, the Olson 30 races best at the extremes of wind conditions—under 10 knots and over 20 knots. Although her masthead rig may appear short, it is more than powerful enough for her displacement. Owners tell us that she accelerates so quickly you can almost tack at will—a real tactical advantage in light air. In winds under 10 knots, they say she sails above her PHRF rating, both upwind and downwind.

In moderate breezes it's a different story. Once the wind gets much above 10 knots, it's time to change down to the #2 genoa. In 15 knots, especially if the seas are choppy, it's very difficult for the Olson 30 to save her time on boats of conventional displacement, according to three-time national champ Kevin Connally. The Olson 30 is always faster downwind, but even with a crew of 5 or 6, she just can't hang in there upwind.

In winds above 20 knots, the Olson 30 still has her problems upwind. But when she turns the weather mark the magic begins. As soon as she has enough wind to surf or plane, the Olson 30 can make up for all she looses upwind, and more. The builder claims that she has pegged speedometers at 25 knots in the big swells and strong westerlies off the coast of California. That is, of course, if the crew can keep her 1800-pound keel under her 761-square foot spinnaker.

The key to competitiveness in a strong breeze is the ability of the crew. Top crews say that because she is so quick to respond, they have fewer problems handling her in heavy air. However, an inexperienced crew which cannot react quickly enough, can have big problems. "The handicappers say she can fly downwind, so they give us a low (PHRF) rating. But they don't understand that we have sail *slow*, just to stay in control," complained the crew of one new owner.

Like any higher performance class of sailboat, the Olson 30 attracts competent sailors. Hence, the boat is pushed to a higher level of overall performance, and the PHRF rating reflects this. An inexperienced sailor must realize that he

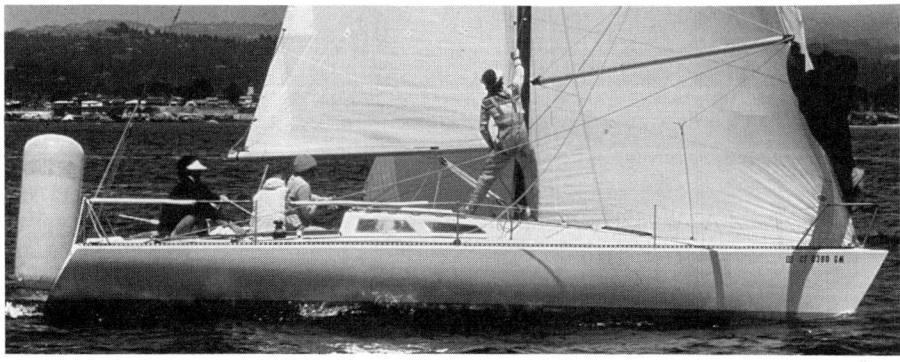

may have a tougher time making her sail to this inflated rating than a boat that is less "hot."

The two most common mistakes that new Olson 30 owners make are pinching upwind and allowing the boat to heel excessively. ULDBs cannot be sailed at the 30 degrees of heel to which many sailors of conventional boats are accustomed. To keep her flat, you must be quick to shorten sail, move the sheet leads outboard, and get more crew weight on the rail. You can't afford to have a person sitting to leeward trimming the genoa in a 12-knot breeze. To keep her thin keel from stalling upwind, owners tell us it's important to keep the sheets eased and the boat footing.

Being masthead-rigged, the Olson 30 needs a larger sail inventory than a fractionally rigged boat. Class rules allow one mainsail, six headsails (jibs and spinnakers) and a 75-percent storm jib. Owners who do mostly handicap racing tell us they often carry more than six headsails.

Handling Under Power

Only a few of the Olson 30s sold were equipped with inboard power. This is because the extra weight of the inboard and the drag of the propeller, strut and shaft are a real disadvantage when racing against the majority of Olson 30s, which are equipped with outboard motors.

The Olson 30 is just barely light enough to be pushed by a four to five horsepower outboard. It takes a 7.5 horse outboard to push the Olson 30 at 6.5 knots in a flat calm. The Olson's raked transom requires an extra long outboard bracket, which puts the engine throttle and shift out of reach for anyone much less than 6 feet tall: "A real pain," said one owner. Storage is a problem, too. Even if you could get the outboard through the stern lazarette's small hatch, you wouldn't want to race with the extra weight so far aft. As a result, most owners end up storing the outboard on the cabin sole.

The inboard was an optional, 154-pound, 7-horsepower, BMW diesel. Unlike most boats, the Olson 30 will probably never return the investment in an inboard when the boat is sold. It detracts from the boat's primary purpose—racing.

Without an inboard, owners have a problem charging the battery. Owners who race with extensive electronics have to take the battery ashore after every race for recharging. If the Olson 30 weren't such a joy to sail in light air, and so maneuverable in tight places, the lack of inboard power would be a serious enough drawback to turn away more sailors than it does.

LIVABILITY

Deck Layout

In most respects, the Olson 30 is a good sea boat. Although the cockpit is 6-1/2 feet long, the wide seats and narrow floor result in a relatively small cockpit volume, so little sea water can collect in the cockpit if the boat is pooped or knocked down. However, foot room is restricted, while the width of the seats makes it awkward to brace your legs on the leeward seat. The seats themselves are comfortable because they are angled up and the seatbacks are angled back. There are gutters to drain water off the leeward seat. The long mainsheet traveler is mounted across the cockpit.

The Olson 30's single companionway dropboard is latchable from inside the cabin, a real necessity in a storm offshore. A man-overboard pole tube in the stern is standard equipment. Teak toerails on the cockpit coaming and on the forward part of the cabin house provide good footing, and there are handholds on the after part of the cabin house.

The tapered aluminum stanchions are set into sockets molded into the deck and glassed to the inside of the hull, a strong, clean, leak-proof system. However, the stanchions are not glued or mechanically fastened into the sockets. If pulled upwards with great force they can be pulled out. We feel this is a safety hazard. Tight lifelines would help prevent this from happening, but most racing crews tend to leave them slightly loose so they can lean further outboard when hanging over the rail upwind. If the stanchions were fastened into the sockets with bolts or screws they would undoubtedly leak. A leakproof solution to this problem should be devised and made available to Olson 30 owners.

The cockpit has two drains of adequate diameter. The bilge pump, a Guzzler 500, is mounted in the cockpit. As is common on most boats, the stern lazarette is not sealed off from the rest of the interior. If the boat were pooped or knocked down with the lazarette open, water could rush below through the lazarette relatively unrestricted. As the Olson 30 has a shallow sump, there is little place for water to go except above the cabin sole.

A "paint-roller" type non-skid is molded into the Olson 30's deck. It provides excellent traction, but it is more difficult to keep clean than conventional patterned non-skid.

The Olson 30 is well laid out with hardware of reasonable, but not exceptional, quality. All halyards and pole controls lead to the cockpit through Easylock 1 clutch stoppers. The Easylocks are barely big enough to hold the halyards; they slip an inch under heavy loads. Older Olsons were equipped with Howard Rope Clutches. The Howards had a history of breaking (although the manufacturer has now corrected the problem).

The primary winches, Barient 22s, are also barely adequate. Some owners we talked to had replaced them with more powerful models. Schaefer headsail track cars are standard equipment. One owner complained that he had to replace them with Merrimans because the Schaefers kept slipping. Leading the vang to either rail and leading the reefing lines aft is also recommended.

The mast partner is snug, leaving no space for mast blocks. The mast step is movable to adjust the prebend of the spar. The partner has a lip, over which a neoprene collar fits. The collar is hose-clamped to the mast. This should make a watertight mast boot. However, on the boat we sailed, the bail to which the boom vang attached obstructed the collar, causing water to collect and drain into the cabin.

The yoked backstay is adjustable from either quarter of the stern, one side being a 2:1 gross adjustment and the other side being an 8:1 fine tune. A

Headfoil II is standard equipment. There is a babystay led to a track with a 6:1 purchase for easy adjustment. The track is tied to the thin plywood of the forward V-berth with a wire and a turnbuckle. On the boat we sailed, the padeye to which the babystay tie rod is attached was seen to be tearing out from the V-berth.

There is a port in the deck directly over the lifting eye in the bilge. This makes for quick and easy drysailing. The Olson 30, however, is not easily trailered; her 3600 pounds is too much for all but the largest cars, and her 9.3-foot beam requires a special trailering permit.

Belowdecks

The Olson 30 is cramped belowdecks. Her low deckhouse and substantial sheer may make her one of the sexiest-looking production boats on the water, but the price is headroom of only four feet, five inches. There is not even enough headroom for comfortable stooping. Moving about below is a real grind for an average-sized person.

To offset the confinement of the interior, the builder has done everything possible to make it light and airy. In addition to the Lexan forward hatch and cabin house windows, the companionway hatch also has a Lexan insert. The inside of the hull is smooth sanded and finished with white gelcoat. There are no full-height bulkheads dividing the cabin. All the furniture is built of light-weight, light-colored, 3/8" Scandanavian, seven-ply plywood.

The joinerwork is above average and all of the bulkhead and furniture tabbing is extremely neat. There isn't much to the Olson 30's interior, but what there is has been done with commendable craftsmanship. The cabin sole is narrow, and with the lack of headroom, the woodwork is susceptible to being dinged and scratched from equipment like outboard motors. Once the finish on the wood is broken, it quickly absorbs water, which collects in the shallow bilge.

The Olson 30 is not a comfortable cruiser. Even after you've taken all the racing sails ashore, the belowdecks is barely habitable. To save weight the quarterberths are made of thin cushions sewn to vinyl and hung from pipes. These pipe berths are comfortable, but the cushions are not easily removed. Should they get wet it's likely they would stay wet for some time. Two seabags are hung on sail tracks above the quarter berths, which should help to insure that some clothes stay dry.

Just forward of each quarterberth is a small uncushioned seat locker. Behind each seat is a small portable ice cooler. In one seat locker is the stove, an Origo 3000, which slides up and out of the locker on tracks. The Origo is a top-of-the-line unpressurized alcohol stove, but to operate it the cook must kneel on the cabin sole. To work at the navigation station, which is in front of the starboard seat, you must sit sideways. In front of the port seat is the lavette, with a hand water pump and a removable, shallow, drainless sink. Drainless sinks eliminate the need for a through-hull fitting—a good idea—but they should be deep, not shallow.

The head is a portable toilet mounted under the forward V-berth, which we think is totally unsuitable for a sailboat. Who wants a smelly toilet under his pillow? Although there are curtains which can be drawn across the V-berth, we think human dignity deserves an enclosed head, especially on a 30' boat. The V-berth is large and easy to climb into, but there are no shelves above it or a storage locker in the empty bow. In short, if you plan to cruise for more than a weekend, you'd better like roughing it.

CONCLUSIONS

A completely equipped Olson 30 ran about $35,000. Today, a used one will cost from $24,000 to $28,000. What do you get for this? You get a boat that's well built, seaworthy, and reasonably well laid out. You get a boat that, in light air, will sail as fast as boats costing nearly twice as much. Downwind in heavy air, you have a creature that will blow your mind and leave everything (except a bigger ULDB) in your wake. If you spend all of your sailing time racing in a PHRF fleet in an area where light or heavy air dominates, the Olson 30 will probably give you more pleasure for your dollar than almost anything afloat.

However, if you race in moderate air or enjoy more than an occasional short cruise, you are likely to be very disappointed. Before you consider the Olson 30, you must realistically evaluate your abilities as a sailor. There's nothing worse, after finding out that you can't race a boat to her potential, than realizing that she is of little use for any other aspect of our sport.

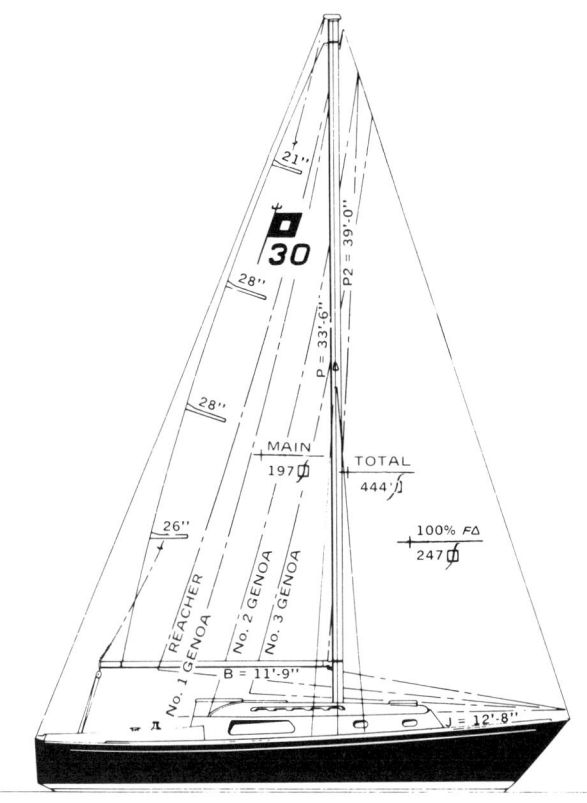

Specifications
Pearson 30

LOA	29'9"
DWL	25'0"
Beam	9'6"
Draft	5'0"
Displacement	8320 lbs
Ballast	3560 lbs
Sail area	444 sq ft

Pearson Yachts
West Shore Road
Portsmouth,
Rhode Island 02871
(401) 683-0100

The Pearson 30:
Moderation in All Matters

THE BOAT AND THE BUILDER

The Bill Shaw-designed Pearson 30 entered production in late 1971. Ten years later, when production ended, well over a thousand of the fin-keeled, spade-ruddered sloops had been built in the company's Portmouth, Rhode Island plant. Peak production years were 1973 and 1974, with about 200 boats produced in each of these years. Production tapered off to about 70 boats per year in the last three years of production, and the P30 was discontinued with the 1981 models, to be replaced in the Pearson line by the Pearson 303.

The Pearson 30 was designed as a family cruiser and daysailer with a good turn of speed. The boat is actively raced throughout the country, however, with about 20 holding IOR certificates, and many more racing in PHRF, MORC, and one-design fleets.

The P30's swept-back fin keel and scimitar-shaped spade rudder are fairly typical of racing boat designs from the late 1960s and early 1970s, but look somewhat dated next to today's high-aspect-ratio fin keels and rudders.

The boat's underwater shape is somewhat unusual. The hull is basically dinghy-shaped. The sections aft of the keel form a deep "V," so that deadrise in the forward and after sections of the boat is similar. Coupled with a fairly narrow beam by today's standards, this provides a hull form which is easily balanced when the boat is heeled—an important consideration in this relatively tender 30-footer.

Above the water the Pearson 30 carries out the standard Pearson credo— moderation in all matters. The hull has a moderate amount of conventional sheer curvature, with modest overhangs at bow and stern. The cabin trunk is well proportioned but is, of necessity, somewhat high to achieve headroom in a small boat without excessive freeboard. Styling is clean and modern with (thankfully) no attempt to incorporate "traditional" detailing. The boat's appearance may not stir the soul, but neither will it offend the eye.

The Pearson 30 has a well-proportioned masthead rig. The mainsail comprises 44 percent of the working sail area, more than is found on many modern racer-cruisers, but a reasonable proportion for a true multi-purpose boat.

Base price in 1971 was $11,750. By November 1979, the base price had jumped to $28,300. The builder's option list included about $8000 worth of goodies for the gadget addict, including wheel steering, a LectraSan toilet system, and a $500 stereo system. The average 1979 sailaway price was about $35,000. In 1987, a good, well equipped 1980 Pearson 30 was bringing more than this.

After years of using the Palmer 22-horsepower and 30-horsepower Atomic Four gasoline engines, the Pearson line is now entirely diesel powered. Late model Pearson 30s came with a two-cylinder Universal diesel, which weighs about the same as the Atomic Four.

CONSTRUCTION

Pearson is one of the oldest fiberglass boatbuilders in the country. Their Triton and Alberg 35 are two of the classic "modern" boats. With over 20 years of fiberglass boatbuilding experience, Pearson has solved most of the construction problems that seem to plague some builders.

The layup schedule of the Pearson 30 did not change during the production life of the boat. The hull structure is a hand layup in a one-piece mold of alternating plies of 1-1/2-ounce mat and 18-ounce woven roving. Two layers of

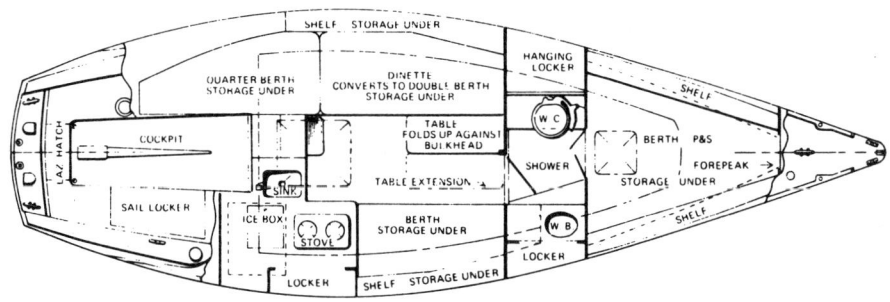

The Complete Book of Sailboat Buying, Volume II

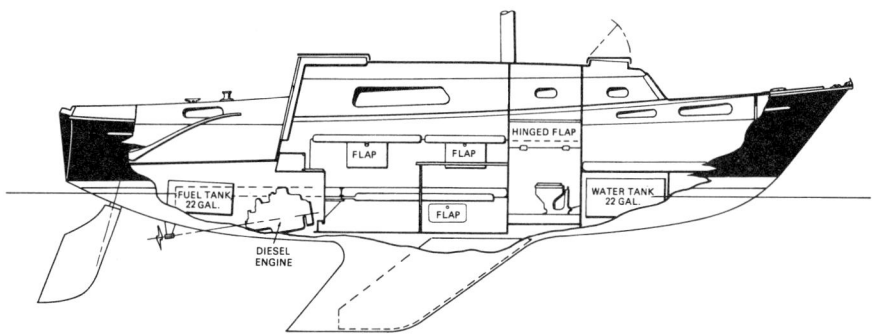

mat are used beneath the gelcoat to prevent "print-through" of the first roving layer, an unsightly and unfortunately common problem with some builders.

Below the water line, the Pearson 30 hull is a solid seven-ply layup, yielding an average bottom thickness of .29 inches. Along the keel, the plies from each side are overlapped, doubling the thickness in this critical area. The topside skin is five plies of mat and roving with an average thickness of .21 inches. The deck is a fiberglass-balsa sandwich. The hull to deck joint is made by glassing together the external flanges of the hull and deck. This chemical bond is backed up by stainless steel self-tapping screws at intervals of approximately 4 inches. The flanges are covered by an extruded plastic rubrail holder, covered by the familiar Pearson soft vinyl rubrail. One Pearson 30 owner who races his boat reported that the hull to deck joint had opened slightly at the bow from excessive headstay tension. No other owner reported this problem, and examination of a large number of Pearson 30s failed to reveal another hull with this problem. Excessive headstay and backstay loading is often found in racing boats and can damage any boat not designed for this type of loading.

The Pearson 30's spade rudder has provided the only recurrent problem with the boat. The rudder stock consists of a thick-walled stainless steel pipe. The stock enters the hull through a slightly larger diameter fiberglass rudder tube, which projects above the waterline to the cockpit sole, eliminating the need for a stuffing box. The rudder stock rides in two Delrin bushings, one at the top and one at the bottom of the fiberglass rudder tube. Wear in these Delrin bushings causes play to develop in the rudder stock. This wear can be accelerated by failing to tie off the tiller when the boat is at rest, thus letting the stock turn from the natural motion of the boat. The bushings are owner-replaceable when the boat is hauled out, requiring removal of the tiller fitting and dropping the rudder through the bottom of the boat. The bushings can then be pried out and replaced.

The frequency with which rudder bushings must be replaced varies with the amount of use the boat receives. Pearson considers the bushings an item of routine maintenance. We would recommend that they be replaced whenever any slop develops. About 30% of the boats we examined showed significant bushing wear.

We also found annoying and excessive play in the tiller fitting, which might sometimes be confused with bushing wear. Correcting this requires shimming or bushing the cast aluminum tiller socket.

The first Pearson 30s had an aluminum pipe rudder stock rather than stainless. Several rudders broke off as a result of corrosion at the narrow gap between rudder and hull. To Pearson's credit, the firm recalled and replaced the rudders on approximately 200 boats built with aluminum stocks.

The Pearson 30's 3,560 pounds of lead ballast is encapsulated in the fiberglass keel molding. This avoids the necessity of keel bolts, but makes the keel more vulnerable to grounding damage.

The deck-stepped, polyurethane-painted aluminum mast is supported by the main cabin bulkhead and an oak compression column. This column is glassed into the top of the keel.

If coaming-mounted genoa turning blocks are installed (they are necessary for genoas larger than 150 percent) it is essential that large backing plates be used. Some of these blocks, which were improperly installed by owners, have pulled through the coamings, which are a relatively thin, solid fiberglass molding.

Through-hull fittings appear to be bedded with silicone, a less-than-ideal choice for underwater fittings. Proper seacocks, or gate valves, are installed in all underwater openings, although none are installed with backing blocks, which are highly recommended. Chainplates, where visible for inspection, are properly bolted to primary structural bulkheads.

Much of the interior construction is bonded to the hull, including the molded fiberglass floor pan and the molded headliner. Molded headliners are relatively expensive and are seen less and less in modern production boat construction. Interior surfaces are of teak- or Formica-covered plywood. Exposed plywood edges are covered with glue-on plastic trim, which we noted, has often pulled off, even on newer boats.

Seatback lockers have friction catches which, if not properly aligned, can let the seatback locker doors come open when the boat is heeled. The cabin sole is non-skid fiberglass. Exposed interior fiberglass surfaces on later models were covered with tan, foam-backed, basket-weave vinyl, which enhances the appearance.

The Pearson hull strength has never been questioned. Their boats tend to have slightly heavier scantlings than average, which is hardly a point to be criticized. The construction of all their boats, including the Pearson 30, is of above average production boat quality.

PERFORMANCE

Handling Under Sail

The Pearson 30 is an active sailor's boat. We find it responsive and a pleasure to sail. It is also tender and very sensitive to proper sail combinations. All owners responding to our survey consider the boat to be somewhat "tippy." The P30 does, in fact, tend to put the rail under more easily than some boats. In a 15-knot apparent wind, the boat is almost overpowered with a 150-percent genoa. Gusts of 12 to 14 knots bury the rail and slow the boat's progress. The P30 does not, however, carry any substantial weather helm, even when over-powered. Any tendency to round up or spin out can usually be controlled by a strong hand on the tiller, and easing the mainsail.

As you would expect in a dinghy-hulled, spade-ruddered fin-keeler, the boat is quick in tacks. It is so quick, in fact, that the headsail winch grinder is likely to be reprimanded for being too slow. The winch grinder is also handicapped by difficulty in bracing himself to exert full power on the winches—a common problem on production boats of almost any size. We strongly recommend the optional Lewmar #40 jib sheet winches, whether the boat is used for racing or cruising. The standard halyard winches are perfectly adequate. The optional roller-bearing mainsheet traveler is practically a must for effective trim of the mainsail, although it does reduce cockpit room.

Although the Pearson 30 was not specifically designed for racing, some of the boats have had very successful racing careers. Pete Lawson's *Syrinx* won the Three-Quarter Ton North American Championship in 1972. Under IOR Mk IIIA, the boat's average rating has dropped nearly two feet, making the boat rate just over half-ton. The boat is still a successful club racer and is hotly raced as a one-design class in some areas, including Chesapeake Bay. Pearson 30s also race in MORC classes, and the boat has been measured for USYRU-Measurement Handicap System (MHS) for hull standardization.

Owners report that, typically, only about 10 percent of their sailing time is devoted to racing. Another 10 percent is spent cruising, while fully 80 percent is taken up with daysailing. The boat will be sailed quite differently by racers and cruisers. Experienced Pearson 30 racers keep the boat moving by reefing the main and carrying on with larger headsails as the breeze pipes up.

Cruisers will find it more comfortable to sail with smaller headsails and more mainsail, even though there will be some sacrifice in performance on the wind. A good selection of headsails (at least a 150-percent genoa, a number three genoa, and a working jib) is necessary. A small heavy-weather jib would be a good idea for boats that cruise in exposed waters.

Handling Under Power

The Pearson 30's underwater configuration creates a boat that maneuvers re-markably well under power. The P30 turns in a circle of its own length. The standard two-cylinder Universal diesel pushes the boat well, albeit with some vibration, although it lacks the authority of the old Atomic Four when punch-ing through a chop.

A strong arm on the tiller is required when backing down under power. "It's a tough boat to handle in reverse. It can tear your arm off," said one experi-enced Pearson 30 sailor. The aft-raking unbalanced rudder will easily go hard over if too much helm is applied while backing down, and an unprepared or off-balance helmsman could be thrown off his feet by the tiller under these conditions. Applying minimum rudder corrections reduces this tendency, but

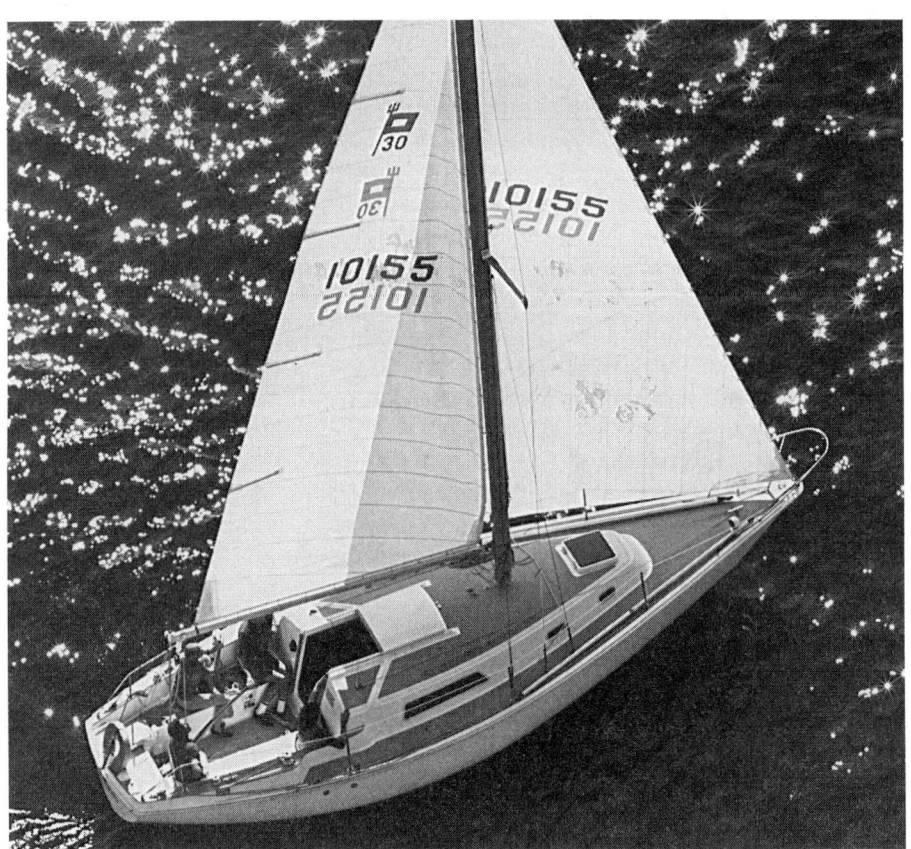

a rudder of this type, which is free to rotate through 360 degrees, can pose a real threat to the unwary.

LIVABILITY

Deck Layout

Certain compromises in deck layout are inherent in almost any 30-footer; the Pearson 30 is no exception. The shrouds hamper access to the foredeck, so it is easier to walk on the cabin top to go forward than along the sidedecks. This is almost a universal shortcoming in boats of this size, as the requirements of interior living space necessitate a large cabin trunk and relatively narrow side decks.

The bow cleat is located well forward and is adequate for the size of lines likely to be used on the boat. However, we would prefer two bow cleats, nearly side by side, in the same location. This is particularly useful on boats that spend a major portion of their lives tied to docks. The rule of thumb is that the dockline which needs adjustment is always the bottom line on the cleat.

The vinyl rubrail around the hull to deck joint presents a problem when anchoring the Pearson 30. It will undoubtedly be chafed by the anchor line.

Redesign or relocation of the bow chocks would be necessary to correct this potential chafe problem.

The large starboard cockpit locker is designated as the boat's sail locker. We recommend that the locker be put to its intended use. The locker is so deep that small items would end up in a heap in the bottom almost out of reach if they were stored here. Space in the lazarette locker—a natural place for fenders, docklines, and sheets—is limited by the engine exhaust hose. Rerouting this hose would increase the usefulness of this space.

The large cockpit seats four adults comfortably for daysailing, and six if they are active enough to stay out of the way of the tiller and mainsheet. The four-foot-long tiller encroaches on the cockpit living space. We might be reluctant to recommend wheel steering for a high performance 30-footer, but it would allow more cockpit space, and would help to reduce the idiosyncrasies created by the spade rudder when under power in reverse.

Belowdecks
The Pearson 30 has a light, roomy interior for a boat of its size. After 1980, all four ports in the head and forward cabin were of the opening type, greatly improving ventilation, particularly when coupled with the optional (and recommended) foredeck-mounted cowl ventilator.

The overhead hatch in the forward cabin is basically a ventilation hatch and is too small for either sails or emergency exit. Anchor storage is awkward without a foredeck anchor well, a welcome addition to many more recently designed boats the size of the Pearson 30.

The 22-gallon water tank and the standard holding tank occupy much of the space under the forward double berth. This double berth is actually the entire forward cabin, and can be closed off from the full-width head by double doors. The standard marine toilet is equipped with a proper vented loop. The discharge line incorporates a Y-valve for overboard discharge of sewage when pump-out facilities for the holding tank are unavailable. This is a practical solution to the MSD boondoggle. The head wash basin is tucked under the deck and is somewhat difficult to use. The location of this wash basin is the only serious flaw in the otherwise functional head compartment.

The P30's main cabin is large and comfortable, with capacious storage above, behind, and below the settees. Owners may find these storage spaces more useful if they are subdivided by partitions to prevent gear stored in one locker from migrating to another. The under-settee and under-galley lockers cannot be considered dry storage unless the bilge is kept bone dry. Although the lockers are sealed to the bilge at the bottom, owners report that, with their boat heeled, bilge water finds its way into the lockers by running up the inside of the hull behind locker partitions, then down into storage spaces. Most dinghy-hulled boats lack real bilge space or a sump, and as little as a few gallon of water in a boat of this type can be annoying.

It is unfortunate that large berth capacity has become the criterion for livability on modern boats. In the past, a 40-footer was likely to have four or five berths. Now, six berths have become standard on a 30-footer (including the Pearson 30); seven on a 35-footer; and eight on a 40-footer. Cruising longer than overnight, with six bodies on a boat the size of the Pearson 30, is a sure way to terminate friendships and wreck marriages. No Pearson 30-owner responding to our survey reported cruising with more than four people on a regular basis.

The standard fold-down cabin table is a practical solution on a boat of this size. The optional slide-out chart table limits room over the quarterberth and lacks the fiddles which are necessary because of its slanted surface.

The Pearson 30 galley is typical of 30-footers. As much as possible is jammed into a necessarily small space. The deep lockers behind the stove and icebox will probably be partitioned into several smaller compartments by the moderately handy owner. Annoyingly, a short person has a hard time reaching the depths of the icebox, particularly if the stove is in use.

We cannot recommend the self-contained alcohol stoves so commonly installed on the Pearson 30 and other boats of this size. There is a very real and well-documented risk of explosion if the stove must be refueled while hot. Liquid-fuel stoves should have a separate fuel tank with the fill located far enough away that there is no possibility of overflow onto a hot stovetop or burner surface.

The galley sink and spigot partially block the companionway. The top companionway step is actually the lid of a nifty storage box, handy for winch handles, spare blocks, and tools.

Engine access is via the companionway steps, which lift out to expose the front of the engine. Two louvered doors in the quarterberth provide additional, if awkward, access to the engine and fuel tank under the cockpit. There is no soundproofing in the engine compartment. The newer, smaller, diesel engine is more accessible than the old Atomic Four. It has molded fiberglass engine beds and a drip pan—an excellent idea—although some engine vibration is transferred to the hull, despite the flexible engine mounts and shaft coupling. It is rare for a 30-footer to have good engine access and the Pearson 30 is no better than average in this respect.

Despite her shortcomings, the P30 is highly livable. Its advertised six-foot, one-inch headroom is really an honest five feet, eleven inches in the main cabin. Achieving good headroom in a 30-footer, without serious compromises in appearance, is nearly impossible. The Pearson 30 comes as close to achieving this as any boat we've seen in its class.

CONCLUSIONS

The Pearson 30 is an industry success story. The boat is fast and responsive. Finish quality is above average. The interior is comfortable and reasonably roomy within the limitations inherent in a 30-footer. Many of the minor design problems can be corrected by the imaginative and handy owner who enjoys tinkering.

Pearson has a reputation for building solid, middle-of-the-road boats; a deserved reputation well in evidence in the P30. Although she is now out of production, the Pearson 30 would be an excellent choice for the aggressive and self-confident beginning sailor who desires high performance for daysailing or club-level racing, as well as for reasonably comfortable short-term cruising. It is not, however, a boat for the timid sailor. The family with two children will find it a comfortable cruiser. Sailors with friends who enjoy spirited sailing, and who don't mind frequent sail changes, will also find it a good choice for daysailing and local racing.

The long production run and continued popularity have created a boat with few inherent problems and a high resale value. The Pearson 30 is a good investment.

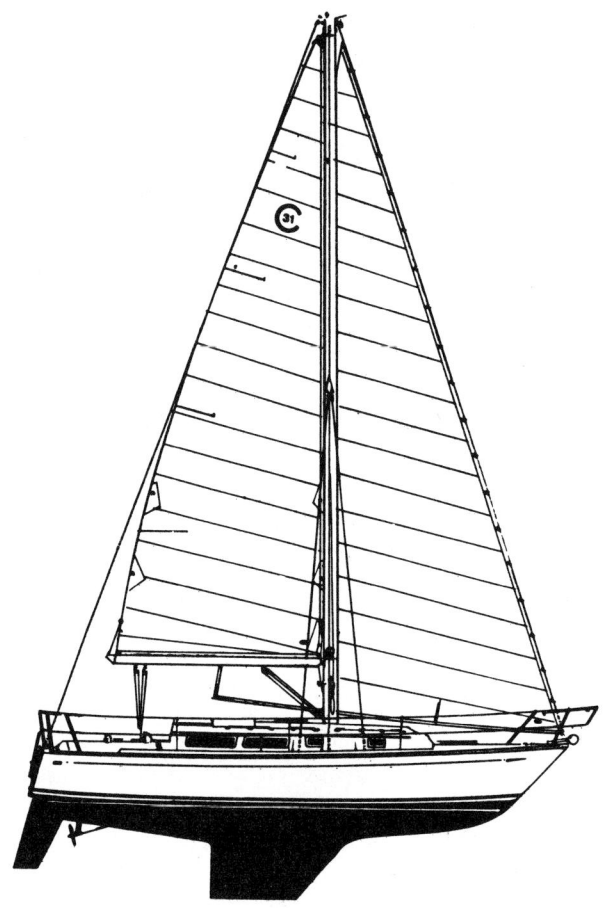

Specifications
Cal 31

LOA	31'6"
LWL	25'8"
Beam	10'0"
Draft	5'0"
Displacement	9170 lbs
Ballast	3600 lbs
Sail area	490 sq ft

Cal Division of O'Day
848 Airport Road
Fall River,
Massachusetts 02720
(617) 678-5291

The Cal 31:
A Pricey Racer-Cruiser

THE BOAT AND THE BUILDER

The Cal 31 was the thirteenth Bill Lapworth-designed boat built by Cal between 27 and 34 feet. Cal and Lapworth were perhaps best known for their breakthrough Cal 40, which began the trend toward today's moderately light displacement, fin keeled, spade rudder ocean racers.

The hull configuration of the 31 is typical of Lapworth designs: shallow-bodied and round-bilged, with a fairly short fin keel, a shallow skeg, and a well faired, high-aspect-ratio spade rudder. The Cal 31 was the middle boat in the Cal production line, which included boats from 25 to 39 feet. Production of the Cal 31 began in the fall of 1978 and 130 boats were built in the first three years. Production ended with the 1984 model.

Cal heavily promoted their entire line as dual purpose boats, the ubiquitous "cruiser-racer" which came to dominate the sailboat market. The company's catchy, colorful ads were prominent in all the sailing magazines and were geared toward the affluent 30- to 40-year-old consumer with lots of sailing experience.

Surprisingly, many Cal 31 purchasers were buying their first cruising sailboat. One Cal 31 owner reported that the 31 was his fourth Cal boat. Cal 31 owners typically spent 70 percent of their sailing time daysailing, 20 percent short term cruising, and 10 percent club racing.

Owners report relatively few defects requiring warranty claims, but the ones they do report are recurrent, and almost exclusively associated with water getting where it's not supposed to be—inside the boat. The most common problems with the Cal 31 are leaking stanchion bases, leaking chainplates, and leaking hatches. These are probably the most common warranty claims throughout the industry and are generally the result of the fact that adequate bedding to prevent leaks requires fairly careful work, can be messy, and takes time to clean up. Owners reported that their dealers were prompt in settling any warranty claims.

CONSTRUCTION

The hull of the Cal 31 is a solid hand layup. The hull weight of the Cal, less ballast, is about average for performance cruisers of comparable length and beam, although total displacement tends to be lighter than average.

Exterior cosmetic finish is good. There is slight print-through of the first layer of roving, and some pinholes appear in the gelcoat in many boats where surface blemishes have been patched.

The deck molding is plywood-cored in areas where heavy hardware is

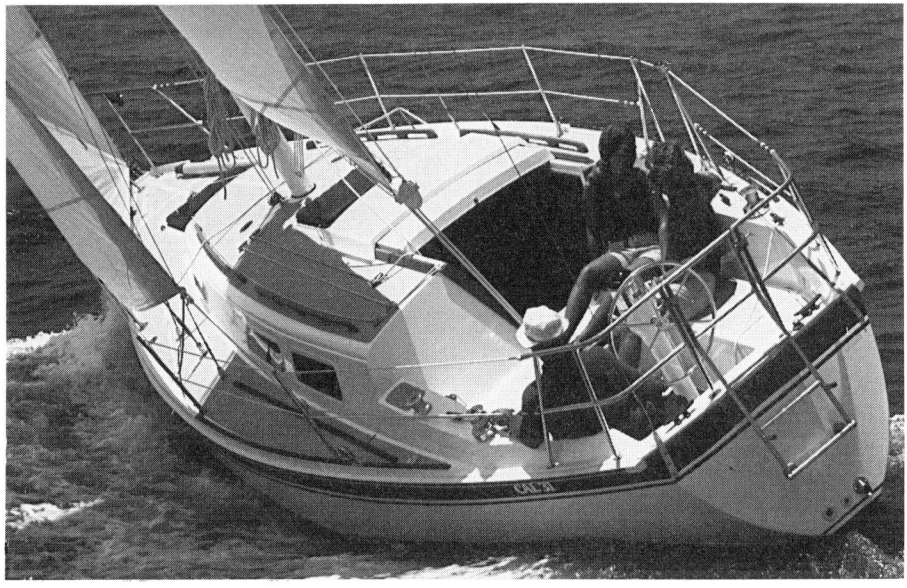

The Cal 31

mounted. The cabin top is sandwich construction; Klegecell foam, cored with plywood inserts in the mast partner area. The cabin top under the deck-stepped mast is solid 3/4-inch fiberglass.

The companionway of the Cal 31 is about its weakest design point. It is too wide and has a strong taper which allows drop boards to be removed by lifting a little more than an inch. The mating surface between the two solid teak drop boards is a simple square butt. In every Cal 31 we examined, daylight was visible between the two boards—in one case, almost 1/4 inch. Simple reverse bevels, or preferably, a stepped joint, would take about two minutes more to make, and would be infinitely better in terms of watertightness.

The companionway slide design is not waterproof. The optional seahood is essential on any boat going offshore, or that will be sailing in areas with boisterous conditions.

The split backstay arrangement allows the use of an integral centerline swimming ladder incorporated in the stern rail. Backstay chainplates are through-bolted, but fiberglass backing plates are used where we would prefer aluminum or stainless steel. The welded combination stemhead fitting is through-bolted but lacks a backup plate. In fact, the only deck fittings, including winches and cleats, which utilize backup plates are the lifeline stanchions and bow pulpit.

Dick Cumiskey, Research and Development Director of Bangor Punta Marine, said that backup plates were not necessary because the deck was plywood cored in areas where hardware was likely to be mounted. As a rule, we prefer to see metal backup plates on through-bolted fittings, even cleats and winches which are normally only subjected to shear loads. Overkill in the mounting of hardware is cheap insurance.

The hull to deck joint is made by chemically bonding the two moldings together. An extruded rigid plastic rubrail holder and soft vinyl rubrail insert cover the hull to deck joint on the outside of the hull.

The ballast keel is an encapsulated lead casting. The fiberglass-covered, high density, foam-cored rudder utilizes a stainless steel rudder stock.

The main structural bulkhead is of teak-faced plywood, bonded to the hull with fiberglass fillers. To avoid hard spots, the bulkhead itself does not touch the hull. The mast is supported by a teak compression column. This rests on a

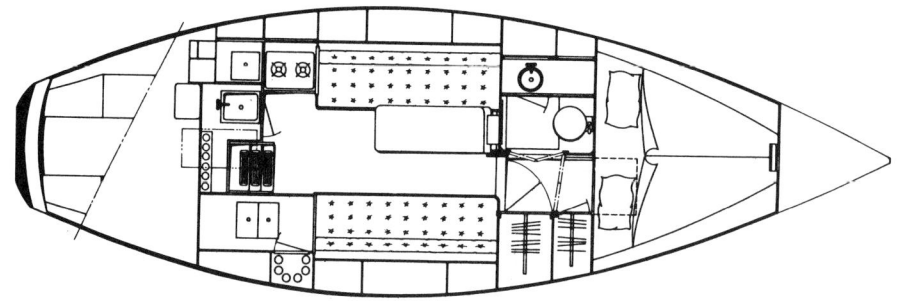

deep molded fiberglass floor timber, part of the molded floor pan which is bonded to the hull.

The chainplates for the inboard shrouds are heavy stainless steel flat bar, properly bolted to the main bulkhead and other plywood webs. Inside the head locker, the chainplates are bolted through a web which is covered with the carpet-like hull liner before installation of the chainplates. We would prefer to have the chainplate and backup pads bear directly on the wood or fiberglass web, rather than on the hull liner.

The rig is a masthead sloop with single airfoil spreaders and double lower shrouds. Lower shroud terminations are inboard and about a foot from the molded fiberglass toerail. The Cal 31 utilizes a polyurethane-coated Kenyon aluminum mast and boom. Although rope-to-wire tailspliced halyards are listed as standard, the boat we sailed had eye-spliced halyards. The wire portion of the main halyard was too short to allow an adequate number of wire wraps around the winch. Other boats we examined had properly spliced halyards.

Water tanks are cast polyethylene, with flexible plastic hose piping. A definite plastic taste is imparted to the water by this system. The fuel tank is welded aluminum. Tanks and batteries are mounted under the cabin settees, below the waterline with the weight concentrated in the middle of the boat. This location utilizes a space often given over to locker which, in many boats, tends to be wet from bilge water. The battery boxes are well secured, but it is difficult to remove the box covers to inspect the battery electrolyte level.

The Cal 31 was one of the few current production boats with a real bilge sump. Unfortunately, both the icebox and the shower drain through the bilge to this sump. Organic matter and food particles in the icebox water quickly leads to smelly bilges. Soap residue from showers can gradually clog impeller-type bilge pumps—which could be a problem in the event of a serious hull leak.

Through-hull fittings below the waterline are bronze, recessed flush with the hull surface, and well bedded, but without backing blocks. Shut-off valves are glass-

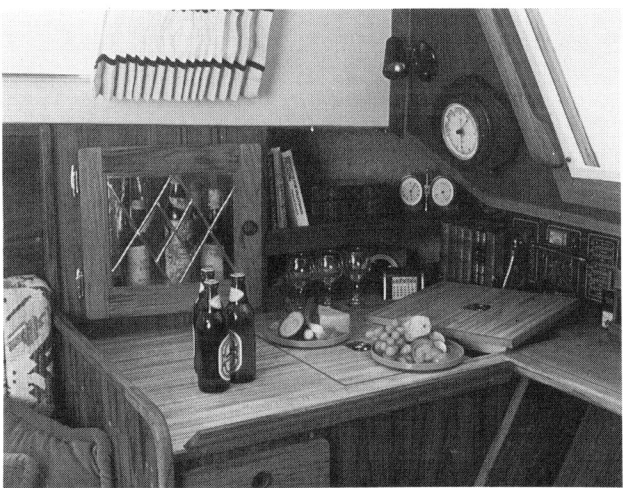

Typical of the attention to detail in the Cal 31's interior are the lead glass liquor cabinet, well-insulated icebox lids, and plenty of room for books and instrumentation in the nav station.

filled nylon ball valves originally developed for the chemical industry. Above-water through-hulls are nylon, with no provision for emergency shut-off. One owner we contacted had bronze seacocks installed on underwater openings, as he was leery of the standard nylon valves.

PERFORMANCE

Handling Under Sail

Sailing performance of the Cal 31 is consistent with her performance-cruiser image. Most owners consider the boat somewhat tender. The boat does tend to bury the rail quickly in gusts about five knots above mean wind speed. On the wind, with 14 knots of breeze over the deck, the boat is on the verge of needing a short reef when sailed with a 145 percent genoa and full main.

The Cal 31 is not particularly wide, but her beam is carried well forward and aft. She therefore develops less weather helm when overpowered than a comparably sized racing boat. She will be a bit more forgiving of improper sail combination than a wider boat whose ends are more pinched.

The Cal 31 is a comfortable boat for a couple to handle. The boat we sailed had Barient 23 self-tailers instead of the standard Barient 21s. We would recommend the larger self-tailers instead of the standard winches on a boat that will be used for shorthanded cruising.

The Cal 31 will hold her own with other performance cruisers of comparable size. She is closer-winded and faster than the Cal 29 in light air. Most owners consider the boat faster than similar boats, but few Cal 31s have raced enough to make a comparison meaningful. Tentative PHRF rating is 150 in southern California, 156 in San Francisco. This implies that the boat will be at her best in light air.

The Cal 31 has generally good handling characteristics under sail. She balances well and can be made to sail herself on the wind with the judicious use of sail trim. The boat has a good, solid feel under sail, more like a 35-footer than a 31-footer.

Handling Under Power

The standard engine in the Cal 31 is a two-cylinder, 16-horsepower Universal diesel. Earlier models were equipped with two-cylinder Volvo diesels. Owners consider the engine adequate power for the boat.

The instrument panel is mounted on the forward end of the cockpit and includes gauges for alternator output, water temperature, and fuel level. There is an oil pressure warning light. An oil pressure gauge and tachometer would be welcome.

The boat handles well under power, but the engine transmits substantial vibration to the hull. This vibration could be tiring if long periods of motoring were required.

Handling in forward gear is uncomplicated. Like most fin-keel boats, the Cal 31 turns in a very tight circle. Handling in reverse is more complicated. With the Volvo engine, owners report that the stern of the boat pulls sharply to starboard. Some owners of Universal-powered boats also report uncertain steering behavior in reverse. We find the steering reasonably predictable, but she does require a firm hand on the tiller or wheel to keep the rudder from going hard over once sternway is made. Gradual application of rudder in reverse prevents rudder stall, which could cause unpredictable steering.

LIVABILITY

Deck Layout

The initial reaction of most owners to the cockpit of the Cal 31 is that it is too small. Their response, after living with it, is that it is just about the right size. With either the wheel or the tiller, it is comfortable for a maximum of four when sailing.

There is a wide bridgedeck at the forward end of the cockpit. The roller-bearing mainsheet traveler, with its essential athwartships control lines, is located on the bridgedeck.

There are two huge cockpit lockers. These would be more useful if divided into smaller spaces and if partitions were inserted to prevent gear from slipping under the cockpit where it might fetch up against the engine.

The cockpit lockers have an excellent molded-in scupper arrangement which allows the leeward seats to drain at all angles of heel. Unfortunately, the boat has an inexplicable method of securing the locker lids. A line is attached to the underside of the starboard lid. This leads under the cockpit to a jam cleat which is reached through the port cockpit locker. The port locker has a similar arrangement which can only be released from belowdecks, in the galley. If the lockers are secured, one must go below, release the port locker hold-down, go back on deck, open the port cockpit locker, and release the starboard hold-down to get into the starboard cockpit locker. The logic of this escapes us.

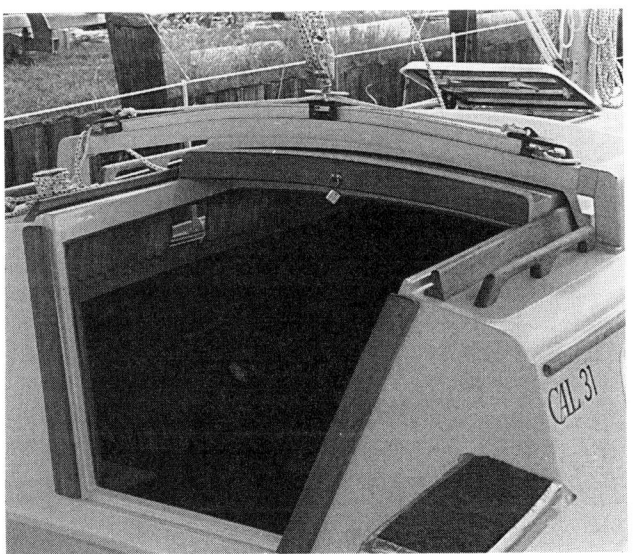

Access to the head of the rudder stock in wheel-steered boats is via a deckplate in the cockpit sole. If the plate were removed in order to rig emergency steering, a substantial amount of water could find its way below in rain or heavy weather.

The rig's inboard shrouds provide a narrow sheeting base for jib leads, but make it almost mandatory to go over the cabin top to go forward of the mast. There is an anchor well at the forward end of the deck. This well contains a strong eyebolt for securing the bitter end of the anchor rode, an excellent idea. Connections for the pulpit-mounted running lights are under the deck, immediately forward of the lid to the anchor well, and will be subject to rapid corrosion from water finding its way below, as well as to mechanical damage when stowing the anchor rode.

The stemhead fitting incorporates a roller, handy for stowing an anchor. There are no bow chocks. The anchor roller can be used as a starboard chock, although the lack of a fair lead to a bow cleat is a serious shortcoming. Anchoring with two anchors would be problematic without good bow chocks.

The long inboard track for jib leads provides for flexible sheet leads, but should be augmented by a toerail-mounted track for greater variety. If genoas larger than 150 percent are used, the stock track will prove too short for optimal leads.

Belowdecks

The Cal 31 has perhaps the most spacious and attractive interior in its class. It is the boat's most outstanding feature. Belowdecks, it is hard to believe you are aboard a boat only 31 feet long. "The interior sold us on the boat" was the most common owner response.

The forward cabin has a large V-berth with an insert to form a huge double. There is a good sail bin under the port berth, and shelves at the foot of the berth. Most owners find the short hanging locker in the forward cabin useless. Most would prefer drawers instead.

The foredeck-mounted hatch provides good ventilation and is big enough for sail bags, but its location requires that it be tightly secured when sailing to prevent water from getting below. Close attention will have to be paid to the water-tightness of the hatch if the berth below is to be kept dry.

The large head is comfortable and incorporates a shower. An overhead deadlight augments the light provided by the opening port. The door to the head also serves as the door to the forward cabin. When this door is used to shut off the forward cabin, the door to the large starboard hanging locker can be used to separate the head from the main cabin.

The main cabin interior is rather dark due to the abundance of teak. This is somewhat offset by a bright carpet. The cabin would be much brighter if a lighter wood, such as butternut or ash, had been used below.

The main cabin is huge. There is good storage in bins and alcoves behind the settees. A large magazine and book rack on the bulkhead behind the fold-up table is inaccessible without folding down the table.

There is no means of positively securing the table's fold-down leg to the cabin sole. The leg could be accidentally kicked out of place when the table is in use, allowing it to fall down. The table is too small to accommodate even four with real comfort. The cabin is wide enough to utilize a permanently fitted table.

The main cabin sleeps three in a large single berth and an extension double.

The deeply-tufted settee cushions look rich and are comfortable for sitting but are miserable to sleep on.

Cooks will appreciate the galley, which is excellent for a boat of this size. There is a large gimballed stove with oven, well secured and capable of being latched in place in port. It is available in both alcohol and gas models.

The icebox top is one of the few we have seen which can reasonably double as a chart table. The icebox lids are insulated, but are poorly fitted, allowing a large gap (over 3/8 inch) between the two trap-type lids. The lids are also usually not flush with the icebox top, a complication for doing smooth chart work. There is a large-diameter tube for rolled charts which extends under the cockpit.

The engine is reached for service by lifting out the companionway steps. The steps should have a positive latch to prevent their bouncing out of place in rough conditions. Engine access for maintenance is excellent.

Selection valves for the water tanks are located under the deep galley sink. This is typical of the well-thought-out plumbing and wiring systems, which are generally well bundled and usually protected from chafe when passing through bulkhead cutouts.

The interior of the Cal 31 is one of the most livable and attractive we have seen in a boat of this size. Interior finish works is of very good production boat quality.

CONCLUSIONS

The Cal 31 is one of the best designed and better executed 31-footers we have seen. Her interior is remarkable. She has broad market appeal, selling to first-time sailboat buyers as well as to the more experienced. She is a reasonably good club-level racer, yet a comfortable cruiser for up to four adults. Realistically, the boat will be used more for cruising and daysailing than for racing.

To those not familiar with what inflation has done to boat prices, the price of the Cal 31 could come as a rude shock. With a 1980 base price around $43,000, the delivered price ran close to $50,000. A well-equipped Cal 31 could easily top $55,000, making the Cal 31 almost the "priciest" 31-foot stock boat on the market. Today, a used 1984 Cal 31 (the last year produced) will run from $40,000 to $45,000.

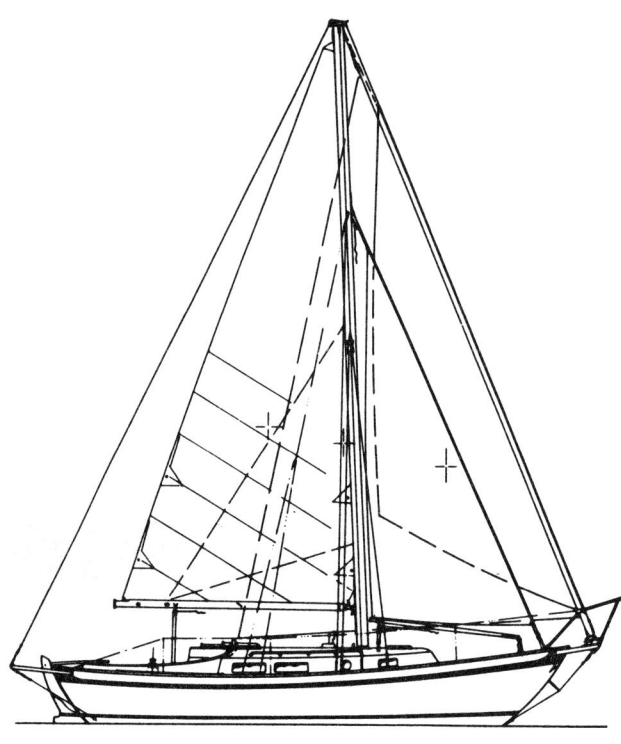

Specifications	
Southern Cross 31	
LOA	31'0"
LWL	25'0"
Beam	9'6"
Draft	4'7"
Displacement	13,600 lbs
Ballast	4400 lbs
Sail area	353 sq ft

The Southern Cross 31:
An Ocean-Going Dream Machine

THE BOAT AND THE BUILDER

The Southern Cross 31 might best be described as a double-ended ocean-cruising cutter of moderate beam, moderate draft, moderate-to-heavy displacement, and moderate sail area. She has a pronounced sheer, moderately cutaway forefoot, and outboard rudder. To many she would embody the ideal ocean cruising hull form.

The Southern Cross 31 might also be termed a dream-machine. She is a boat pitched to those sailors whose idea of sailing—whether they achieve it or not—is palm-fringed islands, the ink-blue of the sea off-soundings, and long trade-wind passages. She is the type of boat to make accountants from Iowa run away to the South Seas.

In the early 1970's, an effective promotional campaign by Westsail rekindled a relatively dormant interest in the wide, heavy, double-ended hull form of the Norwegian rescue boat for long-distance cruising. Since then, that hull form has proliferated to the point of faddish absurdity. Arguing whether the double-ended hull form (whether the stern be of the "cruiser," "canoe," or "Baltic" variety) is better than all others for seakeeping ability dominated conversation among would-be long-distance cruisers in much the way that the cutter cranks and the sloop supporters fought it out in the late 19th century. A generation of cruising boats, many over-heavy, under-canvassed, poorly designed, poorly built, and with all the windward ability of a sand barge flooded the market. If it wasn't pointed at both ends, or at least rounded, it wasn't a world cruiser, the thinking went.

In 1976, in the midst of the double-ended doubletalk, Clarke Ryder, who had set up a fiberglass molding company for industrial parts, began building the Southern Cross 31. In the next 10 years, over 165 hulls were built, many finished off by their owners.

At first glance the Southern Cross 31 might appear to be another boat designed to leap upon the Colin Archer bandwagon, because of the double-ended hull, long keel, and outboard rudder. With those characteristics, the resemblance of the Southern Cross 31 to most of the "modern" offshore cruising double-enders ceases.

The Tom Gillmer-designed Southern Cross 31 is similar to another of his designs, the Allied Seawind. The original Seawind was the first fiberglass sailboat to circle the world. The Southern Cross 31 is basically the same hull as the original Seawind with the stern redrawn from transom-type to a canoe-type, the beam increased by three inches, and the displacement increased by 1500 pounds.

For the singlehanded or doublehanded world cruiser who tends toward the conservative, the Southern Cross 31 may appear to be the ideal combination: a proven cruising hull design combined with a pointed stern.

CONSTRUCTION

The Southern Cross 31 is one of the few Airex-cored production boats built. The hull is molded in one piece, with solid laminate along the centerline, and is Airex-cored from the turn of the bilge nearly to the sheer. The glass laminate is solid abreast the mast where the chainplates are attached.

The deck is a one-piece molding, balsa-cored for rigidity. The cabin top is also balsa-cored, although the area around the mast step is cored with plywood rather than balsa for greater strength in compression.

Airex and balsa coring relieve the Southern Cross 31 of some of the least desirable characteristics of fiberglass construction. Coring greatly reduces the pronounced tendency of fiberglass to sweat in cold weather, deadens the notorious sound transmission of glass construction, and provides strength and rigidity without either a heavy solid layup or a complicated system of internal framing. Coring also functions as an insulator, making a glass hull cooler in the summer and easier to heat in the winter.

We have some reservations about the Southern Cross hull to deck joint. There is no doubt that it is simple and strong. At the sheer the hull molding turns outward 90 degrees. The deck molding drops down into the hull, with an external flange overlapping the hull flange. The hull and deck are bolted together, the joint filled with a polyester compound. Our reservation is that the

The Southern Cross 31
233

flange sticks outboard of the hull more than an inch, almost at right angles to the hull. Not only is this hard to finish off neatly, but also it is somewhat vulnerable.

Ballast of the Southern Cross 31 is an internal lead casting glassed into the keel cavity. This obviates the need for keelbolts and the attendant possibility for leaking. It has the disadvantage that should the vessel run aground—a not infrequent event for the long distance cruiser who frequently enters unfamiliar ports—the hull rather than the lead keel takes the brunt. We have seen other internally-ballasted fiberglass hulls so abraded by a few hours on rocks or coral that the ballast literally fell out of the hull. For our world cruiser, we'd prefer an externally bolted-on lead keel, which should be capable of surviving a severe grounding without damaging the fiberglass hull.

The rudder of the Southern Cross 31 is set well up from the bottom of the rudder post, protected from grounding damage. Rudder design has been changed from a traditionally-shaped rudder to a more modern design with greater area near the bottom of the rudder blade.

Pintles and gudgeons are heavy stainless steel weldments. We prefer castings to weldments for use under water, particularly if the metal chosen is stainless steel. Bronze is usually considered superior to stainless for underwater fittings due to the greater susceptibility of stainless steel to some types of corrosion.

Bulkheads are glassed directly to the hull using Airex fillets. Tanks are of molded fiberglass, set deep into the bilge. There are bronze seacocks on all through-hull fittings.

In 1986, for another $2000 above the base price of $79,500 for the finished boat, the standard anodized aluminum or epoxy-coated deck hardware could be replaced with all bronze hardware. For the person simply seeking a boat to get away in, this may be an extravagance. For the person seeking to keep a very traditional looking boat completely in character, the bronze option may be worthwhile.

The Southern Cross 31 is neither a cheaply constructed—nor cheaply priced—imitation of an ocean-going sailboat. In general, her construction characteristics are up to her billing as a real offshore cruiser.

PERFORMANCE

Handling Under Sail

A boat designed for offshore passagemaking is not likely to have the windward performance of a modern fin-keel racing boat. At the same time, she should be able to claw off a lee shore in a gale—something that many of the so-called "world cruisers" would be hard pressed to do.

In many ways the all-around performance of the long-distance cruiser must be better than that of the coastal cruiser or daysailer. She must be able to sail in light winds, for few small offshore cruisers can carry enough fuel to motor to distant ports. She must have a motion that doesn't tire her crew. Her rig must be easy to handle and must offer sailing versatility without the huge sail inventory of the racing boat.

The Southern Cross 31 can be expected to meet most of these requirements. A huge masthead genoa can be carried in light air, but a staysail and double-reefed main should carry her to windward in heavy going. The hard turn of her bilge implies good initial stability.

There is nothing in the hull form of the Southern Cross 31 that implies poor sailing characteristics. This is borne out by the record of the prototype, which finished third-in-class in the 1977 Marion-Bermuda Race. Her displacement of 13,600 pounds on a 25-foot waterline is a little heavy by modern standards, but is certainly not excessive by any traditional standard.

The standard rig of the Southern Cross 31 is that of a modern masthead cutter. The anodized aluminum mast is stepped on the cabin top. Compression is transferred to keel via a wood compression column securely glassed to the hull structure.

At least one owner who had a taller than standard rig reported a depressed cabin top in the area of the mast step. Ryder repaired that with an oversize load-distributing steel plate attached to the cabin top. If the boat is to be owner-finished, care must be taken to be sure that the compression column adequately bears the load of the mast.

The standard boat shows intermediate shrouds led slightly aft of the after lower shroud. Both the main boom and the mainsail will bear on this intermediate shroud when running before the wind. Care must be taken to protect the main from chafe. We would prefer running backstays, which would lead further aft, giving a better angle for tensioning the forestay. With the run-

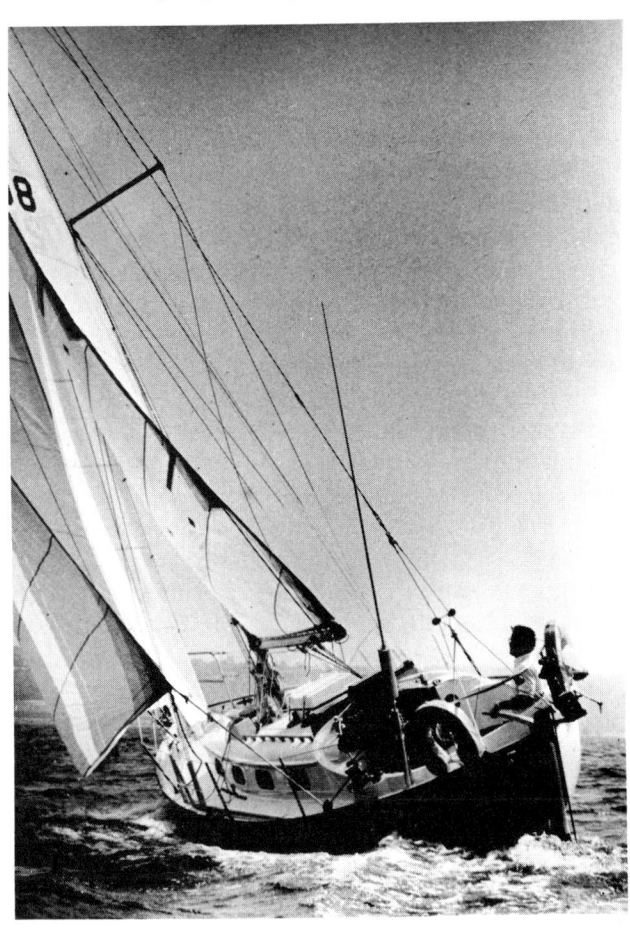

The Southern Cross 31

ners set up, mast pumping in a seaway—a problem not uncommon with deck-stepped rigs—could be pretty much eliminated.

Originally, the boat was drawn with a short boomkin to accommodate the standing backstay. This complicated the mounting of a vane steerer. The backstay is now split, carried to chainplates at either side of the cockpit. The mainsail should be cut with little or no roach to avoid fouling on the backstay with this arrangement.

While a cutter rig may seem unnecessarily complicated on a boat this small, it does allow strength and versatility. These are definitely desirable characteristics in the shorthanded cruiser.

Handling Under Power

With a 22-horsepower diesel to push just short of seven tons, the Southern Cross 31 is adequately powered. The fuel capacity of 34 gallons should give about 65 hours of powering at five knots, for a range of about 325 miles under power. This provides very adequate crusing range under power without the need to carry extra fuel in cans in the cockpit which is always a nuisance, and can be dangerous.

LIVABILITY

Deck Layout

The deck layout is clean and functional. Her sidedecks are fairly wide and unobstructed. The low bulwarks provide a feeling of security when working on deck. We would prefer all halyards led aft to the cockpit for shorthanded sailing, and we would make all winches self-tailing.

A molded seahood is standard, and is an absolute must for any offshore cruiser. A molded-in spray rail will accommodate a cockpit dodger, another useful piece of gear for the offshore sailor.

The cockpit is small and fairly deep, with a good bridgedeck. The deck mold was retooled beginning with hull 85. The crown of the deck was changed slightly, provision was made for a hatch over the main cabin, and the cockpit was lengthened about six inches aft. Cockpit scuppers were moved from the after end of the cockpit to the forward end, and the pitch of the cockpit sole changed slightly to facilitate draining.

A life raft can be carried on top of the main cabin—a little high for such a substantial weight, but perhaps the best solution on a boat this small. We

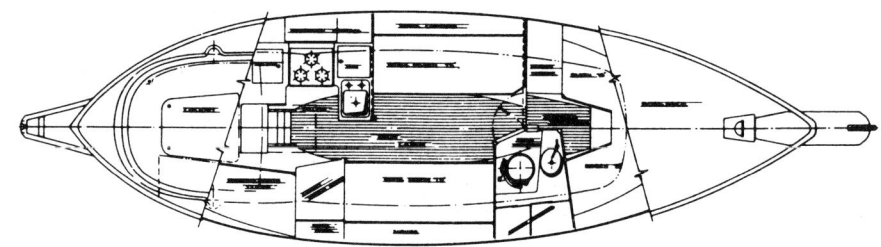

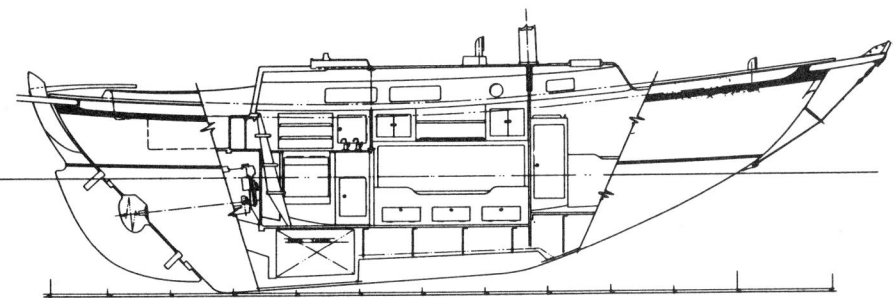

would prefer that the winch islands be big enough for a set of secondary winches.

The small cockpit gives a great feeling of security. This is a very important characteristic in a boat designed to carry her crew to distant places. Big cockpits may be nice in port, but at sea all you can think of is the amount of water they could hold if the boat were to be pooped. We'll take a small cockpit for offshore use.

Belowdecks

The Southern Cross 31 has what is really the minimal amount of interior volume for one or two people for long distance cruising. There are two standard layouts—one with a fixed chart table over storage space, the other with a folding chart table over the quarterberth. Although as a rule we are partial to quarterberths, the space in this case is best given over to storage space, and the larger fixed chart table is more useful.

With this arrangement, the main-cabin settees must be used as berths at sea. This is not really an inconvenience for the shorthanded sailor. The windward settee, fitted with a lee cloth, would keep the sleeper's weight high and on the proper side of the boat for going upwind, while the leeward settee will provide secure sleeping if upwind performance is not a consideration. The forward cabin would be used for sails and other storage when passagemaking.

The galley is small, as it must be on a boat of this size. Double sinks are now standard rather than the single sink of earlier models. The standard stove is a two-burner Shipmate with oven, alcohol-fueled. With eight opening ports and two hatches plus the main companionway, ventilation is not a problem. At sea the main-cabin overhead hatch could be left open if fitted with a small dodger.

Those who finish off kit boats frequently have weird ideas of what the interior of a boat should look like. If you are contemplating finishing a Southern Cross 31 from one of the unfinished versions, think long and hard before making major alterations to the standard layout. A boat which you think is ideally suited to your needs in terms of interior layout frequently proves to be a white elephant if you ever decide to sell her. The standard interior of the Southern Cross 31 is a good, if prosaic interior. We think this may well be better than a highly personalized, but perhaps offbeat interior when the time comes to sell the boat.

The Southern Cross 31
237

CONCLUSION

Is the Southern Cross 31 a good boat for offshore cruising? Most definitely so. We would, however, change some of the details of her construction, as outlined above.

We have carefully avoided a discussion of whether or not you should consider buying such a boat in unfinished form for owner completion. Our opinions on this subject are expressed in the chapter, "So You Think You Want To Build A Boat?" About half of the Southern Cross 31s sold have been "stage" boats, rather than factory completed. No one really knows how many of those have actually been completed and how may still rest in driveways and back yards. We suspect that a fair number are still in the unfinished stage.

For this reason, there is no real established market value for owner finished boats. With the base price of a factory-completed boat at almost $80,000, the "stage two" (sailaway, less engine) starts to look pretty good at half that price. You would think that such a boat could easily be finished off for the $40,000 difference in price. Perhaps so. But in boatbuilding, as in most other ventures, there is rarely—if ever—a free lunch.

She is no doubt a very expensive 31-foot boat when finished off by the factory. In cruising trim, you could easily have $95,000 invested without being extravagant. How much is your dream worth to you, and how soon do you want it?

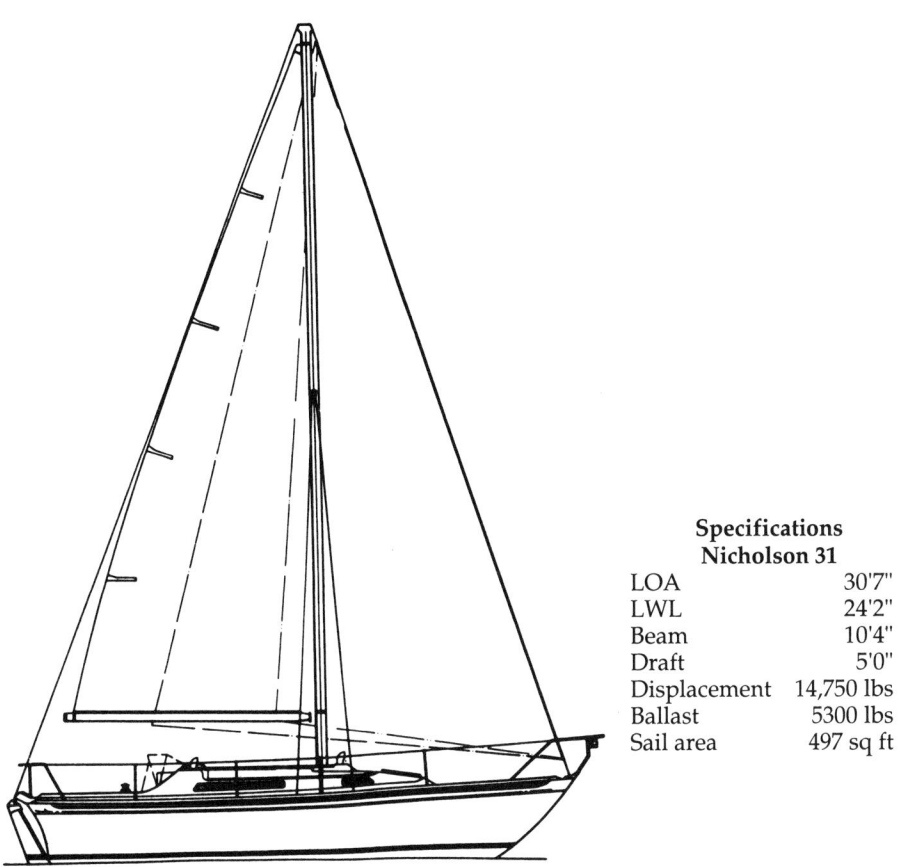

Specifications
Nicholson 31

LOA	30'7"
LWL	24'2"
Beam	10'4"
Draft	5'0"
Displacement	14,750 lbs
Ballast	5300 lbs
Sail area	497 sq ft

The Nicholson 31:
A Go-Anywhere Boat

THE BOAT AND THE BUILDER

Few British sailboats have been a success in the U.S. market. The traditional strength of the British pound against the dollar has meant that British boats have been inordinately expensive compared to American boats of similar quality, and even when the dollar was strong in the mid-1980s the French made more in-roads into the U.S. market than did the English. Coupled with the design eccentricity of some imports (for example, the smaller Westerly boats with their bilge keels and bulbous deckhouses) the high price has been a formidable obstacle to a successful invasion.

Nicholson yachts are well-known for quality construction. The firm was a pioneer in British fiberglass boatbuilding. If experience counts, then Nicholson must be somewhere near the top of the list; the firm of Camper & Nicholsons, Ltd., has been building yachts since the days of Lord Nelson.

The Nicholson 32 was an archetypical boat of the British boatbuilding industry, much like the Triton in this country. Despite a long and successful production run, the Nicholson 32 was starting to look dated: narrow, low freeboard, with longish ends. In 1976, the venerable 32 was replaced by the Nicholson 31, maintaining the concept of a real cruising boat on a small scale, but with more modern styling, more volume, and more displacement.

In appearance, the Nicholson 31 is not unlike many of the current generation of production cruiser-racers. She has a straightish sheer, moderate forward overhang, and a low cabin trunk.

Below the waterline, however, there are substantial differences. She has a deep, powerful hull and a moderately long keel with attached outboard rudder. Her displacement of almost 15,000 pounds is fully 50 percent more than that of the typical cruiser-racer, and equal to the heaviest of the pure cruisers currently in production.

Even with the pound at $1.70, the Nicholson 31 costs a heavyweight $70,000, duty-paid and delivered in the U.S. A big chunk of that cost is tied up in shipping. Unfortunately, a 31-foot boat costs almost the same to ship across as a 40-footer. More than 10 percent of the final cost of the Nicholson 31 ($7,500) is simply the cost of cradling and shipping the boat from Gosport to New York. Another $4,500 is eaten up in duty and local shipping in this country.

Before the price scares you away, you must recognize that the boat comes unusually well equipped, including such items as sails, dodger, anchor, chain, docklines and fenders, pressure water, even the dishes in the galley. Oh, yes, and the name and hailing port are painted on the stern.

This is a go-anywhere boat. She is not a teak-veneered Colin Archer copy, and she is not a fast coastal cruiser or racer. She is austere to the point of plainness. External wood consists of a teak toerail, teak grab-rails, a cockpit grate, the companionway dropboards, and the tiller. On the positive side, this austerity means low maintenance for the cruiser.

At the same time, she is no Clorox bottle. Detailing and workmanship are excellent. The boat looks functional and businesslike.

CONSTRUCTION

Like many European boatbuilders, Camper & Nicholsons does not mold its own hulls. Rather, the hulls are subcontracted to another firm which specializes in hull molding.

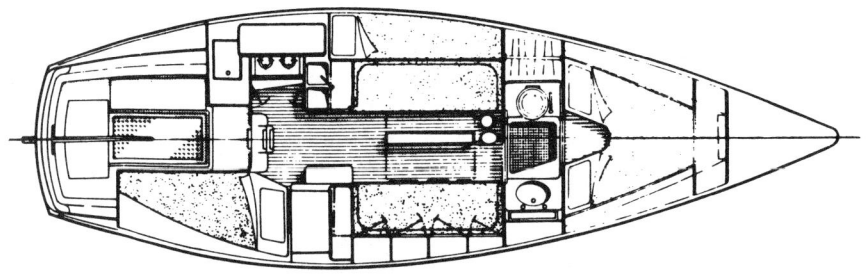

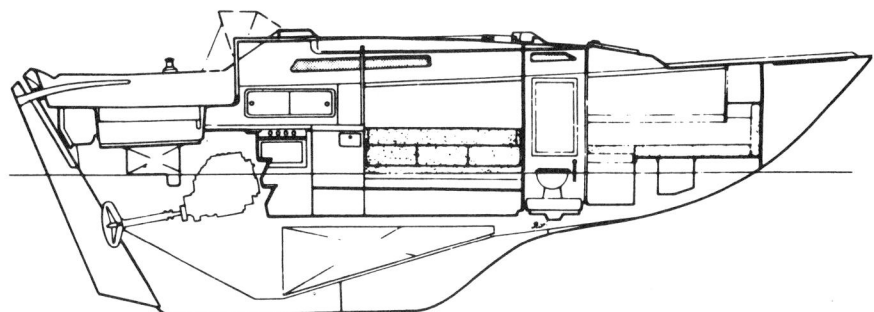

The hull of the Nicholson 31 is a solid glass layup, reinforced with foam-filled longitudinal stringers. Isothalic resin is used in the gelcoat layer to reduce porosity and the subsequent possibility of osmotic deterioration. Deck and cabin trunk are balsa-cored. Molding and gelcoat quality are very good.

The Nicholson 31 is available in a wide range of hull and deck colors at no extra cost. Because the deck molding is a large, unrelieved area of fiberglass, we recommend ordering the deck nonskid in a color contrasting to the base deck color. For those concerned with further improving the aesthetic qualities, teak decks are available as an option.

Hulls are molded to Lloyd's specifications, and Lloyd's hull certificates are available. Full Lloyd's classification of the finished boat requires slight modification of the standard boat, notably the addition of more ground tackle, some alterations to the electrical system, and more ventilation for the battery box. The Lloyd's modifications, additional equipment, and surveys would add about $1,500 to the price of the boat.

Hull and deck are joined with a wide internal flange, bedded with polysulfide and through-bolted at close intervals with stainless bolts. Fit of the hull and deck flanges is excellent, with no gaps or irregularities. A through-bolted teak toerail covers the hull to deck joint.

All deck hardware is properly through-bolted. Removable panels in the interior give access to every part of the underside of the deck.

Ballast is an internal lead casting weighing 5,300 pounds, giving a ballast to displacement ratio of 36 percent. It is ironic that the Nicholson 31, a true cruising boat, has internal ballast rather than an external lead keel. An external keel is less vulnerable to damage in grounding.

Nicholson chainplates deserve comment. They consist of stainless steel rod formed into an inverted V-bolt. The top of the "V" is properly radiussed for the appropriate size clevis pin. The legs of the V-bolt pass through the deck and hull flanges and a heavy backup plate. The hull flange is about one-half inch thick. Two major structural bulkheads and a hanging knee reinforce the hull and deck immediately adjacent to the chainplates.

The same chainplate arrangement is used on larger boats in the Nicholson line. The obvious advantage is that the chainplates are just about leakproof.

The reason that the chainplates work successfully are an exceptionally thick hull flange and local reinforcement with knees and structural bulkheads.

The outboard rudder is attached to the transom by massive nylon-bushed stainless steel pintle and gudgeon castings. Polished stainless castings are infinitely preferable to weldments in a fitting exposed to salt water since they are less vulnerable to corrosion.

A large molded-fiberglass water tank fills most of the bilge space. The tank is gelcoated inside and is equipped with two large manholes for easy cleaning. The manholes are also used to fill the tank as there is no deck fill-pipe. While this is a slight nuisance, it pretty much insures that salt water will not get in the tank. The water tank is properly vented inside the boat, rather than outside. Again, the risk of contamination by salt water is eliminated.

Unlike many modern boats, there is a deep bilge sump aft of the water tank. The bilge slopes sharply aft to the sump, so that any water getting into the bilge will quickly drain to the sump. Bilge water lapping about the cabin sole should not be a problem.

Construction of the Nicholson 31 is strong and heavy, perhaps too heavy for coastal cruising in light air. The boat's displacement of almost 15,000 pounds yields a staggering displacement to length ratio of 468, one of the highest we've ever seen. This figure is misleading, however, since the boat quickly picks up waterline length when she heals, reducing the D/L considerably.

PERFORMANCE

Handling Under Sail

Even with her relatively modern profile, the Nicholson 31 is no racer-cruiser. She's not even a cruiser-racer. Just a pure cruiser, and one close to being underpowered at that. Fully loaded for cruising, she will displace 18,000 pounds or more. At that point the boat will need all the sail that can be piled on in light air

Shrouds mounted at the outboard edge of the deck limit the boat's ability to point. She is most definitely at her best off the wind.

There is a great deal of inherent stability in the hull form of the Nicholson 31. With her relatively hard bilges, wide beam, and reasonable ballast to displacement ratio, the boat is quite stiff, particularly when these hull characteristics are coupled with a fairly short rig.

Spars are by Proctor. The mast is a heavy, untapered section with airfoil spreaders. The boom is equipped for slab reefing. A short mainsheet traveler mounted on top of the transom will help mainsail control. A boom vang is standard equipment.

Lewmar winches are used for sheets and halyards. They are of adequate size for the job, although we would consider slightly larger self-tailing winches than the standard single-speed Lewmar 34 ST's. All sheets are within easy reach of the helmsman.

The boat comes with mainsail and #1 jib. We would rather take delivery of the boat with no sails, then purchase a full inventory from a local sailmaker who understood how we were going to use the boat. On a boat which lacks inherent speed, high quality sails are critical.

The characteristics of the Nicholson 31 that make her such a good offshore cruiser—stability, heavy displacement, and good motion in a seaway—will make her a poor choice for daysailing or even coastal cruising in areas of light air. On a long offshore passage, however, the boat should shine—provided you've got big headsails, including a spinnaker, for light air.

Handling Under Power

The standard engine is a three-cylinder, 22.5-horsepower, raw water-cooled Yanmar. If you want pressure hot water on the boat, it is necessary to order the fresh-water cooled version of the engine. Independent of the hot water system, we'd still prefer the fresh water cooling. The engine is just about the right size for the boat. She should putt along at about five knots using less than a half-gallon of fuel per hour.

The fuel tank is of molded fiberglass mounted under the cockpit sole. The top of the tank, in fact, forms part of the cockpit sole. This means that the teak cockpit grate must be kept in place to keep from walking on top of the tank.

Some sailors are leery of fiberglass diesel fuel tanks. Unless the proper type of resin is used, the tank may be permeable to diesel oil. Fortunately, the fuel tank of the Nicholson 31 is a separate molding and is not integral with the hull. Even if trouble were to develop over time, removal and replacement of the tank would be relatively easy.

The fuel tank is equipped with a small sump on the bottom which is fitted with a drain to remove accumulated water. While this is a good idea, ABYC standards specifically

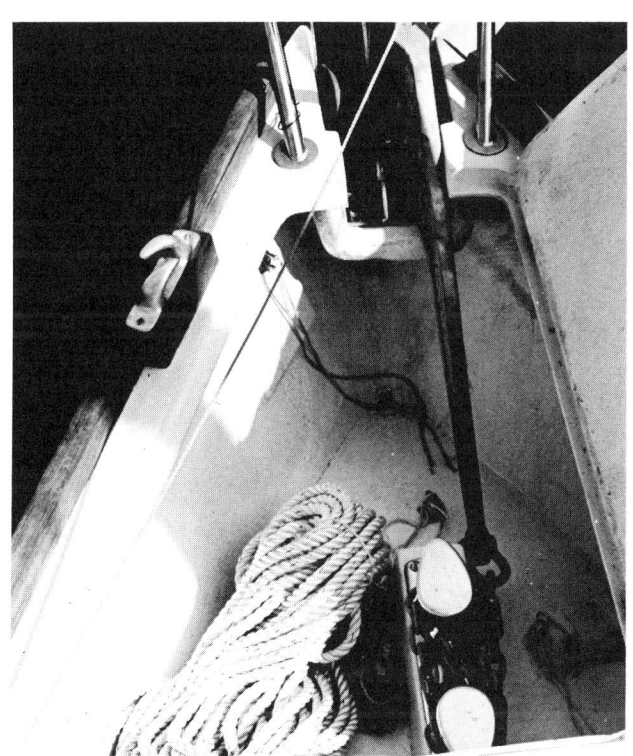

The anchor well is the best we've seen on a small cruiser. The standard 35-pound CQR fits completely below deck level, but can be dropped almost instantly.

The Nicholson 31
243

preclude a drain on the bottom of the fuel tank. Lloyd's is not quite so finicky in that respect.

Capacity of the tank is 25 gallons. This should give the boat a range of 250 to 300 miles under power, perfectly adequate for a 31-foot cruising boat. The location of the fuel fill on the cockpit sole makes it easy to check the fuel level, but a fuel spill could turn the cockpit into a skating rink if the grate were not in place.

For long passages, it is desirable to be able to line up the prop in the aperture behind the deadwood. Unfortunately, access to the stuffing box and shaft requires climbing into the port cockpit locker after removing the access hatch, an exercise most people will find not worth the effort.

The engine installation is a good one. There is a deep molded drip pan under the engine. The shaft is fitted with a flexible shaft log and a flexible shaft coupling as well as flexible engine mounts. This combination of flexible components is essential with a vibration-prone diesel engine.

Access to the engine for service is excellent. The companionway steps remove for access to the front of the engine, and a side panel in the quarterberth removes for access to the rest of the engine. The engine is easily removed through the companionway with no disassembly of joinerwork. However, there is no easy access to the oil dipstick.

The entire engine compartment is equipped with excellent soundproofing. All wiring and plumbing in the engine compartment is neat and workmanlike. Hidden carpentry inside the engine box is as well executed as any finish work in the boat.

LIVABILITY

Deck Layout

The deck layout of the Nicholson 31 is that of a pure cruiser. The recessed stemhead fitting is a massive stainless steel weldment equipped with two heavy bronze rollers. If the rollers are used with a nylon anchor rode they will have to be polished out, as the roller castings are rough enough to damage line. The rollers are designed to stow CQR anchors. Standard equipment includes a 35-pound CQR and a 15-fathom shot of 5/16" chain.

The anchor well is unusual. The lid has a strong, positive latch, and the well contains a large mooring bitt, lashing eyes for anchors and the bitter end of the anchor rode, and a pipe to the chain locker. The chain locker pipe should have been extended higher above the bottom of the anchor well to keep water out of the boat's interior when she takes solid water over the bow.

Because the stemhead fitting and anchor rollers are recessed below deck level, the 35-pound CQR actually stows inside the anchor well, so that sheets and sails cannot snag on it. There is also enough space inside the well to install a windlass, and two different models are listed as factory options. This is perhaps the best anchor well and anchor stowage arrangement we've seen on a small cruising boat.

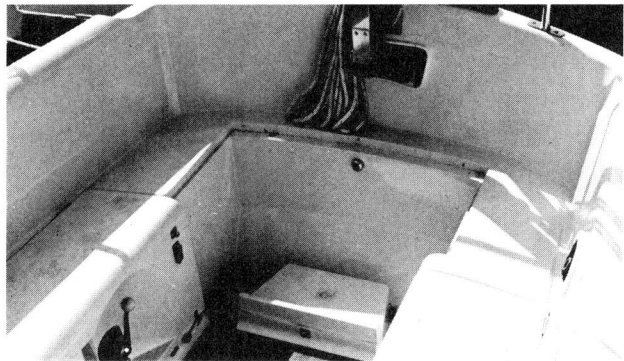

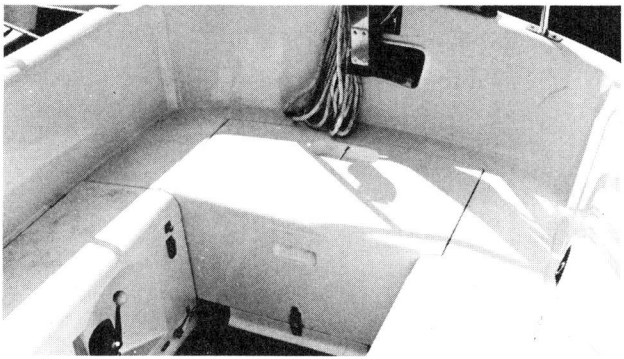

Enclosed storage for a valise life raft is built into the cock-pit, as it should be in every serious cruiser.

There are full length hand rails on either side of the deckhouse. Bow and stern rails, double lifelines, and tapered stainless stanchions are standard. All are properly mounted.

The cockpit is a good compromise for a cruising boat. Seat are narrow, but are over six feet long for comfortable lounging. A high bridge-deck protects the companionway. The companionway is fairly narrow and almost parallel-sided with two drop-boards. Because the companionway sill is well below coaming level, the lower drop board should be left in place for offshore sailing. In accordance with ORC requirements for offshore racing, dropboards for companionway slide have permanent positive inside latches to prevent accident openings in a rollover.

Cockpit scuppers consist of two large holes through the transom, fitted with external flaps to keep following seas from splashing through the scuppers into the cockpit.

There is a shallow locker under the starboard cockpit seat for line and other items. At the aft end of this locker is a molded recess for a single propane bottle. The bottle locker is designed for a European bottle, which may prove difficult to replace if it rusts out.

The scupper for this locker drains into the cockpit. Inevitably, the steel gas bottle will turn into a pile of rust, staining the cockpit where the drain discharges. An aluminum gas bottle or a thoroughly epoxied steel bottle is called for here.

Under the port cockpit seat is a deep locker which can rightfully be called a sail locker. The lid is large enough for the largest headsail on the boat. The locker should accommodate most if not all of the boat's inventory. It is sealed off from the bilge and the underside of the cockpit, and the lid is deeply scuppered.

The Nicholson 31
245

A full-width cockpit dodger is standard. It fits neatly into a plastic extrusion attached to a wrap-around breakwater. The forward end of the cockpit will be dry, even in heavy weather, allowing the upper drop board to be left out until it gets really nasty. The only disadvantage of the molded breakwater and low dodger is that the halyards cannot be led aft without fairly complex modifications to the breakwater.

The cockpit is deep and well protected. It is so deep that a short person will have a hard time seeing over the deckhouse.

All in all, deck layout and cockpit are well suited for serious cruising; simple, clean, and devoid of toe bashers. It is a layout designed not for high performance, but rather for a long haul.

Belowdecks

The interior layout of the Nicholson 31 approaches the ideal for a minimum long distance cruiser for two, but falls short in a few important details. There are a total of six berths, equally divided between the port and starboard sides. Each berth is equipped with a lee cloth.

The forward cabin contains the standard V-berth, with an insert to form a double. Shelves along the side of the hull and a small locker over the foot of the berth are standard. There are large bins under the V-berth with molded drop-in liners. These should provide good dry storage in any conditions.

A Camper & Nicholsons (Canpa) aluminum framed hatch over the berth provides ventilation and can be used as an exit. Teak steps mounted on the bulkhead serve as a ladder for climbing out the hatch.

Aft of the forward cabin is a full-width head, which makes a lot of sense on a small boat. In the attempt to avoid a full-width head in a small boat, builders invariably end up with a cramped compartment barely big enough to turn around in, much less shower or dress in comfort.

The water closet is the unique Lavac design, which uses a separate diaphragm pump in place of a built-in pump. This is an efficient toilet which absolutely will not splash when pumped. Outboard of the toilet is a good-sized hanging locker. It is, unfortunately, the only hanging space on the boat. The lack of a wet locker will be sorely felt by the serious cruiser.

A pressure cold-water shower is standard. The shower sump is fitted with a separate electric pump and does not drain to the bilge.

Opposite the toilet is a huge sink, the largest we've seen in the head of any boat. The sink is fitted with both manual and pressure taps. The head sink has the only manual fresh water pump on the boat. A heavy stainless steel grab rail is mounted horizontally in front of the sink. Above the sink, tucked under the side deck, is a mirror-fronted medicine chest. The mirrors are angled upward so that it isn't necessary to duck to see your face in the mirror when shaving—a small touch but typical of the thought which has gone into the interior.

The head compartment has solid, heavy sliding doors which have positive latches to hold them open. They are held shut only by magnets, which could prove inadequate offshore. Ventilation is provided by a small cowl vent in a molded dorade box. We would replace the cowl with a larger one.

The main cabin has a number of excellent features, not the least of which is a strongly mounted dropleaf cabin table. Bolted to an aluminum plate under the cabin sole, the table is as sturdy as any we've encountered. The folding leaves should be fitted with fiddles, however, for use in a rolly anchorage. (At sea, a lap is more often used than a table. We can recall very few sit-down dinners at sea.)

Settees, port and starboard, are fitted with lee cloths, as are the pilot berth and quarterberth. There is a good dry, compartmented storage below, behind, and above the settees. Footwells under the chart table and galley counter make the settees long enough for sleeping. Both settees pull out to increase width for sleeping.

While the pilot berth and quarterberth afford permanent sea berths on both sides of the main cabin without using the settees, this configuration wastes storage space that the cruising couple would find handy. We doubt if four berths in the main cabin are really necessary.

The galley is the weakest part of the interior. There is one small drawer; the only drawer in the whole boat. Admittedly, drawers are expensive and waste a certain amount of space, but the one place they do make sense is the galley, and one is barely adequate.

A two-burner, gimballed, strongly-mounted propane stove with oven and broiler is standard. The stove is a simple enameled steel model and will probably last for only a few years of hard service before it rusts out. At the same time, it probably only cost a couple of hundred dollars rather than the $800 or more you would pay for a good stainless model.

The gas system lacks a shutoff valve belowdecks, a violation of ABYC standards for propane installations. We suggest you fit a Marinetics or Bass electromagnetic propane solenoid or a good manual valve somewhere in the galley.

As is typical in many European boats, the icebox is a bit of an afterthought. In much of the world, ice isn't the readily available commodity that it is in the U.S., and people simply learn to do without. When cruising offshore, ice only lasts a few days anyway, so unless you have a refrigeration system, why bother with an icebox? So the logic goes, anyway. In this country, most cruising is well within range of sources of ice, and we'd want a good box to keep it in.

While the icebox of the Nicholson 31 is well insulated including the lid, the lid lacks a sealing gasket. The lid is so small that a 25-pound block of ice must be broken in half to pass through, and a gallon jug of milk would be a close fit. In addition, the rounded cabin trunk liner protrudes so much into the space over the icebox that access is difficult. The icebox also lacks shelves to keep food off the ice, and it drains into the bilge sump.

There is fairly good storage outboard of the stove in well-fiddled shelves behind sliding doors. Crockery and glasses are provided as standard items.

Treadmaster is used on the cabin sole in the galley and at the aft end of the main cabin. This is an excellent nonskid surface which is, unfortunately, very difficult to clean. The rest of the main-cabin sole is varnished teak and holly plywood.

On the starboard side opposite the galley is an excellent navigation station with a huge chart table and plenty of bulkhead space for radios, instruments, bookcases, and other goodies. The electrical panel—again typical of European boats—lacks adequate circuits for the addition of many extras. The electrical system does have a built-in ground system utilizing an external ground plate, which greatly improves the functioning of SSB radios, shortwave receivers, and Loran.

The navigator sits at the head of a large, comfortable quarterberth. Batteries mount under the quarterberth in the best battery box we've seen, with a positively latched lid. Two heavy-duty, 95-amp-hour batteries are standard and should be adequate for the electrical needs of a 31-foot boat. The battery box does lack adequate ventilation to disperse charging gases, an easily remedied problem.

Ventilation of the main cabin is provided by a large aluminum-framed hatch in the middle of the cabin, and two small cowl vents in molded dorade boxes at the aft end of the cabin.

The ventilation hatches in both the main and forward cabins open aft. When fitted with side curtains, they can be left open at sea for additional ventilation. Forward-facing hatches are fine in port, but cannot normally be left open at sea.

The interior of the Nicholson 31 is clearly that of a seagoing boat. There are full-length hand-rails along each cabin side, and vertical posts in the galley and nav station. Interior workmanship is excellent, with a good blend of very light teak and off-white molded components. The interior is cheery and homelike. It's easy to imagine a long cruise aboard.

CONCLUSIONS

The Nicholson 31 is a well-designed, well-built cruising boat. Her somewhat modern appearance above the water may confuse those who connect serious cruising boats with lots of teak, bowsprits, sweeping sheers, and "traditional" appearance.

The Nicholson 31 is not a copy of any "ideal" cruising hull form. She is, rather, a well thought-out answer to the problem of putting a lot of carrying capacity, volume, and comfort in a minimum-sized boat for extended cruising.

If the British pound were valued at much above two dollars, the Nicholson 31 would be prohibitively expensive. At current exchange rates, however, she represents an excellent value for someone willing to go through the logistics of importing a boat.

The prohibitive transatlantic shipping cost of a boat as small as the Nicholson 31—about $7,500—tempts us to offer an alternative. Arrange to purchase a boat through one of the U.S. agents or through the builder (the price is the same either way). Take delivery in England in the spring. Spend the summer cruising England and perhaps some of northern Europe.

In the fall, begin the migration south with other European boats, arriving in the Canaries in late fall. When the northeast trades fill in and the hurricane season is past, depart the Canaries for the long, downwind passage to Barbados. Spend the winter working north through the Caribbean. In late May, depart north toward Bermuda and the East Coast of the U.S. or west toward the Panama Canal.

The money you've saved on transatlantic shipping will have gone a long way toward paying for your year of cruising. And you'll have a good solid boat under your feet, a few thousand miles of cruising under your belt, and some memories you'll never forget. Just hope that your boss understands when you ask for a year's leave of absence. And hope you can make the right decision when the time comes to either go home, or sail on.

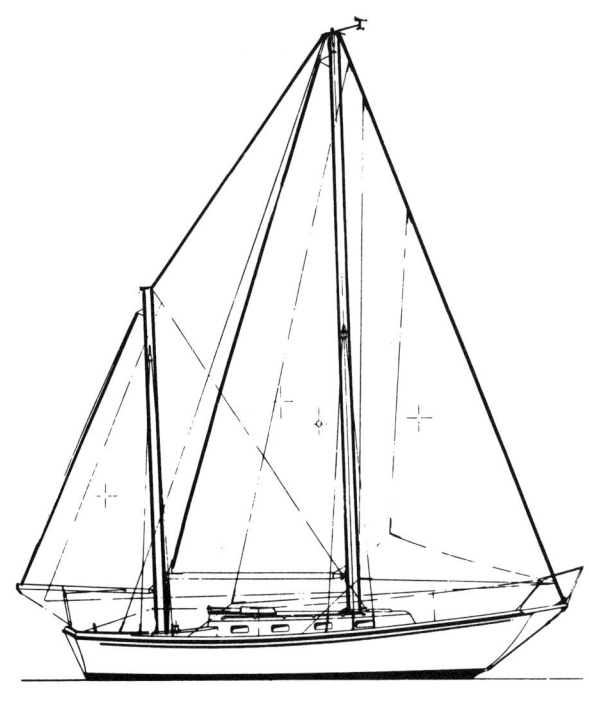

Specifications	
Allied Seawind II	
LOA	31'7"
DWL	25'6"
Beam	10'5"
Draft	4'6"
Displacement	14,900 lbs
Ballast	5800 lbs
Sail area	
ketch	555 sq ft
cutter	512 sq ft

The Allied Seawind II: Staying Power

THE BOAT AND THE BUILDER

When Allied Yachts went out of business for the fifth—and last—time at the end of 1981, they did so in a rather messy fashion. At least two potential owners were left holding the bag, having made down payments of about $20,000 each for boats that were never built. The manager of Allied seemed to disappear, along with the dreams of the would-be owners of the unbuilt Seawind IIs.

One of Allied's dealers took over the management of Allied Yachts in the spring of 1980, when the firm was on the verge of financial disaster for the fourth time in less than 20 years. Over the years, Allied had suffered from mediocre management, severe under-exposure, and the vagaries of the boat buying public—a not unusual story in the boatbuilding industry.

Allied had the reputation for fashioning solidly built (if uninspiringly finished) boats, unabashedly oriented toward cruising—with the exception of a single foray into the world of racing yachts with a Britton Chance 30-footer.

Allied had already secured its place in the boatbuilding pantheon with the original Seawind ketch, which became the first fiberglass boat to circumnavigate, and the Luders 33, recognized as a classic design of the era preceding the introduction of the fin keel racer-cruiser. Unfortunately, while its products were heading for glory on the high seas, the company was repeatedly headed for the boneyard.

In 1975, Allied began building the foot-longer, foot-wider, Gillmer-designed Seawind II as a replacement for the original thirty foot, six inch Seawind. The extra foot of length and beam, 1-1/2 feet of waterline length, and 2,700 pounds of displacement add up to make the Seawind II a significantly larger boat than her predecessor.

Like its cousin the Southern Cross 31, the Seawind II is a cruising sailor's dream machine, but these dreams can come with a hefty price tag. Base price for a new Seawind II with its extensive standard inventory was $75,000. For this you got a well-equipped, well-built, proven world cruiser with such standard features as hot and cold pressure water, shower (in both cockpit and head), shore power, and wheel steering. In the last years of production, Allied attempted to overcome its dowdy image. Older Allied boats were heavy on woodgrain Formica, bland expanses of fiberglass, and mediocre woodwork. Allied actively sought to overcome this hard-to-shake reputation by using large expanses of interior wood (which hid most of the interior glass), good hardware, and the perceptions of new management with a great deal of cruising experience.

CONSTRUCTION

The hull of the Seawind II is a solid layup. The deck and cabin trunk are balsa cored. The top of the coachroof, in the way of the deck-stepped mast, is cored with solid, filled epoxy for greater compression strength.

The hull to deck joint is complex, expensive, time-consuming to make, and extremely strong. In this day of simple, through-bolted inside flanges, it is an anachronism. Both hull and deck have outward flanges at the sheer line. These flanges were coated with 3M 5200 adhesive sealant, and a teak batten placed between them, laid on the flat. Hull, deck and batten were then through-bolted vertically with stainless steel bolts. After the sealant cured (which took several days) the joint was ground flush on the inside and heavily glassed over.

On the outside, a heavy aluminum extrusion was filled with bedding, slipped over the flange, and fastened horizontally with screws into the teak batten. (Now you know what the teak batten was for.)

This is an incredibly labor-intensive joint, substantially improved over the old Seawind joint which was the same basic design but had a reputation for developing small leaks. The aluminum extrusion makes an excellent rubbing strake, but damage to it would require getting a replacement piece from the builder, rather than a patch job with resin, putty, and a little teak. Needless to say, with the builders long gone, this could present a problem. This joint may look a bit massive for a boat of this size, but it is an excellent idea for a serious cruising boat.

The ballast is lead, molded to shape and glassed into the keel. While this technique eliminates keel bolts, it also makes the fiberglass hull more vulner-

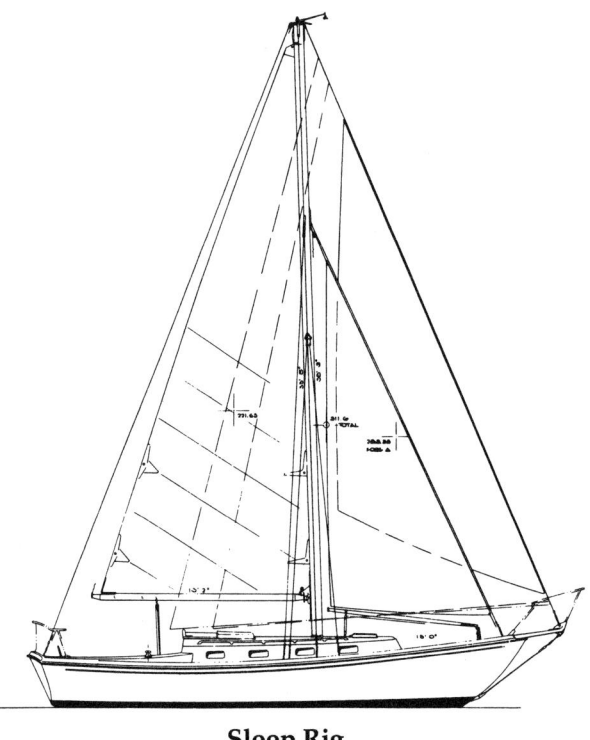
Sloop Rig

able to grounding damage.

The Seawind II's mast is stepped on deck, and uses a massive oak compression frame under the cabin trunk for support. This frame forms the head door framing, and is solidly, though a little crudely, attached to the top of the ballast.

Seacocks are used on all through-hull fittings. These are through-bolted to the hull and have double-clamped hoses that are cheap insurance for any boat.

All deck hardware is through-bolted and reinforced with fiberglass backing plates. We prefer aluminum backing plates for their greater strength and rigidity for a given thickness and area.

There is very little exterior wood on the Seawind II. The molded toerail is capped with teak. There are teak hand rails on the cabin top, and teak trim around the edge of the cabin. That's all. Even the dorade boxes are molded in. This results in low maintenance, a highly desirable characteristic on a serious cruising boat, but one that leads to an appearance of austerity that can border on plainness. The austere appearance of the Seawind II is greatly relieved by contrasting cockpit, deck, and deckhouse molded-in non-skid surfaces. The Seawind II will never look as flashy as a Taiwan-built teak plantation, but neither will her owners have to make the decision between endless wood maintenance or the drabness of unfinished "natural" teak (mildewed gray).

PERFORMANCE

Handling Under Sail

The standard rig of the Seawind II is a masthead ketch. The ketch rig is not particularly desirable for a boat of this size. The mizzen adds considerable weight and windage and almost no drive upwind, since the mizzen sail acts almost completely in the backwind of the mainsail. The real purpose of a mizzen upwind is to balance the boat, and for this purpose the smaller, more out-of-the-way mizzen of the yawl is equally useful.

Off the wind, the area of the mizzen, plus the added bonus of a mizzen staysail, do provide considerable drive. The mizzenmast clutters up the cockpit, although it does provide a good handhold. Its position, five feet forward of the helmsman, is guaranteed to make him cross-eyed if he is in the habit of sitting directly behind the wheel.

The sail area of the Seawind II is small enough that the oft-cited advantage of the ketch rig (smaller individual sails) is rather unimportant. A mizzen is useful for heaving to, for anchoring and weighing anchor, and to enable the boat to weather-cock in a rolly anchorage. It is, however, a most inefficient rig upwind.

An optional cutter rig was available. It uses the same mainmast as the ketch rig, but shifts it aft about a foot. The mainsail is longer on the foot and the base of the foretriangle is a little longer than that of the ketch rig. The total sail area of the cutter rig works out to slightly less than that of the ketch rig, but the reduced windage and slightly increased stability probably make up for the loss of sail area. For tradewind passages, the double headstays on either rig allow the use of twin downwind jibs. With a working sail area of just over 500 square feet for a displacement of 14,900 pounds, the Seawind II is not under-rigged as are many cruising boats.

The Seawind II's rudder is a rather large, old-fashioned design of the barn door variety. It would be interesting and not at all difficult to change it to a more modern Constellation-style rudder, which would slightly reduce wetted surface and perhaps give a little better performance with no loss of control.

With the cutter rig that we prefer, twin running headsails, and sails built for speed as well as durability, the Seawind II should have good performance for a pure cruising boat. Without a large genoa she will not be at her best in light air, although owners report that she is surprisingly spirited under these conditions. Unfortunately, she will not be able to use a genoa to its full potential upwind, due to the wide shroud base and wide spreaders.

Handling Under Power
The Seawind II is powered by a lightweight, four-cylinder Westerbeke 27-horsepower diesel. This is plenty of power for the Seawind II's displacement. A welded aluminum fuel tank is located in the bilge.

The standard propeller is a fixed, three-bladed bronze prop in an aperture. Rather than being burdened by the considerable drag of such a propeller, we would install a two-bladed model that could be lined up behind the deadwood to reduce drag under sail. Alternatively, a two- or three-bladed feathering propeller could be installed. On a boat with the considerable wetted surface of the Seawind II, reducing drag becomes critical to performance in light air. No matter what the builders of ocean-going dreadnoughts may tell you, much of the sailing in the world—even on the ocean—is in light air.

Do not expect the Seawind II to maneuver like a modern fin keeler under power. Despite her cutaway forefoot, there is enough lateral plane here to

The Allied Seawind
253

require a little planning ahead in a tight situation under power. But then, you should always plan ahead, no matter how well your boat handles.

LIVABILITY

Deck Layout

An unusual feature of the Seawind II is the lifeline stanchions and pulpits. They stand 30 inches off the deck, rather than the more common 24 inches. Coupled with a fairly high toerail, these give the foredeck hand a real feeling of security. Unfortunately, they also require that a long tack pennant be installed if you want to get the foot of the jib above the lifelines. The cutter rig is an advantage here, for a high-cut yankee jibtopsail will easily clear the lifelines.

The bowsprit is a massive teak platform with attached rail. There are double bow rollers at the end of the bowsprit, but these are so far outboard that the anchor rode chafes against the forward pulpit stanchion when the rollers are used. This defect also prevents secure storage of an anchor in the roller, as the stock would bear against the pulpit. The pulpit is a comfortable and secure place to handle sails or ground tackle.

The Seawind II is one of the few boats we've seen with properly sized bow cleats. There are two 12-inch foredeck cleats, with hawsepipes to the divided anchor rode locker outside each cleat. An anchor windlass is optional, and will fit nicely between the cleats.

Because of the width of the cabin trunk, it is easier to get to the foredeck by walking over the cabin top than by squeezing inside the shrouds. Good non-skid on the cabin top makes this fairly easy.

Unfortunately, it's not particularly easy to hoist the sails on the cutter rig, because the two dorade boxes fall exactly abreast the mast, making it necessary to straddle them awkwardly. This is less of a problem with the ketch rig, whose mast is stepped farther forward.

A variety of mainsheet leads have been used on the Seawind II. One version uses a traveler mounted over the companionway seahood. In this version, the blocks are located far apart on the boom, giving poor mechanical advantage. The best of the Seawind II's mainsheet arrangements consists of a traveler mounted on the bridgedeck, which reduces seating but gives much better sail control. This should be used on either the ketch or the cutter, as the old end-of-

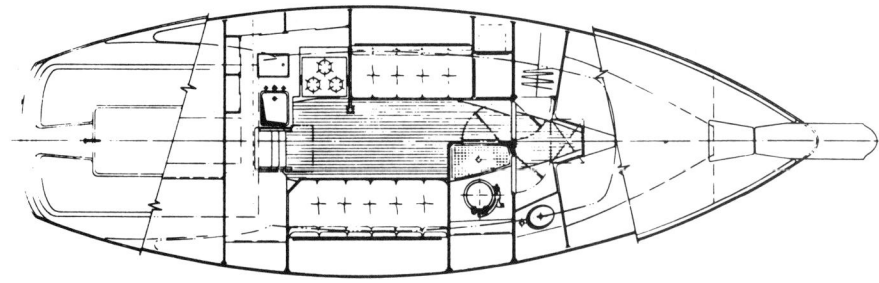

boom arrangement was only necessary with a roller furling mainsail, which should appropriately be considered a thing of the past.

The standard steerer on the boat is an Edson rack and pinion model that is mounted directly on the head of the rudder stock. This is the only steering placement possible with the ketch rig.

There are more possibilities with the cutter rig. The most appealing would be to mount an Edson pedestal steerer at the forward end of the cockpit. Then the helmsman could reach the mainsheet on the bridgedeck, the headsail sheets, and even the halyards if they were led aft. If a cockpit dodger were also installed, the helmsman would be protected from all that nasty spray when going upwind.

The cockpit is large and reasonably comfortable. It was probably made so large to accommodate the mizzen mast, which also serves as a handy foot brace. Without the mizzen, the cockpit looks rather large and empty. It is too wide, in fact, to adequately brace your feet on the opposite cockpit seat when the boat is heeled over.

There is a deep gutter at the back of the cockpit seats on either side. This is a good feature, for it means that water will not collect in a puddle against the leeward coaming on a long, wet beat to weather.

Be sure to check the fit of the emergency tiller. The rudder stock of the new boat we examined had been improperly machined, and the emergency tiller was overly sloppy in its fit.

A large underseat locker on either side of the cockpit will hold a lot of gear, and is equipped with drop-in dividers to keep items from the depths of the bilge. Another unique feature of the cockpit is a fresh water shower, whose spray head and hose are recessed into the side of the footwell. This means that it isn't necessary to track saltwater belowdecks after a swim.

The companionway is narrow, with almost parallel sides. While this may make it a little less convenient to get below, it is far more seamanlike than most companionways. Coupled with a molded seahood, and a good bridgedeck, it provides well designed access for people, but not water.

Belowdecks

On the latter day Seawind IIs we were pleased to find the best finished interiors of any Allied boats we'd seen. The layout is conventional, and as befits a serious cruising boat, there is tremendous storage throughout. There were also a number of storage options, such as bureau, extra drawers, and extra cabinets that allowed the new owner to tailor the boat to his or her individual needs.

The forward cabin contains a V-berth, a hanging locker, and a wash basin. There are drawers and bins under the berths, and a large stainless steel holding tank. We would replace the holding tank with a fresh water tank to greatly increase water capacity.

A door from the forward cabin gives access to the head without entering the main cabin. The primary door between the main cabin and the forward cabin does double duty as a door which shuts the head off from the main cabin.

The head is small, containing only the toilet and the shower. The head doors are extremely narrow, since their heavy framing also carries the compression load of the rig.

Because the settees in the main cabin are asymmetrical, it is not possible to accommodate more than four people at the fold-down dining table. Since, quite rationally, there are only four berths in the boat, this should rarely be a problem. The space behind the settees is given over to storage, rather than attempting to cram more berths into the boat.

A number of galley stove options might be found on Seawind IIs on the used boat market, including surface-mounted kerosene and alcohol stoves, and gimballed LPG, kerosene, or alcohol stoves with oven. Alcohol should not be considered as a cooking fuel for a serious cruising boat, and kerosene, while hot, soon turns the galley overhead to a dingy greyish-brown. We would prefer the LPG gas option.

The icebox is insulated with four inches of urethane foam, and has a tight fitting, well-gasketed top. It is second only to the icebox of the CSY 37 for efficiency. The large, deep sink is equipped with both pressure fresh water taps and a manual pump—absolutely essential as a backup, or to save electrical power at sea.

Although there is no navigation station—which would be a little too much to expect on a boat of this size—there is a large dresser surface on the starboard side aft of the settee. Like most boats, there really isn't enough room at the table for navigation electronics, a sextant, and the navigator's pile of books.

Engine access is poor. The engine is tucked away under the cockpit and it is necessary to remove both the companionway ladder and the bulkhead panel behind, in order to check the oil. Needless to say, this is not conducive to good engine maintenance. There is an oil pan under the engine, so spilled oil will not drain into the bilge sump. Neither the shower nor the icebox drain to the bilge either, a welcome feature.

With its wide cabin trunk, good headroom, and no attempt to sleep an army in tiny, uncomfortable berths, the Seawind II provides excellent accommodation for a couple, either living aboard or for extended cruising. That is what the Seawind II is all about.

CONCLUSIONS

The Seawind II is truly a boat that can call herself a world cruiser without apology or explanation. Her construction is strong without being inordinately heavy. She makes no attempt to be all things to all people. It would be a shame to see her tied up to the dock in a marina.

She deserves better.

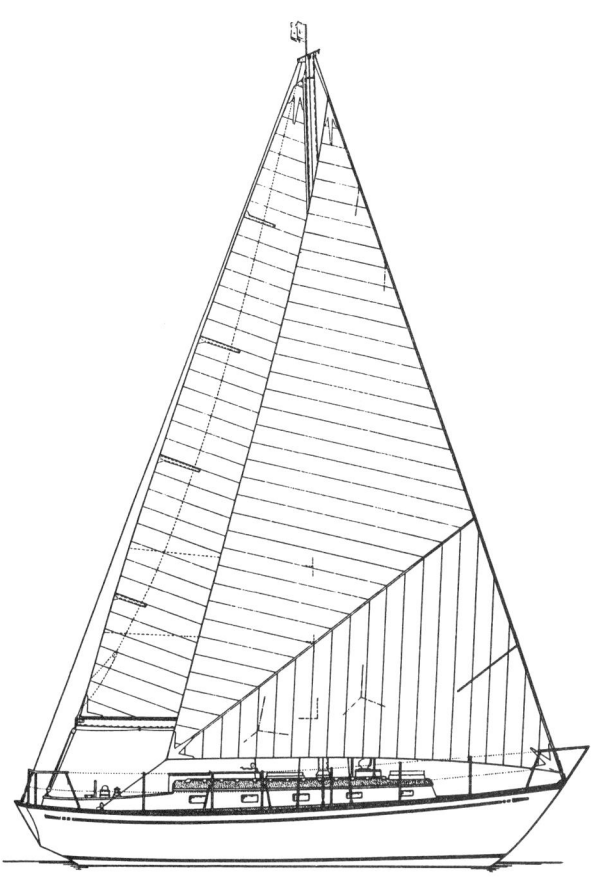

Specifications
Mason 33

LOA	33'9"
DWL	25'5"
Beam	10'10"
Draft	5'0"
Displacement	14,020 lbs
Ballast	5320 lbs
Sail area	602 sq ft

Pacific Asian Enterprises
Box F-A
Dana Point,
California 92629
(714) 496-4848

The Mason 33:
The Cruising Dream Fulfilled

THE BOAT AND THE BUILDER

Pacific Asian Enterprises (PAE) is a small California company that likes to think of itself as more than an importer. "Yacht developers" is a term the firm frequently uses. The term refers to the total process of producing the Mason line of sailboats, from inception of the design, through having the boats built to its own specifications, to import and sales.

PAE got its start in the early 1970s when Kettenburg Marine closed its sales office in Dana Point, California, and temporarily put its boat salesmen out of work. Three of them—Jim Leishman, Joe Meglen, and Dan Streech—decided to fill the resulting void by opening their own brokerage business, Lemest Yacht Sales. Though they started by mostly selling used boats, they also "inherited" some importing businesses, involving CT and Tradewind boats, built in Taiwan. They also sold a few 38-foot wooden boats built in the Orient, designed by Al Mason, a journeyman designer who at various times has worked with

Carl Alberg, John Alden, Philip Rhodes, and Sparkman & Stephens, as well as in his own independent design office.

After several successful years in the booming boat business, the three partners decided to develop their own boat, and to capitalize on their Taiwan connections, so they established Pacific Asian Enterprises.

They commissioned Al Mason to design a fiberglass 40-footer similar to the wooden 38, but with a more elaborate list of specifications to appeal to the American market. By the time all the specifications were fitted in, the boat had grown to 43 feet.

In Taiwan, they contracted with Ta Shing boatyard to build the Mason 43, PAE's first boat, introduced to the U.S. in 1978. At the time, Ta Shing was a small yard generally recognized as one of the quality builders in Taiwan. PAE ordered the hull and deck molds and other tooling for the boat from Ta Shing and maintains ownership of them while Ta Shing builds the boats. (In this practice, they are fundamentally different from companies which are only importers.)

Over the years, the company's relationship with Ta Shing has changed considerably. Originally, PAE (and Al Mason) specified in elaborate detail how the boats were to be built, finished, and equipped. As Ta Shing has grown and learned the demands of PAE, and as PAE gained confidence in Ta Shing, the builder has increasingly attended to the details without specific direction from PAE itself.

In general, the change reflects a change in Taiwanese boatbuilding in the past 15 years. Whereas in the early 70s, Taiwanese boats tended to be either very bad or very good, the country now has the work force and the industrial base to build the best fiberglass boats, and the Taiwanese builders who wish to do quality work are no longer prevented from it by circumstance.

A decade ago, problems often showed up in the metal parts (poor casting, fabricating, or finishing) and many importers were specifying only American-made hardware on the best boats. The watershed occurred for PAE when they discovered that some American blocks they were specifying for deck hardware were actually being made in Taiwan and shipped to the US—before PAE re-shipped them to Taiwan.

Ta Shing still uses some American-made hardware, and PAE continues to manufacture its own electrical panels in California and ship them to Ta Shing

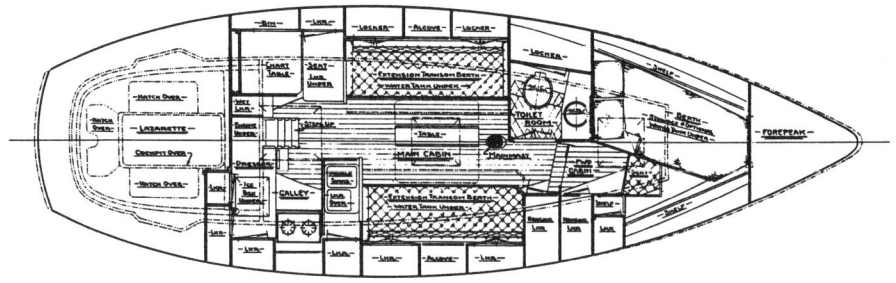

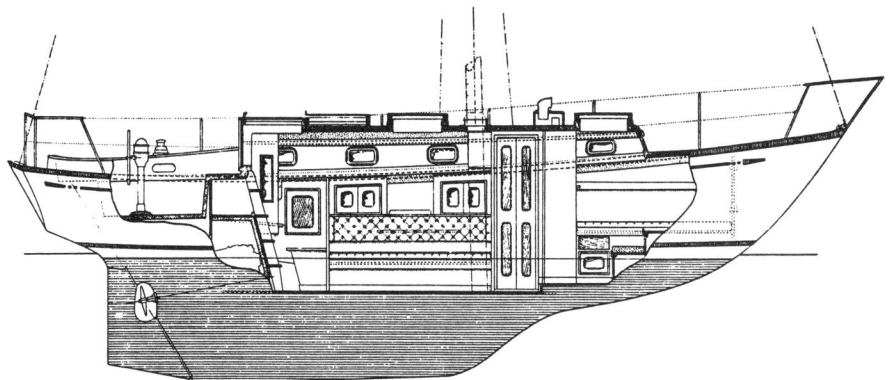

for installation. Otherwise, most of the equipment is Taiwanese, and the custom-made fittings—like bow pulpits, bow chocks, and portholes—are generally as good as can be had anywhere.

Boats are built complete in Taiwan but without the Forespar masts and rigging, which are added after the boats arrive in the U.S. A good indication of the cooperation between PAE and Ta Shing is that all pieces of deck hardware, such as the turning blocks that lead the halyards back to the cockpit, are put on the boat per specification in Taiwan. When the spar is added, everything matches and fits. As most people who have commissioned a new boat will tell you, components often don't match even when the boat and spar come from the same factory.

The Mason 43 was successful enough that PAE commissioned the design for a 53-footer from Al Mason, and then, before the 53 was in full production, the design for a 63-footer. The first boats appeared just as the sailboat market was going flat in the early 1980s, and the two new models were not initially a financial success for the company.

PAE then decided to develop a smaller boat, and the Mason 33 was introduced late in 1984. By 1987, 24 hulls have been sold, a modest number by comparison to high-volume production lines, but respectable on the quality end of the sailboat spectrum.

The 33 is a moderate traditional design that harks back to the CCA handicapping rule of the 1960s. It might best be described as a modern full-keel hull with a cut-away forefoot and sharply turned bilges to reduce wetted surface. Though narrow and short on the waterline compared to modern lightweight fin-keelers, she is beamier, with shorter overhangs that you would find on a typical 1960s design. If that racing rule had survived into the 1980s, we suspect the Mason 33 would be a typical, if conservative, specimen.

PAE's requirements to the designer were for a seakindly hull with the capability for carrying ample stores and an ability to take a couple or small crew anywhere. The company makes no bones about their distaste for contemporary fin-keelers which it condemns as limited-purpose boats with too many berths and totally inadequate storage space. They believe the moderate traditional

The Mason 33
259

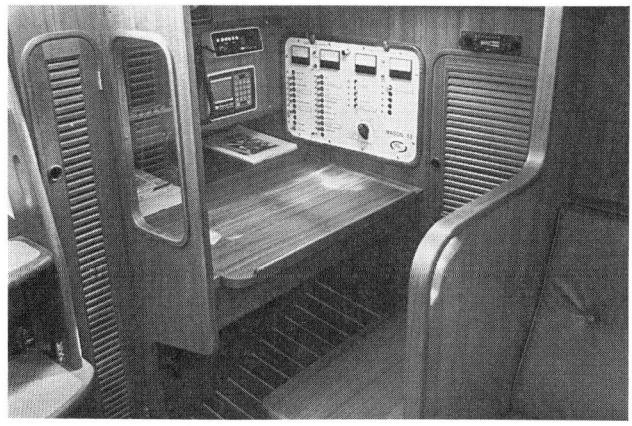

design of their 33 makes for not only comfortable coastal cruising and daysailing, but also bluewater passagemaking and living aboard. And it's conceivable you could even race one in PHRF.

CONSTRUCTION

The nav station has a screen to protect from spray from the companionway. The electrical panel is well crafted and folds down to give easy access to the connection blocks.

The hull is a standard solid fiberglass, hand-laid laminate. It's different from others in a couple of respects. The company specifies a somewhat heavier than normal laminate, and the hull also has four full-length longitudinal stringers to give additional support to the bulkheads and floors.

Isophthalic resin is used in the laminate. The theory is that iso resins are less water permeable and hence less likely to allow hull blistering to develop. PAE is also recommending that buyers have an epoxy coating put on at the factory. The $840 option (which includes bottom painting) is probably a worthwhile investment.

The ballast keel is iron, placed inside the hull molding in two pieces, taped into place, and sealed to minimize rust or leakage problems in case of a hard grounding. Americans are more accustomed to lead keels, which are unquestionably preferable for exterior ballast, but iron internal keels are fairly common in the Oriental boats, and we don't hear of many problems. (The external iron keels common on European boats are more rust-prone and a higher maintenance item.)

The full keel gives a roomy bilge, and there's a 20-gallon sump tank as well as a good, deep bilge sump. The interior of the hull itself is generally hidden by joiner work, but where it shows, it is sealed with resin and painted. The hull is reinforced in the way of seacocks. A neat touch is that each of the through-hulls has an identifying nameplate so visitors and guest can follow your instructions without your having to go through elaborate descriptions of what they should be turning off, turning on, or plugging up in case of an emergency.

The deck molding is a standard glass layup with balsa core, with plywood in the cabin trunk and other spots to provide additional backing strength and attachment points for the interior joinerwork. The non-skid on deck is satisfactory, but the optional teak overlay is generally preferable. While it does cost $2,280, the price seems reasonable, especially considering the quality of the workmanship and the finished appearance it gives the boat. Further, the hull

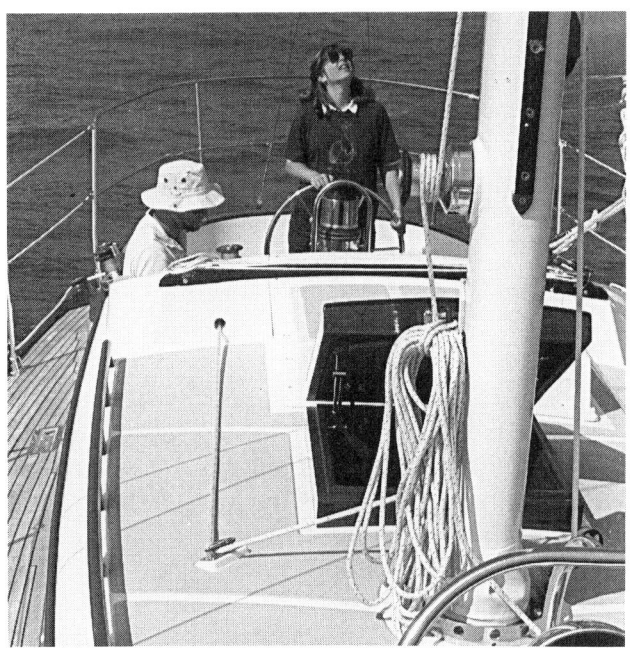

The mainsheet leads forward and down from the mast, then aft through the dodger coaming. Adjusting most sail trim gear requires a trip to the mast.

has the displacement, ballast, and form stability so that the additional weight of the teak deck won't be the problem it could be on a lighter design.

The hull to deck joint is a standard inward-turning hull flange on top of which the deck rests. It's somewhat unusual in that the teak toerail sits on top of (and hides) a stainless steel flat bar on top of the deck. Inside the hull there's a matching stainless flat bar. The flat bar then acts as an extended washer for the through-bolts which fasten the joint together, with every other bolt going through the toerail as well as through the joint. About the only complaint we have heard about the older Masons was some leaking in the hull to deck joint, but it's hard to see how the joint could leak on the 33.

The exterior finish of the hull and deck is generally good with no evident hard spots to mar the fairness of the hull in any of the three boats we examined. The gel-coat work also appears good. Although we went over the topsides and cabin house of one of the three boats carefully, we found no flaws—a rarity in fiberglass boatbuilding.

The boat has fairly extensive teak trim on the exterior, most notably the heavy-duty toerail, cockpit grates, and deckhouse trim. The standard hatches are teak with Lexan tops. Optional Goiot or Taiwanese "Manship" hatches are also offered. (The Taiwan hatches look like knock-offs, as well made but cheaper than the Goiot.) Having the exterior teak varnished is a $625 option. The result is the look of real quality, but many people will not be inclined to get involved with the continuous maintenance required of varnished teak.

One of the things that marks the construction as good quality is the exterior detail. The custom-made cleats and chocks, for example, are well done and well fitted to the teak trim, and the little stainless steel chafing strips to protect the teak around the stern chocks are just one of the many touches.

Although we might have preferred some things to be different (like using

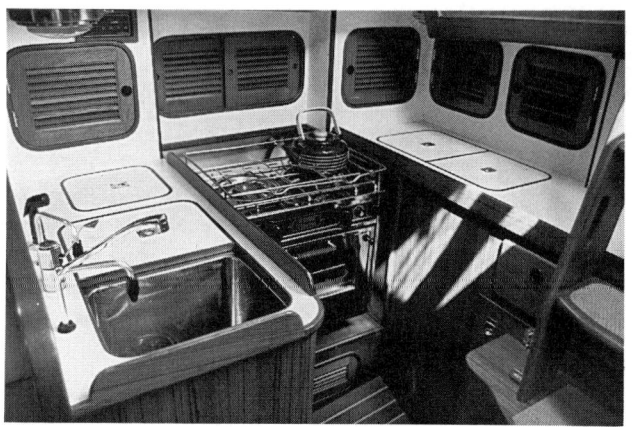

Galley features storage space and fiddles galore. Unfortunately, the cabin sole rises to follow the hull contour, for uncomfortable footing at anchor.

lead ballast rather than iron), it is clear that the developers and builder have given thought to all details of the boat's construction. Overall, it is hard to find fault with any aspect of it.

PERFORMANCE

Handling
Under Power

Early models of the boat came with a 21-horsepower Westerbeke engine, normal for an offshore cruiser, but probably near the minimum size for the American market. Later boats have a Yanmar three-cylinder diesel, at 27 horsepower, a motor adequate for the boat and more in line with what most Americans like in a coastal cruiser. The fuel tanks hold 35 gallons for a good powering range.

Standard is a three-bladed propeller. A two-bladed prop would be preferable for performance under sail since it could be positioned upright in the aperture between the aft end of the keel and the forward edge of the rudder to reduce drag. However, under power, the two-bladed "hammers," that is, it creates a sharp vibration because the two blades are alternately in the water flow but then "hidden" behind the keel and not pushing any water when vertical. The hammering is a minor irritant, but we can imagine it becoming major during long motoring sessions. Unfortunately, it is inherent in the hull design.

The company recommends buying both a three-bladed and a two-bladed wheel, using the three-blade most of the time but putting on the two-bladed prior to long passages under sail. We would be inclined to go with a two-bladed and put up with the vibration, but that's a choice each owner will have to make.

The boat we sailed had a two-bladed prop and the Westerbeke diesel, and we found that the boat generally behaved well under power, being just a mite disinclined to back up in a straight line. Otherwise, she tracks and turns well, although boats with a long keel and attached rudder always have a greater turning radius than the fin keel/separate rudder models most people are accustomed to these days.

The engine installation is well done. There is a good drip pan under the engine and everything is neat and tidy. Full access to the engine, however, requires not only removing the companionway steps, but also taking out a drawer assembly. It's not a complicated job—you have only to remove two wing nuts—but it takes some time.

Handling Under Sail

The Mason 33 is heavy by comparison to most boats her size, and she definitely has a different "feel." We sailed her on a fairly calm day on the Pacific, but it was easy to sense that she would handle rough conditions in a more sedate fashion than typical modern lightweights.

Given that the 33 is a long keeled boat with lots of wetted surface, she probably will not be a sprightly performer in lighter airs, but she has a powerful enough sail plan that the boat moved well in the 8-10 knots of air that we sailed in. Our sense was that the hull must be quite efficient for its type, since the boat sailed better than we expected in the conditions. Though we did not try her in heavy air, we suspect that the boat will be at her best sailing in a good breeze.

The Mason 33 points well enough considering her outboard shrouds and her hull design, but windward work is not her strong point. She does her best with the wind slightly ahead of the beam and next best from a beam reach to a broad reach. It is likely that she would roll heavily dead downwind in heavy air.

Compared to modern racer-cruisers like the Pearson 33 or Beneteau 345, she will be fairly slow for typical coastal cruising, especially in light air and to windward, but she was obviously designed for long distance passages at which she should be respectable.

The boat comes with a mainsail and a working jib as standard equipment, so most people will want to add a genoa and spinnaker. The boat we sailed had a roller-furling jib of about 130 percent, which would be right for moderate-to-heavier air locales. For light-wind areas, a 140 would probably be better. The boat should handle a reefable 150-percent genoa if one chooses not to add furling gear.

The standard sails are made by Sobstad Watts. The mainsail on the boat we sailed was good, the jib average. If we had a sailmaker whom we knew and trusted, our inclination would be to try to negotiate a purchase so we could have the sails made by our own sailmaker. However, the standard sails are good enough that we wouldn't feel "stuck" if we got them. That's not common when stock sails come with a boat these days.

LIVABILITY

Deck Layout

The teak decks, high toerail, and grabrails on the cabin top make movement around the deck easy. The walkways are plenty wide, and even the outboard shrouds require only a small duck and dodge when going forward.

We like the deep cockpit of the boat, with its high coaming and comfortable seats, but it is somewhat smaller (more suited for seagoing) than is common nowadays. It's definitely a cruising cockpit, but it works well for a couple. Tiller steering is standard, but most buyers opt for the wheel which does

The Mason 33's Sisters

In addition to the 33, PAE's line includes the Mason 43/44, Mason 53/54, and 63/64. All are similar in design concept, are built by Ta Shing, and generally show the same attention to detail and finish as the Mason 33.

The company is not currently projecting additional models; instead it has modified its original 43, 53, and 63, calling them the Mason 44, Mason 54, and Mason 64. Most of the redesign work has been handled inhouse, primarily by designer Jeff Leishman, younger brother of company founder. The new versions are referred to as "Mason/PAE" designs.

The Mason 43/44

The 43 was the first PAE boat and was a successful model with 92 boats sold to date. Unlike the 33, which seems "small" for her size, the 43 looks big, roomy, and powerful.

The 44 has basically the same hull as the 43 (a heavier keel is used) and only some minor changes to the interior arrangements. The major change is a redesign of the cabin house/deck/cockpit mold, with the shape and size of the portholes changes, the angles softened to look a bit more "modern."

The interior is a "tri-cabin," with an aft owner's cabin, a forward V-berth cabin, and a big main saloon with galley and navigation area.

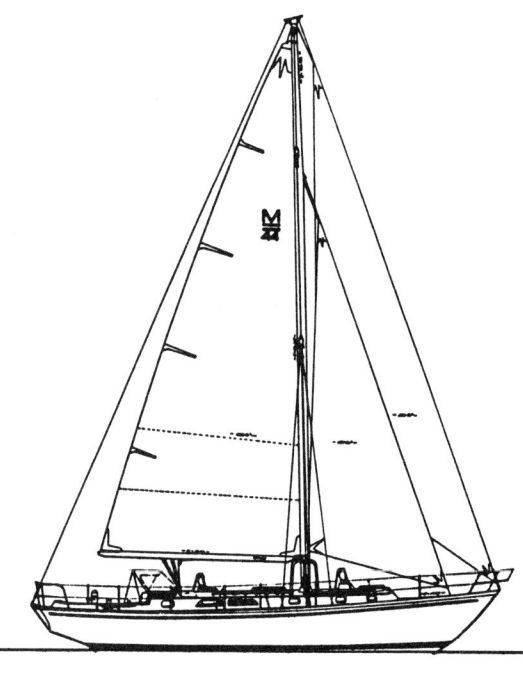

There's ample room for cruising with four people with some occasional guests, and the boat would be spacious for a liveaboard couple. Some sailors might object that there's only one head, but the head is not cramped as it usually is on a two-head 44-footer.

We examined two different 44s and, if anything, we would say that the 44 is better finished than the 33.

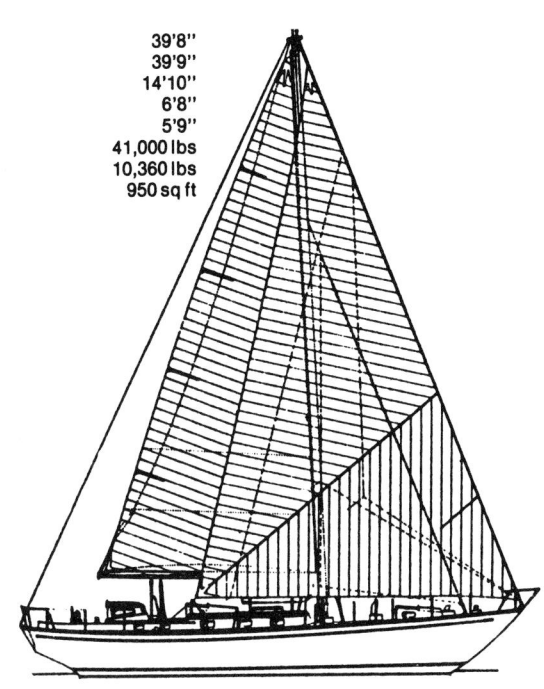

```
39'8"
39'9"
14'10"
6'8"
5'9"
41,000 lbs
10,360 lbs
950 sq ft
```

The exterior is well done, but plain—especially so without the optional teak decks. The interior is executed as well as any production boat we've seen.

The 44 is not a cheap boat. With a good standard equipment list, base price is around $150,000 (varying slightly depending on the shipping destination). With the teak-deck option, electronics, and other equipment of personal choice, the price will probably end up over $160,000. Still, when compared to other boats in her class like the Hinckley 42, the Alden 44, or the Swan 43, she is a bargain.

Mason 53/54 and Mason 63/64

The big Masons are members of a rare class of luxury yachts. We are impressed with them and think they tend to be good values. In this size and price range, most boats are at least semi-customized, and it is difficult to make meaningful comparisons with other manufacturers.

The 54 and 64 (modified along lines similar to the 44) were just becoming available at the time of this printing. The boats have been finished in a variety of ways: ketch and cutter, aft and center cockpit; with many modifications to the basic interior plans.

The price is well over $300,000 for the 54. For the Mason 64? If you have to ask...

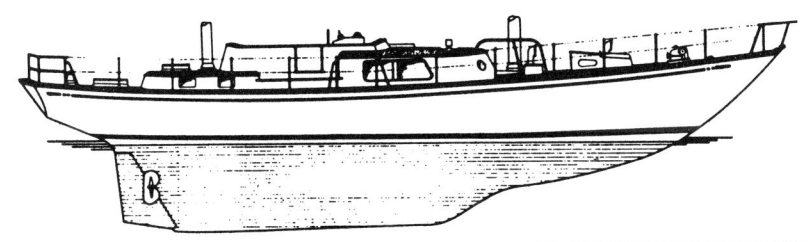

The Mason 33

provide more room. The cockpit lockers are enormous. They're actually too big in the new boat configuration, and most owners will want to subdivide them with partitions so things can be kept orderly.

The Lewmar #40 self-tailing primary winches are adequate, with easy access, but 43s are optional for weaker or harder-driving owners. A set of secondary winches is available; however, there's scarcely enough room on the coaming top—we would probably try to get by without them, even when flying a staysail or spinnaker. The standard mainsheet winch is a Lewmar 16. The optional self-tailing #30 would be preferable, since the traveler is ahead of the companionway, and the sheet is not only loaded up, but also prone to plenty of friction as it leads forward to the mast before turning down to the deck and back underneath the dodger coaming. Sail controls are minimal—you have to go to the mast to adjust the cunningham, outhaul, or vang, so you won't do much tweaking of sail trim.

The foredeck is small, adequate for sail handling and anchor work, but without much room for sunbathing or lounging. The bow anchor roller is set up for a CQR. The forepeak is called a chainlocker. We would consider stowing nylon anchor rode there, but chain would put way too much weight forward. One problem to solve is where to put the anchors and rodes necessary for serious cruising. In this, the 33 is typical of most boats her size.

One shortcoming on deck—again inherent in the design of the boat—is that there is no good way to permanently install a swim ladder. The conventional transom mount does not work well because of the traditional slope of the transom, and a permanent mount has not been devised for the port or starboard side gates. The company sells a handsome teak ladder as an option, but it has to be removed and stowed when underway.

Belowdecks

The interior of the Mason 33 does not look spacious. That's partly because it is quite "teaky" and fairly dark, but mostly because everything inside the boat is good sized, especially the storage spaces. We particularly like the roomy forepeak (which has all but disappeared on contemporary boats), the double hanging lockers, and the small hanging locker next to the companionway for wet gear (PAE's brochures say it's for "fowl" weather gear—duck hides, perhaps).

The galley has ample fiddled counters, good storage space, and a deep sink that works well under sail. At anchor, it's awkward in that the sole rises to follow the hull contour. The icebox is big enough and apparently well insulated, hot and cold pressure water are standard, and there are two water tanks for a total of 65 gallons. Opposite the galley is the navigation station, with an adequately sized chart table and a sort of "screen" bulkhead to protect charts and electronics from sea or rain water entering through the companionway. The electrical panel is beautiful.

Settees are port and starboard of a centerline table, and a pilot berth is available portside, though most owners will likely use the space for storage.

The head has a shower which drains into the sump tank, good storage space, and a decent wash basin.

The forward cabin is the owner's cabin, and the portside double berth is big and roomy. It should be comfortable at anchor or in mild conditions, but during heavy air passagemaking, the settees will have to be used for sleeping. The berthing arrangement makes it clear that the boat is primarily designed for a couple, with perhaps one or two children and only occasional guests.

Notable below is the joinerwork which is uniformly of good quality. Teak is almost everywhere—either veneered plywood or solid—with white Formica for contrast. Hatches and portholes provide excellent natural lighting, augmented by deck prisms. Ventilation is adequate, with a large dorade box and cowl forward exhausting the forward cabin and head, and ten opening ports as standard equipment. For passagemaking, a few more deck vents would be desirable.

CONCLUSIONS

While it is true that some people may not like the full-keel design of the boat, preferring a lighter, high performance hull; there is little to criticize in the Mason 33. Her construction is solid, her deck is well laid out with good equipment, her spars and sail-handling equipment are good quality, her interior is well laid out and well finished, the machinery and mechanical systems are made well and installed properly, and she's a good looking boat.

We can't even object to the price. She is expensive—the price will be well over $90,000 by the time you sail her away—but you will be buying a quality boat that should retain her value. When you look at her current French and American cousins coming off the production line at $70,000 to $80,000, it makes her price seem reasonable. There are few, if any, other boats of comparable quality in her size and price range.

For a sailor wanting a serious bluewater cruiser or a liveaboard boat in her size range, she is the logical choice. For others, wanting a coastal cruiser or a weekender/daysailer, she may be less practical—probably more boat than would be needed. Of course, many people buy not just a boat, but the dream of being able to take off at any moment and leave the boss and the rat race behind. The Mason is one of the few boats we've seen recently that is capable of fulfilling the dream.

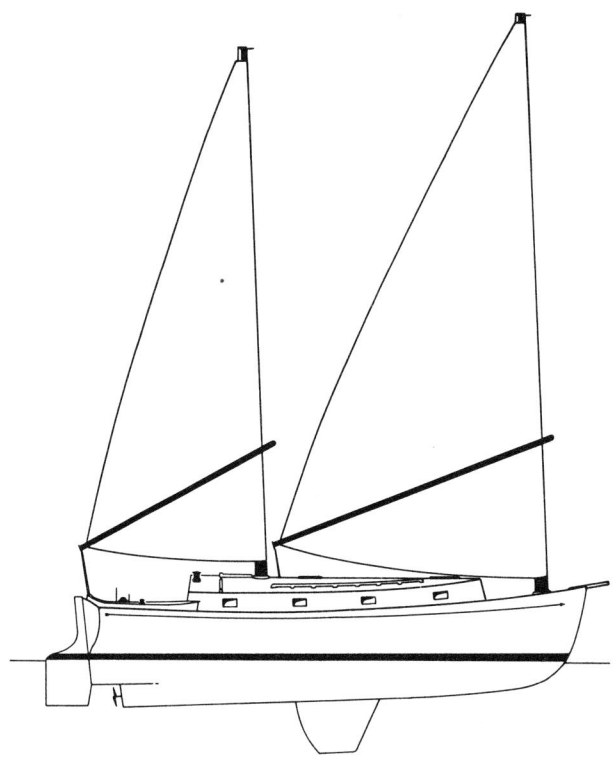

Specifications
Freedom 33

LOA	33'0"
LWL	30'0"
Beam	11'0"
Draft	
board up	3'6"
board down	6'0"
Displacement	12,000 lbs
Sail area	516 sq ft

Freedom Yachts
Bend Boat Basin
Portsmouth,
Rhode Island 02871
(401) 683-3500

The Freedom 33:
Selling a Concept

THE BOAT AND THE BUILDER

When a restless 40-year old advertising executive with a background in one-design sailing (1970 World Sunfish Champion) went shopping for a cruising boat some years ago, he could not find one that made him happy. He felt that conventional cruisers were poor performers, needlessly difficult to sail short-handed with their big headsails and complicated rigs, and with hull forms that demand auxiliary power any time the wind is forward of abeam.

It was in 1972 that this sailor, Garry Hoyt, set about to develop an alternative. His alternative was the original Freedom 40. Discarding conventions one by one, he came up with a long-waterline, quasi-traditional hull form, and a wishbone cat-ketch rig. Then, to prove he had something, he took his proto-type to Antigua Race Week and decisively out-performed the cruising boats with which he had been so unhappy. Granted, his talents as a sailor were considerably better than those of his competition, and granted, his prototype (without an engine) had no propeller or aperture drag. Nevertheless, his idea gained credibility.

In the intervening years, Hoyt refined his rig and developed a whole line of boats: a 21, 25, 28, 33 (express and pilothouse models), and the 44. The Freedom 33 is no longer produced, having been replaced in the lineup by the 32, a single masted "cat sloop" with a self-tacking jib and gun mount spinnaker. Today (fall of 1987) Freedom is building its line: the 28, 30, and 36, and planning to introduce a 42.

Good luck led Hoyt to Ev Pearson of Tillotson-Pearson when he went looking for a builder, and his background in advertising led him to create attention-getting explanations of his concept. His one notable weakness was in marketing. He tried to bring potential buyers to the boat, rather than putting together a dealer network which takes the boat to the public. Freedom later signed on dealers from coast to coast.

The U.S. builder, Tillotson-Pearson, was one of the most successful, low-profile boatbuilders during the 1970s. They put together such popular boats as the J-Boat line, and the Etchells 22 one-design. The firm was a leader in the development of balsa coring for hull structure, and carbon fiber for light, stiff laminates.

Unlike the situation with more conventional craft, selling the sailing public on the concept behind the Freedoms was a stiff challenge. The rig, in particular, was unfamiliar to most cruising sailors, and for the concept to gain acceptance, they needed education. Not only did they have to be convinced that stayless masts, wishbone booms, and wrap-around sails are durable, they literally had to be taught how to use them advantageously. For this reason, acceptance of the idea was mixed, and the appeal of the Freedom line was mainly to sailors a little more adventuresome than traditional.

CONSTRUCTION

The construction of the Freedom 33 hull and deck is, in our opinion, among the best in the production boat building industry. From our observation, as a result of examining boats both finished and under construction, we can detect no serious cost-cutting or scrimping in the way of materials or techniques.

The Freedom 33 (as with other boats in the Freedom line) has a balsa-cored hull and deck. There are advantages to this typical construction—hull rigidity, thermal and acoustical insulation, weight savings—that we believe recommends it for hull structure *provided it is properly engineered*. In the case of the Freedom 33, we believe it is.

Lead ballast, 3800 pounds, is cast in wedge-shaped pieces and fiberglassed in to the bilge. The aluminum fuel tank (25 gallons) is also deep in the bilge. The centerboard, a combination of lead and fiberglass, is a hefty 1200 pounds, also contributing to stability. The centerboard is the product of perhaps the most thoughtful design and engineering on the boat. It is pivoted in a channel, eliminating the need for a pin that breaches the hull. Hoyt, with his eye firmly on performance, adopted an idea of designer Jay Parris for a centerboard configuration having a triangular profile and a constant chord. The design permits a centerboard with a shape that gives lift at any angle and, more importantly in reducing drag, a centerboard that fits its slot closely.

The Freedom 33

If the centerboard is not the most extensively engineered feature of the Freedom 33, then the spars are. Initially the Freedom 33 had two-part aluminum tubular masts that were heavy, reducing stability and increasing pitching moment. To help cure this weakness, Tillotson-Pearson undertook a research program into building one-piece spars using a carbon-fiber laminate. The result is an approximate 30 percent savings in weight, and a considerably stiffer spar. The savings translated itself into markedly better performance, so much so that we suggest that any buyer considering a boat with stayless spars should look into spar weight and stiffness. And, incidentally, we also think stayless spars are the next most significant development in sailboat design.

Additional construction details of note on the Freedom 33 include a hull to deck joint through-fastened with 5/16-inch stainless steel bolts, and bonded with 3M 5200 adhesive sealant, a technique we recommend. Bulkheads are tabbed to the inside fiberglass skin, leaving the core intact to prevent hard spots from showing up on the topsides. The interior joinerwork, of attractive oak, ash, and spruce, is done to a high quality.

PERFORMANCE

Our evaluation of the performance of the Freedom 33 is, in part, the product of having spent a week sailing aboard the boat during Antigua Race Week. For comparison with that experience on the prototype, we recently sailed a production version, as well.

For those sailors used to masthead headsails and conventional mainsails with their sheeting, reefing, and halyard systems, the rig of the Freedom 33 does require some re-education. Initially one has the impression that the boat is under-rigged and that the sailplan is inefficient. That impression is, however, deceptive. The boat does have speed and liveliness that exceeds that of most out-and-out cruising boats of her size. In many conditions, she can rival the performance of the so-called racer-cruiser or "performance cruiser."

The mainsail and mizzen are efficient in that almost all their area forms an effective airfoil. The wishbone boom permits a longer luff than a conventional boom and does not interfere with the draft at the foot. The wishbone does create windage, though. Draft control is easier with a wishbone boom through either outhaul tension (the Freedom 33 mizzen) or adjustment of the effective

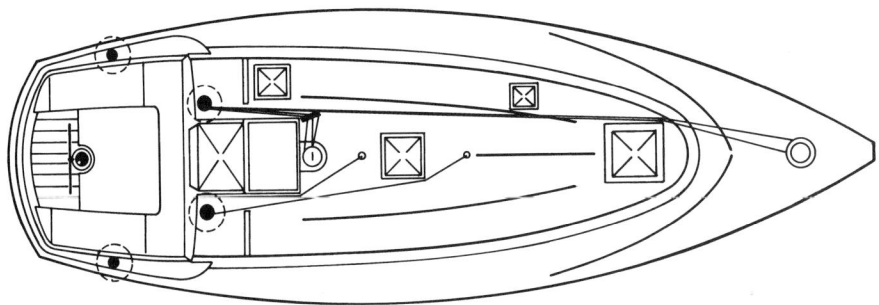

length of the wishbone (the mainsail). Similarly, the wrap-around sails are more aerodynamically efficient than sails set on a mast track or groove, which are, in part, blanketed by the spar section. Given the greater diameter of stayless spars versus conventional spars, the wrap-around system is important in this type of rig.

Proper sail shape, adjustment, and trim are as vital for this rig as for more conventional rigs. There are still some aspects of the Freedom rig about which we have reservations. But we believe the Freedom line has come closer to perfecting the system than any of its rivals boasting similar rigs. Incidentally, Ulmer Sails (in particular Ulmer sailmaker Bob Adams), has worked hard to develop Freedom sail shape, plus reefing and trimming systems, and we therefore urge buyers to order the sails offered as factory options, rather than trying to find another sailmaker who will have to go through the extensive design exercise needed to provide suitable sails.

The Freedom 33 is stiffer (and, we think, foot-for-foot faster) than her sisters in the Freedom line. Her sailplan gives optimum performance in a mid-range of wind strengths, about 10 to 15 knots. In winds below 10 knots, especially to windward in any chop, the stubby hull, with a centerboard and plenty of wetted surface, is sluggish. In fact, no Freedom is as lively as we would wish in lighter winds, a factor to consider in such areas as Chesapeake Bay and Puget Sound. For such conditions, we strongly recommend at least one mizzen staysail. Although we are not sold on poleless spinnakers for conventionally rigged cruising boats, we think they are superb as mizzen spinnakers on a boat like the Freedom 33.

The wishbone booms and stayless masts combine to make the Freedom a delightful boat to sail with the wind from astern. The absence of shrouds lets the mainsail (and boom) swing forward of abeam, encouraging her to sail wing and wing with the wind as much as 25 degrees or so off the quarter. Moreover, the sail stays out to windward in light winds without a preventer. Nor does it need a vang as the angle of the wishbone boom off the mast eliminates any tendency for the boom to lift. On a run, any sailor accustomed to dealing with blanketed headsails, mainsail chafe on shrouds, and the threat of an accidental jibe, will have to appreciate the Freedom rig.

Closewindedness is a relative term, but a major attraction of the better modern designs. The Freedom 33 is not closewinded. This is as much a result of her hull shape as her rig. However, she gives nothing upwind to boats with shallow hull forms and long keels. Boat for boat she will sail by Morgan 41s, Irwin 44s, CSY 44s, Westsails, and their ilk.

The Freedom rig uses a slab or jiffy reefing system. Instead of the reefed portion gathering above the boom (as with conventional sailplans), however, the excess material gathers at the wishbone in aerodynamically messy folds. It just isn't a rig that lends itself to simple, uncluttered reefing. We think finding combinations of reduced sail area (using staysails) would be a better solution than trying to reef main and mizzen. Yet the present rig seems to have proven

The Freedom 33
271

itself in offshore sailing. Several boats have made long passages without difficulty and weathered severe storms at sea with no breakdowns or crises.

The sails are two-ply, loosely connected at the leech. Furling is easy; the sail gathers into a basket formed of shockcord stretched across the wishbone. More shockcord across the top keeps the sail secured. The convenience of this system, obvious as it may be, is one of the major recommendations of the rig, doing away with the onerous chores of conventional mainsail furling and headsail folding and bagging.

In all, we have been favorably impressed with the performance of a boat that experience and instinct tells us should be poor. The wrap-around sails take getting used to, but the more we played with them, the more effective they seemed to be.

LIVABILITY

Deck Layout

There is no reason why anyone has to leave the cockpit of a Freedom 33 under sail. All halyards, sheets, outhauls, reefing pennants, and the centerboard pennant lead aft to the cockpit, where they are handled by a pair of self-tailing winches (Barient 23s) and an array of sheet stoppers. The cockpit is short enough that anyone handling these lines can also keep one hand close to the steering wheel—a boon for short-handed or singlehanded sailing.

The cockpit seating is deep and the coamings are unobstructed. Best of all, the cockpit space is entirely usable. Because the mizzen traveler is mounted aft, the Freedom 33 is a distinct rarity among production boats—a boat in which the traveler does not threaten to mash one's legs or the mainsheet to garrote the crew. This feature alone makes the cockpit of the Freedom noteworthy.

The steering pedestal is mounted well aft, the helmsman sits on a fold-up seat, or stands on a teak grate under which is the steering cable and quadrant for the outboard rudder. This grate also serves as the cockpit drain with scuppers through the transom—a most effective arrangement for quickly draining a flooded cockpit. A sliding door at the after end of the cockpit houses propane fuel bottles.

The deck and coachroof are uncluttered sundecks and lounging platforms. Sailors accustomed to stepping gingerly around a conventional deck may feel

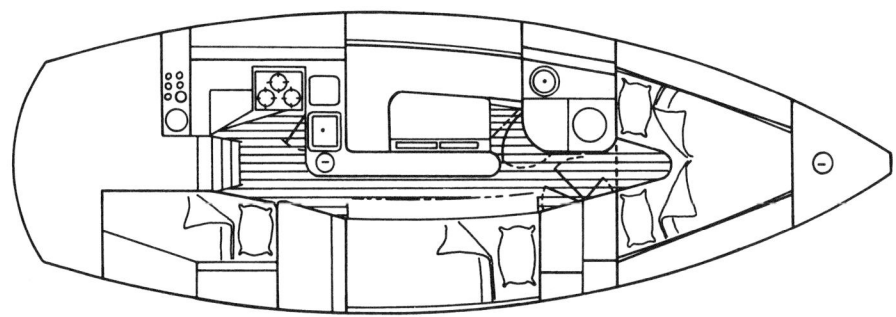

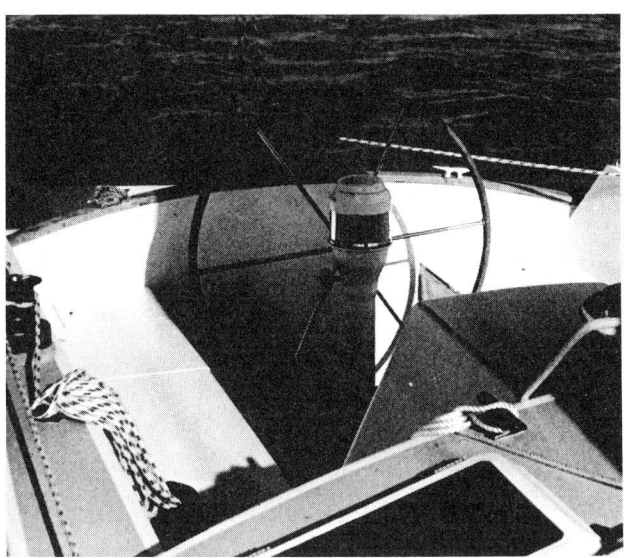
Usable space is a plus in the cockpit.

disoriented; missing are chainplates and shrouds, headsail sheets and blocks, and a spinnaker pole. The anchor cats in an optional fiberglass bowsprit. Good large chocks on either side of the bow, and amidships, are integrally fitted into the teak toerail.

Belowdecks

Garry Hoyt's reputation as a designer clearly lies in his ability to develop performance; it has not been in his ability to design a yacht interior. The 40-foot prototype originally appeared with a midship cockpit and an interior so broken up into sub-sections as to be almost unliveable. The public reaction to the interior layout, understandably, was less than favorable. Marketplace imperatives soon resulted in an alternate version with aft cockpit and a more versatile layout. The present Freedom 40 is a far more marketable product.

Similarly, the Freedom 33 was first designed with an aft cabin that reduced cockpit space, and a main cabin that succumbed to, rather than accommodated itself to, the centerboard trunk dividing it.

The later production version does away with the aft cabin; locates the galley conventionally at the base of the companionway; tucks a dinette (which is convertible to a double berth) to port of the trunk; and has a settee berth to starboard. The result is a main cabin laid out much like other production boats of comparable size.

By having her waterline stretched to almost the overall length of the hull, the 33 has exceptional roominess for her modest deck length. Moreover, with her mast stepped close to the stem, her hull fullness has to be carried well forward to support the weight. The forward cabin, with its V-berths, is the beneficiary. Farther aft, the roominess is deceptive. The main cabin is broken up by a five-foot-long, waist high centerboard trunk running down the middle, with the mizzen mast rising up at its after end.

Had Hoyt not had his eyes so focused on performance, he might have opted for a longer, shallower centerboard, permitting a lower trunk that could be located where it would intrude less into the main cabin. As it is, the centerboard does offer minimum drag, does not "thunk" annoyingly in the trunk, and is rugged. It also requires a trunk that makes casual conversation awk-

The Freedom 33

ward to impossible, and creates a cul-de-sac in the dinette, leaving the person on the inside with no convenient way to get out.

The aesthetic impression created by the interior joinerwork is among the best we've seen on any production boat. All the wood below—and there is plenty— is a combination of oak, ash, and spruce (plus the teak and holly cabin sole). We have long been critical of interior decor relying on dark woods such as teak and mahogany. The mellow warmth and the illusion of spaciousness imparted by these blond woods will appeal to many sailors.

There is a place for teak below. Grab rails, companionway treads, the framing around hatches, and the trim in the head (all areas vulnerable to wear and moisture) would be better in teak than in woods like ash and oak, which are subject to staining. Moreover, oak is less dimensionally stable than teak, so moisture might eventually effect the structure as well as the finish.

The comfortably wide quarterberth to starboard has little overhead footroom. The pilot berth to starboard is accessible only to a person shorter than four feet and weighing less than forty pounds. It is either a luxuriously cushioned shelf, or a berth for an agile ship's cat. Both the chart table and the cleverly designed dinette table need removable fiddles, and the hinges on the chart table lid would be better recessed.

On the positive side, the stowage capacity of the Freedom 33 is far and away the best we've seen on a boat of this size. In particular, the huge galley drywell, incorporating a sliding section for seldom-used items, is unsurpassable. The engine (a Yanmar 3GM diesel) under the companionway is well above average in accessibility. Another nice feature is that the forward cabin can be completely closed off from the rest of the interior (and the head) by its own door.

The Freedom 33 thus offers an intriguing dichotomy—impressive and inventive with innovative decor and layout—offset to a disturbing extent by drawbacks that might justifiably turn off buyers.

CONCLUSIONS

The Freedom 33 is an interesting boat. She is, however, not a conventional boat, and the concept behind her rig takes getting used to. Sailors born and raised in the tradition of headsails, standing rigging, mainsails that ride on tracks, hulls with overhangs and aesthetic proportions (and other such quaint qualities) might feel uneasy.

The base price of $69,900 in 1980 was steep for a 33-foot boat. With sails, plus other options and amenities, the bottom line would have been at least $75,000. However, when measured against other boats of comparable waterline length and displacement, the price is more understandable (but still high). Comparably equipped, a better quality conventional production boat (such as a Sabre 34 or Cal 35) would run $65,000 to $70,000.

With used 1980 Freedom 33s bringing about $60,000, it is clear that the boats in the Freedom line continue to retain their value over the years. As long as the concepts she represents continue to gain new followers, she should be in the forefront of boats of her type.

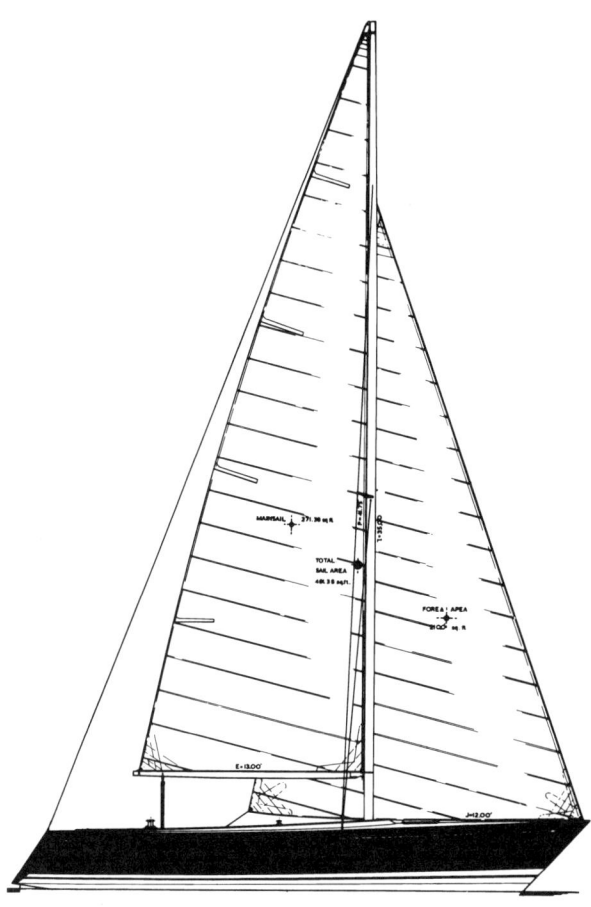

Specifications
Tartan Ten

LOA	33'2"
LWL	27'0"
Beam	9'3"
Draft	5'10"
Displacement	6700 lbs
Ballast	3340 lbs
Sail area	486 sq ft

Tartan Marine
320 River Street
Grand River, Ohio 44045
(216) 354-5671

The Tartan Ten:
A Performance One-Design

THE BOAT AND THE BUILDER

The Tartan Ten was born out of a popular rebellion against the International Offshore Rule (IOR) in the mid-1970's. This was the worst period in the IOR's history, when production sailboats were obsolete, even before their molds had jelled. Although the IOR has since straightened up its act, many of its early supporters had abandoned ship (for good) by 1979. The disenchanted went in one of two directions—PHRF or one-design.

The Tartan Ten is the brainchild of Charlie Britton of Tartan Marine. Britton was one of the first to recognize the market for offshore one-designs. While he was conceptualizing the Tartan Ten, the J/24 (soon to become the most successful offshore one-design) was being tooled up for production—although Britton knew nothing of its existence. He had been impressed by the Danish-built Aphrodite 101 and it's not coincidence that the Tartan Ten bears a resemblance to the Aphrodite. Sparkman & Stevens designed the boat for Tartan in 1977 and production began in early 1978.

Nearly 350 boats were built in the next five years, most of which went to sailors on the Great Lakes, and most of which spend the bulk of their time racing one-design. There are over 200 boats in the national class association, and 80 percent of these race in one-design fleets on Lake Erie and Lake Michigan. According to class secretary David Hamister, there is one-design racing every weekend on Lake Erie, and small fleets at Houston, Long Island Sound, Chesapeake Bay, and Jacksonville. Unlike a great many boats that tout themselves as one-designs, the Tartan Ten is one of the few boats that has accumulated in large enough numbers to actually *race* as a one-design.

When the Tartan Ten was introduced in 1978 (at a base price of $21,500), she sold easily. Several boats a week were produced in the years immediately following. Then, a steady series of price increases, the recession of 1981, and the first signs of a saturated market began to take their toll. For Charlie Britton—a boatbuilder first and a business man second—the problems of running so large a business was more than he wished to handle. So in the spring of 1982, production of the Tartan Ten ceased and Britton put his company up for sale. By the spring of 1983, he found a buyer in John Richards, and production began again at the rate of two Tartan Tens a month. However, only a few dealers are actually stocking the boat. Most boats are built only to order.

Company involvement in the Tartan Ten is, for the most part, exemplary. The only complaints we received were from sailors outside the Midwest who complained that the company's promotional efforts were biased toward the Great Lakes. Both Britton, who stayed on with Tartan as a consultant, and new owner Richards, own and race Tartan Tens. Marketing Manager Pat Black also sails a Tartan Ten. Owners report that Tartan is quick to settle warranty problems and to rectify construction flaws to prevent future warranty claims. Typical of comments from owners are, "I've called for advice on a number of occasions, and was always given courteous and useful information" and "I can't praise the people at Tartan Marine enough."

The 1987 base price of the Tartan Ten is $40,190. With a one-design sail inventory (main, jib, and spinnaker), spinnaker gear, cradle, genoa tracks, compasses, and double lifelines the price climbs proportionally. Most owners report that their used Tartan Tens have appreciated. The exception was an owner in Chicago who said a glut of used boats was keeping the price down.

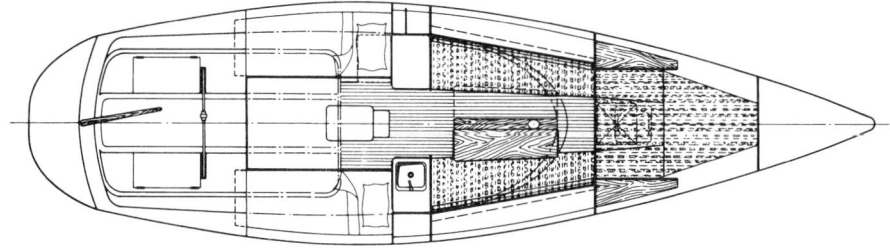

The Complete Book of Sailboat Buying, Volume II

CONSTRUCTION

While we would consider the Tartan Ten to be one of the better built racers, she doesn't have to be. Since she is primarily intended to race against her sisters, consistency between boats is perhaps more important than superior (and hence, more expensive) construction. The major construction criterion she must meet is to be sufficiently seaworthy to endure an occasional short off-shore race. She meets this criterion, although like many production boats, she barely meets it.

There have been a number of problems with the Tartan Ten over the years. Tartan Marine has generally acted responsibly in correcting them. The worst problems occurred in the first 100 boats. For example, the original hollow stainless steel rudder posts were too light and bent too easily. According to Tartan, every boat with that type of rudder post was located and repaired by inserting a second post inside the original one.

A second problem was with the reinforcement of the hull around the keel sump and under the mast step. From 5 feet forward of the transom, the Tartan Ten's hull is cored with 1/2-inch balsa, except in the bilge area, which is stiffened by a grid of hollow, hat-shaped, fiberglass floors and stringers. Because the Tartan Ten has a relatively flat underbody and fin keel, she is more susceptible to flexing of the bilges than a boat with deeper, more rounded bilges.

In the first 90 boats, the grid was neither stiff enough, nor attached to the hull securely enough, to prevent flexing. As a result, the fiberglass tabbing (which holds the grid to the hull) began peeling off. On a few boats, small cracks

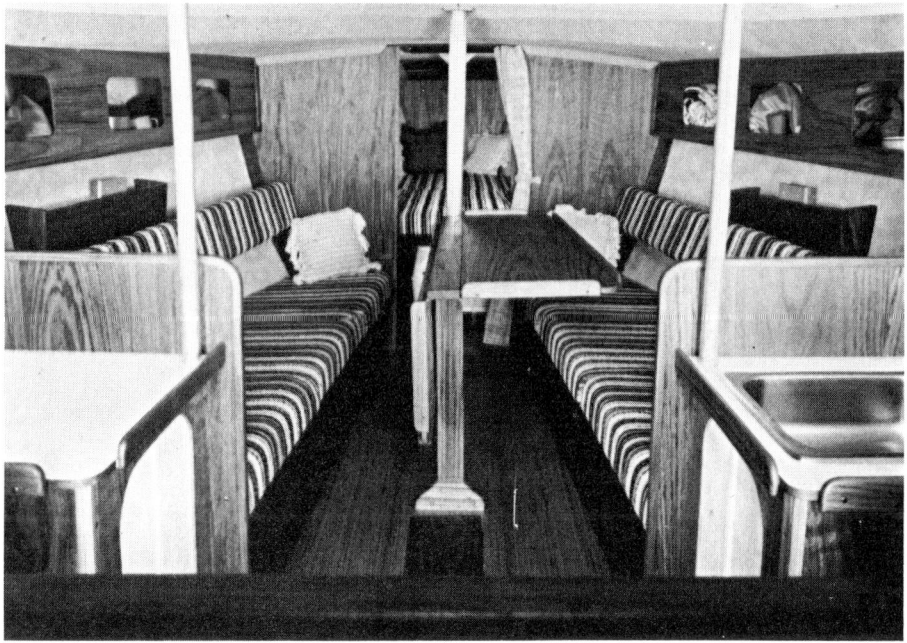

The Tartan Ten

developed in the grid and in the bilges. Tartan claims that it sent repairmen all around the country to track down and fix every boat earlier than hull #84. In most cases, the repair consisted of removing the old tabbing and re-tabbing with a heavier laminate. In cases where the grid or hull actually showed damage, more substantial repairs were made. According to Britton, "We got every one of them."

The mast step has been strengthened several times during the Tartan Ten's history. The Tartan Ten has a deck-stepped mast, rare in non-trailerable racers because they offer less control of mast-bend. They are no less seaworthy than a keel-stepped mast, provided there is adequate support below the mast, such as a compression post, or bulkhead in the cabin.

The Tartan Ten's compression post sits atop the floor grid. After the initial problems with the first 83 boats, a 1/4-inch aluminum plate was inserted under the compression post to distribute the load. The thickness of this aluminum plate was later increased to 1/2-inch. Mast step problems still existed, to some degree, after the first 83 boats. On a hull numbered in the 150s, we observed that the compression post had been moved off the floor grid (presumably because it was crushing it) and lengthened with a threaded extension so it rested directly on the hull.

Unlike most boats, which have chainplates extending above deck, the Tartan Ten's shrouds pass through the deck, to chainplates in the cabin. Although this may reduce windage and genoa chafe, the hole in the deck is difficult to seal. Many owners report chronic deck leaks around the shrouds. The chainplates

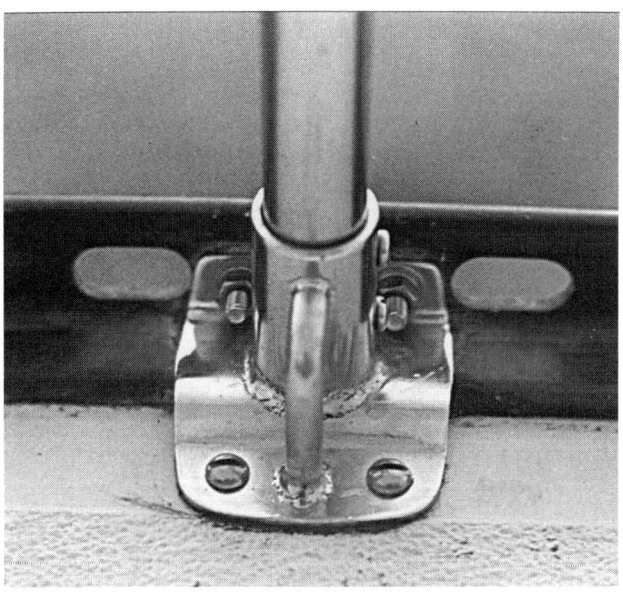

are anchored on a heavy fiberglass "tab" which extends up from the topsides inside the main cabin. According to the manufacturer, there were two chainplate tab delaminations in the first 100 boats. Tartan attributes this to the hull being cored under the tab. Tartan didn't take steps to correct the potential problem until nearly 100 boats later. One owner of a 150-series boat reported that he had reglassed one chainplate tab after he no-

Stanchion bases are rigidly bolted to both the toerail and deck, but several owners reported weld failures where the socket is fastened to the base.

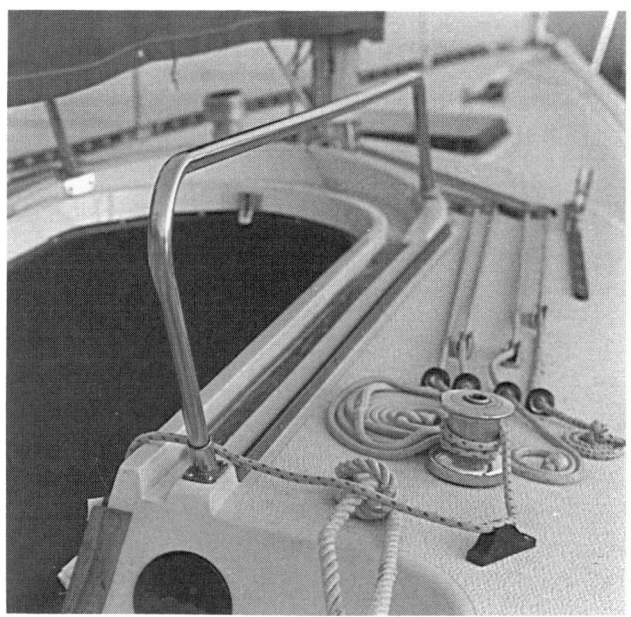

ticed the telltale signs of delamination—the color of the tab changing from dark green to white where it is anchored to the hull.

By hull #200, Tartan had eliminated the core under the tab and began anchoring it directly to the outer skin of the hull. This didn't completely solve the problem, according to Britton. Because the section of the topsides around the chainplates was uncored, that section could dimple slightly inward under heavy rig loads, causing isolated incidences of gelcoat cracking and delamination. Tartan corrected this problem shortly afterward ("about hull #270," according to Britton) by widening the chainplate tab from 12 to 18 inches.

Large companionway is covered by a three-piece removable hatch, and protected from errant feet by full-length handrails. When opened, the companionway provides the cabin with a minimal amount of headroom.

Although the Tartan Ten is cored through 80 percent of her hull, she exhibits a fair amount of structural flexing. As one successful Tartan dealer pointed out, "she's not overbuilt like the rest of the Tartan line." We had several reports of the cockpit flexing noticeably while sailing in rough weather. Part of the reason is that the bulkheads under each side of the cockpit are glassed firmly to the hull, but very poorly to the cockpit seats. Also, the main bulkhead is well forward of the mast, and divided by the forward berth. A bulkhead in two halves, located some distance from the chainplates, is not a very effective means of absorbing rig loads.

The Tartan Ten's hull to deck joint consists of an inward-turned hull flange, overlapped by the deck, and topped by an aluminum toerail. The joint is bedded with butyl tape, which stays soft and rubbery for the life of the boat. It has no adhesive properties but is a good watertight sealant. (We've also seen it melt and bleed out of hull to deck joints on occasion.)

A strip of aluminum is glassed under the hull flange. This allows Tartan to fasten the hull and deck with bolts (but without nuts) by tapping the bolts through the aluminum insert—a real time saver. The bolts must be bedded, though, or corrosion could compromise the integrity of the joint, especially important since there is no chemical bond to fall back on. Tartan beds the bolts with silicone, which is probably adequate, but a chromate paste would be a better (although more expensive) bedding material.

The hull laminate was strengthened when production was into hulls numbered in the early 100's. A heavier mat was added to improve the bond between the balsa core and the laminate. An extra layer of fiberglass was added to the hull laminate as well.

The mast of the Tartan Ten is a "safe" section. It bends easily with the backstay, but is sufficiently strong to sail without running backstays in a strong breeze. The shrouds are swept back.

The mast is not anodized. Until recently it was finished with clear lacquer. Now it is painted black. According to Frank Colaneri of Bay Sailing Equipment—who rigged all early Tartan masts—finishing with lacquer or paint is cheaper than anodizing.

On the first 150 or so boats, the jib and spinnaker halyards were wire, and exited the mast above the hounds. They then led through "bull's eye" fairleads, which have a tendency to chew the wire. (Colaneri called them "wire eaters"). This system was redesigned so the wire jib halyard now exits below the mast without a fairlead, and the spinnaker halyard (still exiting above the hounds) has been changed to rope.

Schaefer booms were used on the first 70 boats, and bent reefing hooks were a problem. Since then, Tartan has used Kenyon booms. The Kenyon booms have no outhaul car, relying instead on clew slugs to support leech tension. According to Colaneri, many booms had to be retrofitted with stainless steel plates over the sail slot because the clew slugs had pulled through the slot.

The mast of the Tartan Ten is currently rigged with a gate to accommodate luff slides. Before boat #175, the gate position accommodated a bolt rope.

PERFORMANCE

Handling Under Power
Since hull #309, the Tartan Ten has been equipped with an 11 horsepower Universal diesel. Before then, a Farymann 7.5 horsepower diesel was standard. On boats prior to hull #200, excessive vibration and shaft coupling failures were a problem. According to Britton, the cause was poor shaft alignment. Britton says flexible shaft couplings were used on the first 200 boats because Tartan was afraid the boat would bend under rig tension. The use of flexible couplings meant less attention was paid to alignment, hence occasional coupling failure and excessive vibration. Solid couplings were used on subsequent boats. "We thought we were bending the boat (by tensioning the rig), but we were wrong. Now we know it's better to concentrate on alignment and use solid shaft couplings," says Britton. Because vibration could be a problem, when considering a used Tartan Ten you should check both the engine mounts and the electrical harness on the back of the engine. The covering of any wires attached to the engine should be checked for wear.

Tartan Ten owners report that the Farymann is relatively trouble-free, runs well, and is easy to hand-start should the battery run down. Owners also say it tends to be underpowered. "Doesn't do well into the wind," reported one owner. A folding prop is standard equipment.

Access to the engine is excellent. The fiberglass engine box is light and lifts off easily, and because it also doubles as the companionway step, slides forward without obstruction. The box is easy to refit and latch in place. With the box off, all engine parts are accessible.

Handling Under Sail

Tartan Ten owners rave about her performance. She may not be a ULDB, but she's fast for a 33-footer. Typical comments are, "Offwind we pass 36-foot masthead rigs," "rides the waves well, good control downwind," and "recorded 15 knots—sustained 10.5 knots."

However, owners do not rave about her handicap ratings. The Tartan Ten was not designed to fit any handcapping rule. She carries an astronomical IOR rating of about 28.5. Under PHRF she rates from 123 to 132, depending on the handicapper. Most PHRF fleets assume that you have a 155-percent genoa, and the most common rating is 126. Some fleets, such as Detroit, allow the Tartan Ten to sail with its one-design inventory (100% jib) at a rating several seconds slower.

Owners report that she will sail to a rating of 126 in light air with a 155-percent genoa. However, with her narrow beam, she is tender and becomes overpowered quickly. In winds over 12 knots, she has difficulty winning with a rating of 126. Using a one-design inventory, the Tartan Ten will sail to a rating of 132 in medium winds. Although she is always fast downwind, owners say she has a difficult time making up what she loses upwind in a strong breeze.

Those who want to race both one-deign and PHRF have several problems. Until 1982, headfoils were illegal for class racing. The class has dropped this rule to encourage Tartan Ten owners to race PHRF. Running backstays are still illegal for class racing. Although they're not necessary to keep the spar in the boat, backstays nonetheless will improve performance slightly without rating penalty. Another, more subtle problem, is that a sailmaker will design the working sails of a class inventory differently than he would for a larger inventory. For example, a 100% jib that must be used for both light and heavy air in one-design racing will be more powerful than a 100% jib for a larger PHRF inventory.

Despite its drawbacks, the Tartan Ten still makes for enjoyable PHRF racing because its sailplan is so manageable, the boat is so maneuverable, and its cockpit is so easy to work when you're racing one. The boat feels much smaller.

As good as PHRF racing can be, one-design racing is even better. Owners report that all boats are extremely well-matched. Before each boat leaves the factory, it is placed in an outdoor pool, and 50 to 100 pounds of lead are glassed to the hull, five inches forward of the mast, to make her float on her lines. Flotation marks are molded into the hull to insure that this lead is not subsequently moved to change the boat's trim. This helps make the boats equal in performance.

The keels are relatively fair from the factory, although most racers will want to spend a weekend making them smoother. The class association has published the keel offsets for those who want to make templates.

Most Tartan Tens race with a crew of 5 to 8. Although she is a light boat, her narrow beam limits the effectiveness of crew weight. Unlike beamier counterparts (such as the J/30) packing on more crew in a strong breeze is not really essential.

For best performance, the backstay and traveler must be constantly adjusted. Some of the more successful racers routinely barber-haul the jib outboard in strong puffs. As with any light displacement boat, you must be quick on sail trim to keep her level and driving.

LIVABILITY

Deck Layout

The Tartan Ten is equipped with a tiller, as any boat this small and light should be. With a tiller, though, you need a larger cockpit. The cockpit of the Tartan Ten is 9-1/2 feet long, which gives the crew plenty of room for racing. The companionway, though, is obstructed by long stainless steel handrails. When tacking, the crew must all pass through the cockpit.

The cockpit seats have short, outward-angled seatbacks with a small coaming. This provides a modicum of daysailing comfort without sacrificing much racing efficiency. The slotted aluminum toerail, does, however, compromise

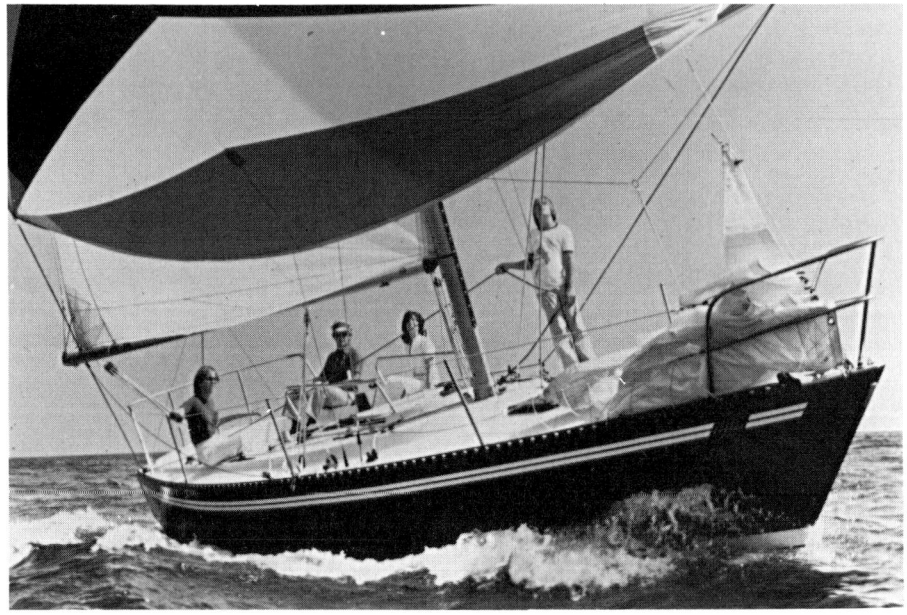

racing comfort. The crew could slide farther outboard for more hiking leverage if it weren't for the toerail painfully biting into the backs of their thighs.

Owners report that the cockpit drains quickly when pooped by a large wave. It nevertheless is worrisome, because its large volume would hold a lot of water, and its 6-inch companionway sill would do little to keep that water from rushing below. We wouldn't race it in rough weather without all companionway drop boards locked in place.

The rudder post exits the deck through a cockpit coaming that wraps around the stern. The tiller is attached to this post. When lifted and lashed to the backstay, it leaves the cockpit unobstructed, for an extraordinary amount of space when moored.

The mast is stepped into a cast aluminum collar on deck. The collar is not hinged. The running rigging exits through the bottom of the mast, then runs through sheaves built into the collar and aft through sheet stoppers to Lewmar 16s on each side of the cabin house. Several owners said they had moved or replaced the stoppers made by Delta. Tartan has plans to begin rigging boats with Easylock clutch stoppers, a far superior choice.

The primary winches are Lewmar 30s. Secondary winches are permitted under class rules, but are not offered as a factory option. Some owners report that larger primary winches are helpful to trim the genoas used for handicap racing. On the boat we sailed, the genoa tracks were backed with strips of aluminum, but the backing plates for the winches were 1/8-inch plywood.

The non-skid on the deck provides good traction, but also makes it more difficult to clean. Stanchion bases, made for Tartan by High Seas, bolt through the deck and through the toerail. On one boat we examined, there were no backing plates on the through-deck stanchion bolts, but bolting through the toerail gives the installation adequate rigidity. Several owners reported that the welded sockets for the stanchions have failed.

The boom vang runs in a single part, up from the mast step to the boom, then forward to the gooseneck, down to the deck via a 6:1 purchase, and aft to a winch. At the gooseneck, it attaches to a small welded eye, which could be of heavier gauge.

The backstay is split with a 4:1 purchase dead-ended on the stern. A crewmember would have to sit aft of the helmsman to play the backstay. The ball-bearing traveler spans the cockpit and is easily adjusted with its 3:1 purchase. The 5 :1 mainsheet dead-ends on the traveler car.

Belowdecks

For a 33-footer, there isn't much to the Tartan Ten's interior. Headroom is only 5 feet, 2 inches. However, the companionway hatch is in three pieces and lifts off for stowage below, opening a 5-foot-long "skylight" in the cabin. This feature provides some amount of standing headroom below without having to sacrifice the clean lines of the deck to a high cabin trunk. Erecting a dodger over the companionway encloses the standing headroom. The hatch cover could be stronger—we nearly cracked it by stepping on it. There is no icebox in the cabin. A portable cooler stores in one of the two cockpit lazarettes. The standard head is a portable toilet, stowed under the forward V-berth. Nearly every owner we talked to complained of its smell and that it is difficult to empty. Most had either discarded it for a cedar bucket or installed a full marine head. There is no built-in stove and the chart table is small.

There is a small sink with a hand pump on the port side. On boats prior to hull #200, the water tank was installed under the starboard quarterberth, with the fuel tank under the port quarterberth. With the water tank and sink on opposite sides, all the water in the tank could drain out through the sink on port tack. Tartan's retrofit was a rubber plug for the sink nozzle. By hulls numbered in the early 200's, they had switched the position of the fuel and water tanks, solving the problem.

The interior of the Tartan Ten is dark. The bulkhead, cabinetry, and cabin sole are teak-veneered plywood. We would paint the settees white. The forward V-berth is a comfortable 6 feet long. The "filler," or section of the berth that covers the Porta Potti, is removable for access to the head. However, the filler sits on very narrow cleats, so when you climb over it to get out of the berth, the filler frequently falls off its cleats and you tumble onto the head.

Vertical posts from the overhead, to both the sink and the navigation station, make good handrails for moving about below in a seaway. Under both the sink and nav station are small lockers with zippered cloth covering instead of doors.

There is further stowage under the settee berths and quarterberths. These stowage bins are not insulated from the hull, but because the boat is cored, condensation should be minimal. The bins are sealed from the shallow sump, preventing water in the bilge from soaking their contents. One owner com-
mented to us, "There should have been no attempt to create six berths at the expense of adequate storage."

On the boat we sailed, the joinerwork and furniture tabbing were mediocre. The overhead panels also were sloppily fitted.

The ceiling is covered with a padded vinyl liner. A strip of wood covers the hull to deck joint.

There were several major changes to the interior after hull

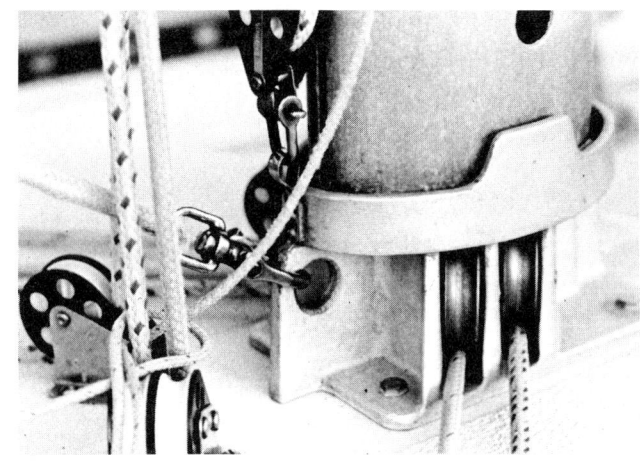

The mast is deck-stepped into an aluminum casting. The step has integral sheaves through which the running rigging exits, eliminating exit holes that compromise the mast's integrity.

#160. In earlier boats, both the settee berths and quarterberths were "root" berths. Root berths are anchored to the side of the hull and slung to a pipe running the length of the berth. The pipe fits into notches so the angle of the berth can be adjusted to suit the boat's angle of heel. Another piece of cloth attaches with Velcro to the pipe to form a seat back. While the root berths make for comfortable sleeping underway, they are far less comfortable than a fixed berth for sitting while the boat is anchored.

After hull #160, the roof berths in the main cabin were abandoned for fixed berths, with a dual purpose design backrest/leeboard. Additional stowage bins were added over the berths. A drop-leaf table was also added between the settee berths. It is doubtful whether it would survive the rough and tumble of hard racing. We suspect most owners remove it for racing.

CONCLUSIONS

Like any boat, the Tartan Ten is built to a price for a particular purpose. She is not built as well, nor laid out as lavishly as a J/30, but she also costs $10,000 less. People don't buy Tartan Tens to make long offshore passages, nor do they buy them for extended cruising. People buy them to day race, either as one-designs, or under one of the handicap rules. Occasionally, they might weekend cruise.

The Tartan Ten is a joy to day-race. It is easy to maneuver and crew on, offers lively performance, and is affordable. We think that one-design racing would be far more fun than handicap racing. At least, under one-design, you are competitive in all wind velocities. The Tartan Ten class association appears to be well organized, which should help keep the resale value of the boat high. If you live near a Tartan Ten fleet, you should give offshore one-design racing a try. But beware: you'll probably get hooked.

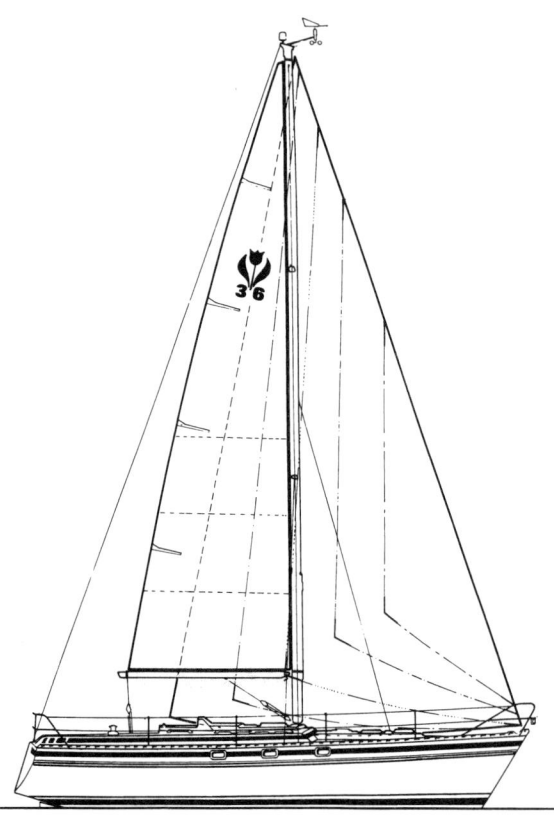

Specifications
Contest 36

LOA	35'10"
LWL	29'2"
Beam	11'8"
Draft	
fin keel	6'3"
shoal keel	5'5"
Displacement	15,969 lbs
Ballast	6475 lbs
Sail area	
masthead rig	733 sq ft
7/8 rig	701 sq ft

Conyplex
Overleek 7
1671 GD
Medemblik, Holland

The Contest 36:
A Dutch Treat

THE BOAT AND THE BUILDER

Contest is the principal brand name for sailboats produced by Conyplex, an old-line Dutch company located in Medemblik, Holland. Originally a supplier of fine woods and marine plywood, Conyplex first became incidentally involved in sailboat production in the 1950s by supplying wooden parts for the 20-foot Flying Dutchman daysailer.

With the advent of fiberglass, Conyplex produced glass molds as well as wood parts for other companies before it started building on its own. The U.S. connection began through exporting the Flying Dutchman to a Connecticut businessman, Arie van Breems. Van Breems has continued the import business since then, now with his son Martinus, and their 25 years as exclusive importer for Conyplex must be an American record for longevity in the boat import business.

The van Breems' association with Contest is more than as an importer: he originally approached Conyplex with plans for a small cruising boat and eventually provided the designs and molds for what became the first Contest—the

25, a roomy (for her era) and ruggedly built sloop that enjoyed a modest, but successful production run in the 1960s.

Since the 25, Conyplex has been building increasingly larger cruising sailboats in a variety of models. Their popularity in the U.S. has been steady, and somewhat less dependent on favorable currency exchange rates than other European boats. Customer loyalty is high with considerable repeat business. The repeat business is apparently based on good service by the importer. For example, the price of a new boat includes commissioning anywhere in the U.S., as well as sail and power trials by van Breems with the owner.

The Contests 29, 30, and 31 (all out of production now) were the most popular models from the late 60s to the early 80s. The current Contest line is made up of 32-, 34-, 38-, 41-, 44-, 48-, 56-, and 64-footers. Conyplex's total production of just over 5,000 Contest boats since 1960 shows that they have continued as a small yard, especially compared to the European megabuilders, Beneteau and Jeanneau.

All of the company's sales brochures state that the boats are "built according to Lloyd's rules in the Lloyd's-approved Conyplex factory," a statement of dubious significance. The company does submit construction drawings and undertakes the other initial steps, but all that is only preliminary to having a boat built under Lloyd's survey. When we contacted Lloyd's about it, their response was unequivocal: "Lloyd's does not approve workshops. We accept workshops as suitable environments in which we would carry out the survey of a hull being molded to our certification. This 'acceptance' is only valid for the hull or hulls actually under survey at the time." The Contests could be surveyed for Lloyd's certification (as *could* most any boat), but the importer said that none of the boats he has sold had ever received a Lloyd's certificate.

The Contest 36 was designed by Dick Zaal, who is responsible for all of the current Contest models. The 36 began life as the Contest 35 in 1982, but a new deck molding and design modifications stretched her overall length to 35 feet, 10 inches, and she was rechristened the Contest 36 in 1985. The boat we examined was hull number 229, which is the 40th Contest 36. (We don't understand their numbering system either.)

The 36 is "conventionally modern;" a bit heavy and full-bodied, but otherwise a moderate cruising design. She is distinctive for having a raised deck with almost no cabin house; the hull-deck joint is nearly a foot below the sheerline. Some people will consider her too high-sided to be attractive. But the flush decks add interior volume, and the boats all come with sheer stripes and rub rails to help diminish the "Winnebago look."

Apparently a selling point for the Contest 36 is the wing keel option, advertised as providing shoal draft without sacrificing performance. The boat is available with a modern fin keel (six-foot, three inches draft) or a longer, conventional shoal draft keel (five-foot, five inches draft), as well as the winged keel (four-foot, six inches draft). The wing keel was designed by Dr. Peter van Oossanen at the Netherlands Ship Model Basin. Not surprisingly, it looks similar to the keel he developed for the Australian 12-Meter which won the 1983 America's Cup.

CONSTRUCTION

The hull is a conventional fiberglass layup of mat and roving, having a core of end-grain balsa, with solid glass where bronze seacocks are installed. Isophthalic gelcoat is used, as is an iso resin for the first layer of glass behind the gelcoat. The isophthalic resins increase the builder's resin costs about 10 percent, but the current theory is that they are more resistant to water, so osmotic blistering should be reduced.

The gelcoat generally looks good and is fair with no evident hard spots. Where the glass is bare inside the hull, it is covered in white resin with blue splatter specks. Although there are a few rough edges inside some of the cabinetry, the glass work throughout the boat seems workmanlike.

As is typical of many European boats, the external keels are cast iron, bolted onto the hull. Inside the hull, the keelboats are glassed over, and most are inaccessible without tearing up the cabin sole—a potential problem in case of a hard grounding. The keel, coated with epoxy paint and anti-fouling, is a bit rough—not as fair as a racing sailor would require—and after one season there will be rust spots that need grinding and refinishing.

In the wing-keel version, the cast iron offers one advantage over lead, which would otherwise be preferable: the boat can stand upright on her keel, the wings serving as supports like training wheels on a bicycle. In fact, during construction, the wing-keel models stand on their keels with only a single poppet supporting the bow.

The deck layup is similar to the hull, with plywood substituting for balsa core underneath deck hardware. The raised deck makes the hull to deck joint peculiar. The deck molding overlaps the hull by about four inches and is mechanically attached to the hull with aluminum rivets. A teak rubrail is put outside the joint and also riveted to the hull/deck overlap. The inside of the joint is then overlaid with fiberglass.

The joint is strong, but there are two problems. First, damage is a bit more likely at the joint because the teak rubrail (and a stainless rubbing strake screwed to it) will take most of the impact of the hull bouncing off pilings and docks. Second, the damage will be difficult to repair.

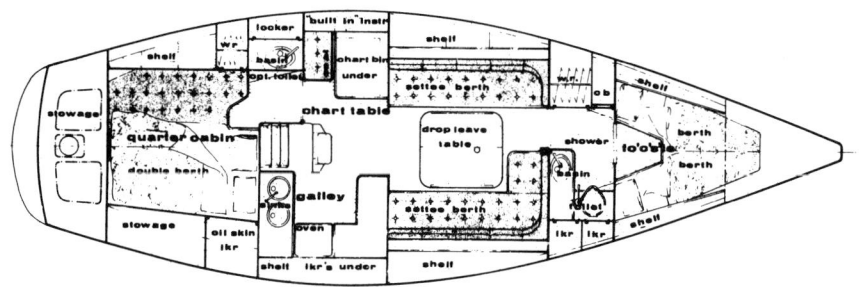

The Complete Book of Sailboat Buying, Volume II

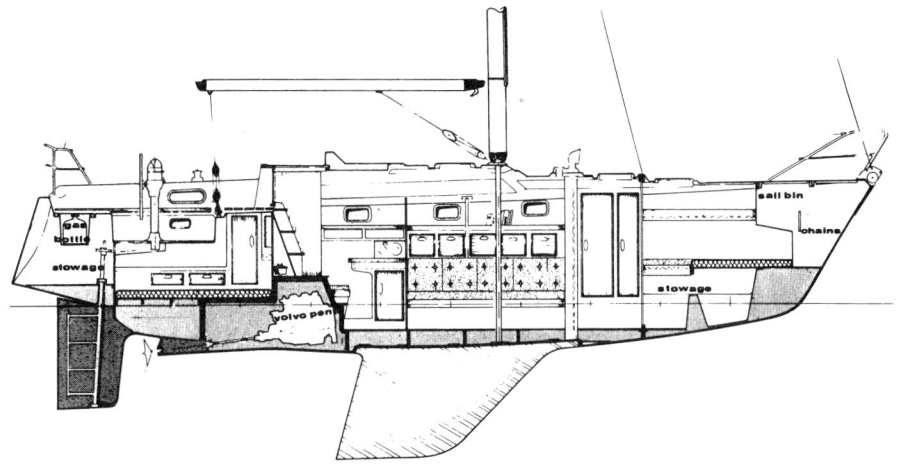

Unlike the more customary procedure, major interior pieces, including the bulkheads, are installed after the deck is attached to the hull and the joint is fiberglassed. The interior of the hull is covered partially by a fiberglass headliner, partially by teak plywood, partially by carpeting. Although sections of the headliner were removable under some of the deck hardware, many of the through-bolts were inaccessible. This might be an acceptable practice under some hardware, but it is disconcerting to note that the bolts for highly-loaded hardware, like the halyard stoppers and the deck-mounted halyard winches, are totally hidden. Any loosening of the bolts will require cutting out and replacing a section of headliner, hardly a good construction practice.

In contrast to what we judge as average hull and deck construction are the mechanical systems which are well above average. Some of the electrical wiring is hidden behind the hull liner, but the electrical work is good with soldered connections everywhere. The water tanks and plumbing systems are neat and secure, and the propane tank and its copper tubing are well installed. The Volvo Penta three-cylinder diesel, stainless steel fuel tank, and muffler are well installed. The Whitlock wheel steering is a bit unusual in that there are solid steering rods with universal joints rather than wire cables.

All the mechanical systems have a general appearance of neatness and craftsmanship. One reason for the good mechanical work may be the long list of standard equipment—you don't end up with different components installed in different ways. For example, two 12-volt batteries are standard, two bilge pumps are standard, the shower sump pump is standard—and all come ready installed. The mechanical work makes the Contest distinctive from most other production sailboats we've seen.

The interior woodwork is also well done in teak-faced plywood. All the wood was varnished, glossy in the head and satin-sheen elsewhere. The joinery is somewhat better than typical American pre-fab work.

PERFORMANCE

Handling Under Power

The 43-horsepower, turbo-charged Volvo Penta is of ample size for the boat. In motoring, we ran aground twice, and the engine was easily able to force the winged keel through mud to deep water.

The engine pushes the boat to hull speed easily, and the boat is under control in reverse as well as forward. We handled the boat only in protected waters, but the high topsides may make maneuvering a bit difficult in strong cross-winds.

The engine compartment is well insulated with a lead/foam sound deadener, and the engine mounting made vibration minimal—tolerable everywhere on deck and below except in the aft cabin where the head of the berth is on top of the engine. If you want to take a snooze while motoring, you'll have to do it in the main saloon or forward cabin.

Access to the engine is good, as the Volvo has dipstick, oil fill, and water pump up front. The companionway steps come off to expose the front half of the engine; the back half is accessible from the aft cabin.

Handling Under Sail

The 36 is available with either masthead or fractional rig, both with deck-stepped aluminum spars by Selden of Sweden. The fractional mast is tapered above the forestay attachment. Most European cruising boats (including other Contests) tend to be undercanvassed, but the rig on the 36 is lofty with ample sail area for the boat's displacement. The rig and rigging are of good quality, however, the mast tangs on the boats we examined were noticeably out of alignment with the shrouds.

Shrouds come down to a common chainplate. Most sail handling lines are led aft to the cockpit.

For the masthead rig, the mast is nearly four feet taller and stepped three feet further aft, with a compression post underneath through the dining table. The result is a much larger genoa on a furler, 431 square feet compared to 296, and a much smaller main, 270 square feet versus 437.

For cruising, the fractional arrangement is preferable because of the division of sail area. The smaller genoa of the fractional rig is easier to tack and winch in, the smaller spinnaker is more controllable, and the larger main provides better performance on reaches and runs as well as when sailing under mainsail alone.

However, mast support on the fractional rig is not quite so good. The rigging is a standard dinghy arrangement with swept-back spreaders for the upper shrouds taking almost all the forestay loads in addition to athwartship loads. Single lowers also run aft to a common chainplate. With the shroud chainplates well inboard, the load on them will be tremendous. (On this type of rig, the backstay provides very little mast support.) Fortunately, the mast section is heavy and rugged, making up for some of the potential weaknesses in the rigging arrangement.

We sailed the boat with the 7/8 rig on a light to moderate day and found the performance satisfactory on all points of sail. (The boat we sailed had a fully-battened mainsail with a new "lazy jack" furling system designed by importer Martinus van Breems.) The modern "cruising" underbody and tall rig should make the 36 a decent performer in all conditions. The only shortcoming we

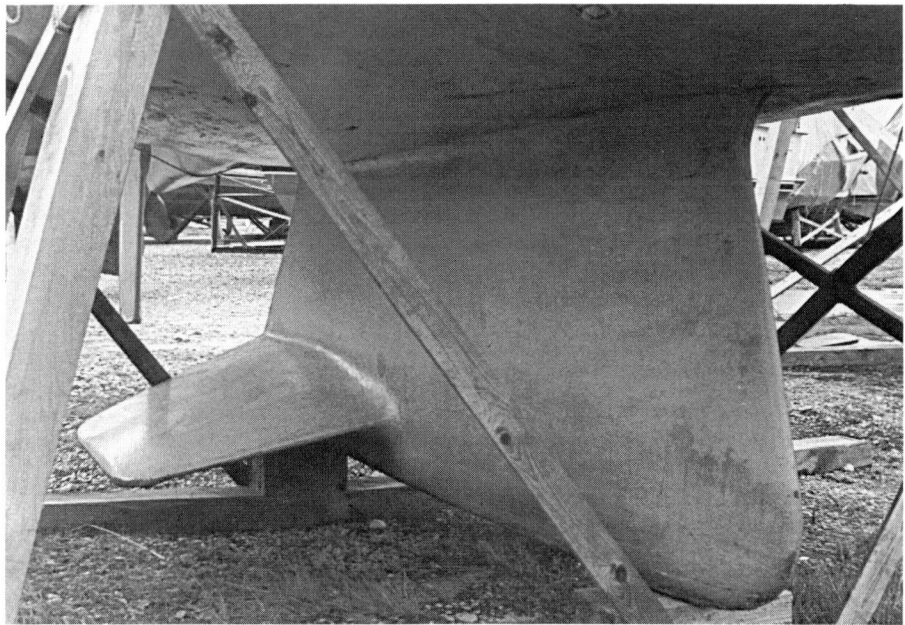

The winged keel is remarkably similar to the keel of the 1983 America's Cup winner, which is no surprise, since the designer was the same.

The Contest 36

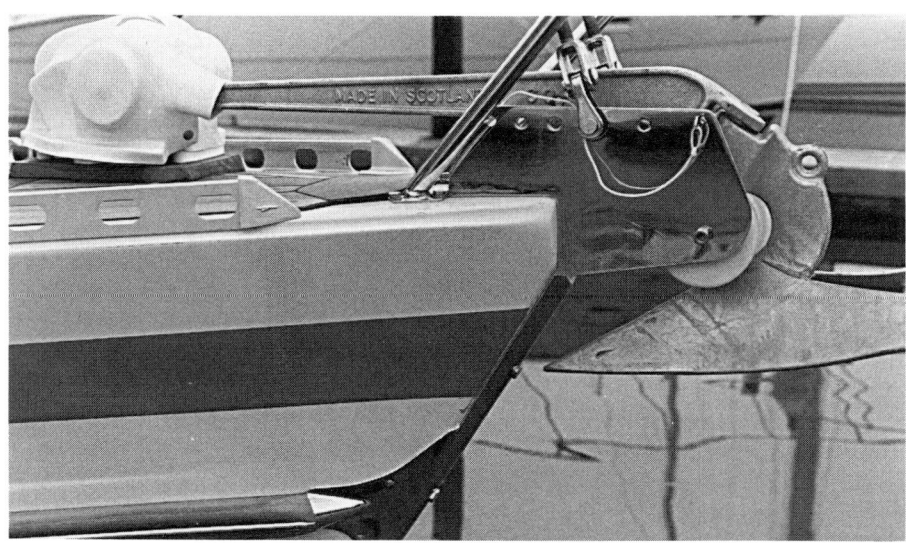

For an advantage that we cannot fathom, the forestay is "split" to allow the anchor shank to be passed through it.

noted was that she was slow to accelerate out of tacks, but this may be the fault of the solid prop that comes standard. Overall, her performance is probably about midway between modern racer-cruisers like the Beneteau 36 and more old-fashioned designs like the Cape Dory 36.

The boat also had the optional wing keel. We had nothing to compare our performance to, but the boat did point well and the amount of leeway did not seem excessive. Tank test figures on the keel suggest that its performance should be nearly equal to the fin keel except upwind in light air and superior to the more conventional shallow-draft keel in all conditions. According to the keel designer van Oossanen, "The tank results show that the 1.40 meter draft design now has comparable performance to the 1.90 meter design. In fact the velocity made good (VMG) is about 0.1 knots higher over a large range of windspeeds." While tank tests are certainly not foolproof, our experience showed us nothing to contradict the tank test findings. We had no sense that the boat's performance was suffering from having a shoal-draft keel.

The value of the wing keel will be for boats moored or docked in shallow water. The wings are of little advantage for sailing in shallow water because, unlike a conventional fin, the wing-keel's draft actually increases when the boat heels. This fact became clear to us during our test sail. When we ran aground, our first inclination—to heel the boat to get off the bottom—proved wrong. We had to release sails and get the boat upright in order to power off the mud. The disadvantage of the keel, with its wings and reverse sloping forward edge, will be in snagging lobster pots and weeds.

The wing keel costs an extra $2,650. Unless you have a particular need for shallow draft, it is probably not a desirable option. Of course, if you're eager to be the first on your block with something new, the wing keel will definitely give you bragging rights at haul-out time.

LIVABILITY

Deck Layout

We looked at two 36's; one with teak decks, one with fiberglass. The fiberglass non-skid seemed mediocre; the teak decks are definitely desirable for good footing as well as appearance, even though they are a $6,300 option.

Generally, the deck is good for working the boat. The deckhouse is minimal, representing at most a four-inch step from side decks to cabin top. The foredeck is wide open, and the sidedecks are wide with inboard shrouds and an aluminum toerail. In heavy weather, there will be little to grab onto—jackstays for a harness would be desirable.

Halyards and reef lines lead aft to the cockpit. The cockpit is comfortable (you will have to get used to the mainsheet traveler on the aft edge of the bridgedeck), but the teak slats for seats will call for cushions. The boat can be ordered with an aluminum-framed windshield which makes the boat look like a motorsailer. Most Americans will probably get a conventional dodger.

There are two big lazarettes aft, and a shallow locker under the starboard cockpit seat. The propane locker, under the helmsman's seat, will hold only one odd-size (8-pound) tank. As is often the case with European boats, the steering wheel (even the optional over-sized one) is too small, making it difficult to steer from the side decks. A good Plath compass comes standard on the binnacle.

There are a couple of peculiar details on the deck. The forestay has a strange "split" at its base, to allow the shank of a plow anchor to fit directly on the centerline of the boat—a complicated arrangement with little apparent advantage. And the cubbyholes in the cockpit coamings are trimmed with cheap plywood roughly finished—quite a contrast to the other joinerwork.

Belowdecks

The interior is a strong selling point for the boat because of its appearance and finish. Though of modest beam by current standards, the 36 is roomy, much of the space achieved through the raised deck. The aft cabin is a bit unusual in that the double berth is almost a triple. In the entryway to the berth, the only spot with standing headroom, there is a washbasin. From the companionway forward, the layout is conventional: chart table and U-shaped galley; settee berths; head; then V-berth. There is good stowage under the V-berths, with cabinets elsewhere throughout the boat. Blue corduroy cushion covers are standard. The cushions fit well enough that there's no need for Velcro or snaptabs to hold them in place.

The cabin ventilation is minimal, depending on three overhead hatches and two opening ports from the aft cabin into the cockpit. The only odd things in the interior are the exposed stainless tubes which anchor the chainplates to the hull sides, and the push-button latches on cabinet doors which look like they are off a tugboat rather than a yacht. All the other detail work is good.

CONCLUSIONS

In general, the Contest 36 seems to be an above average production boat which has come to have a strong reputation, mostly because of considerable attention to detail work and because of unusually good service from her importer.

Besides the good mechanical and woodwork details, the boat has one of the better standard equipment lists we've seen. Among the extras that are options on most boats are lines, fenders, anchors and rode, two horseshoe buoys, flagstaff, bottom paint, and an emergency tiller.

In addition, the optional equipment list is quite complete, including such things as dishware in racks, Dutch tiles in the galley, cockpit tent, and name and hailing port painted on the stern. Prices for all optional equipment and their installation are spelled out in detail. For the sailboat buyer who has been previously stung by sharp dealers or surprised by commissioning costs, the

---

Sisters of the Contest 36

The 36 is Contest's biggest seller in the U.S., but Conyplex makes eight other models, from 32 feet to 64 feet, with the smaller models being most popular.

Contest 32
The 32 is a stubby little boat. Although she has the same general lines as the 36, her raised deck and center cockpit give the 32 a motorsailer appearance, especially in the short-masted ketch version. (A "wheel shelter" option—an aluminum-framed cockpit house—will take you the final step toward the powerboat look.)

If you don't get sleek looks, you *do* get lots of room in the 32, with a big aft cabin, under-cockpit passage, and a tolerable forepeak cabin. In the center of the boat is a roomy head with shower, as well as twin settees opposing the centerline table.

The standard version of the 32 has a long, shoal draft keel and a ketch rig. She is likely to need the big Volvo diesel in most U.S. sailing areas. Both a deep keel and a taller sloop rig are options for the performance-minded, though presumably performance sailors would not focus on the 32 among currently available boats. The winged keel is not available.

Contest 38
Like the 32, the Contest 38 has a center cockpit and a ketch rig. Close in length to the 36 (she's really only 37' 3"), she is quite a bit different—bigger and heavier bodied.

Someone interested in a Contest would likely choose the 38 over the 36

---

straightforward pricing will be welcome. Some people enjoy outfitting a new boat, but those who don't may find the equipment lists irresistible.

The 36 is also getting a lot of attention because of her wing keel. To us, the keel is a feature of doubtful value since it draws less primarily when under power. If you are forced to shallow draft, this particular wing keel configuration does seem to offer improved performance, but we would still be concerned that the keel would tend to foul often with weeds and pot warps.

Overall, we judge the 36 to be moderate and wholesome—a good cruising configuration inside and out. Her base price at slightly over $100,000 is not cheap, but it is the kind of cruising boat that should hold her value pretty well. Her appearance is a potential drawback, but even though the high sheer cannot be called attractive, the boat is not ugly as are some other current imports.

And for those hot after a foreign boat, the importer's longevity and reputation for good service are important. The combination of these two characteristics is not at all common in today's import scene.

---

primarily for her aft cabin, and secondarily for her smaller and handier rig. Although a sloop rig is available, neither version is likely to offer the sailing performance of the 36.

All the extra length of the boat has gone into the aft cabin (the saloon is actually a bit shorter than the 36's). Whereas the 36's under-cockpit aft cabin is mostly for sleeping, the 38's could be regarded as an "owner's stateroom" and offers a settee as well as a double berth. It has a built-in wash basin and (crowded) space for an optional second toilet.

The boats are finished very similarly, with the same mechanical systems and engines. The 38 can be purchased with either teak or mahogany interior woodwork. A winged keel is an option.

Contest 41

The 41 is the newest model imported into the U.S., and many of its design features were aimed at the American market following consultation with the importer.

She is a center-cockpit aft-cabin, with a second head aft that is as roomy as the forward one. The galley is U-shaped and large, and the saloon and forepeak cabin are both enlarged versions of the 38.

To some extent, the interior can be customized. The 41 we looked at, for example, had the aft double berth installed athwartships rather than fore and aft.

A sloop rig is available; however, the standard ketch rig should provide plenty of power, and the ketch's smaller sails should be more manageable for the cruising couple at whom this boat is aimed. The boat is finished like the 36 and is available with the winged keel. We suspect she will become the second most popular of the Contest line.

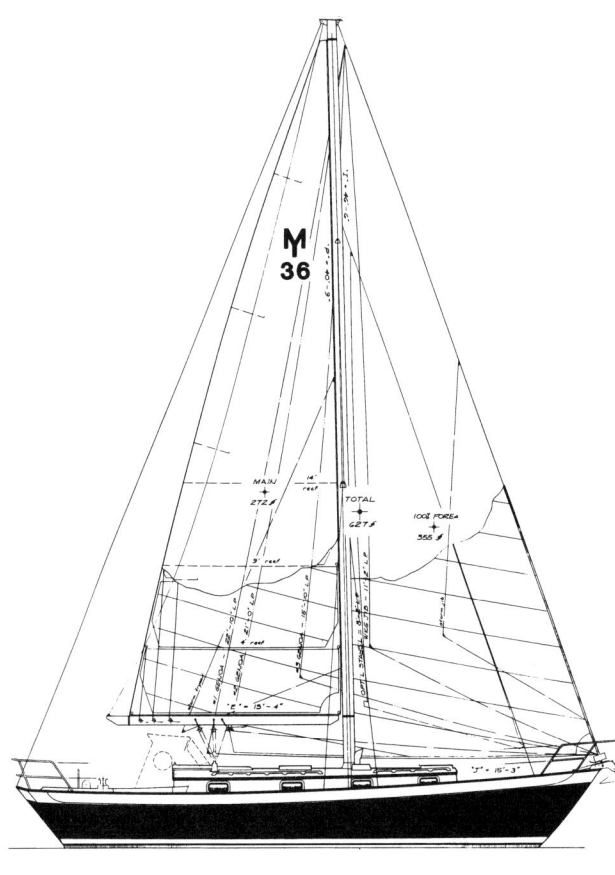

Specifications
Morris 36

LOA	36'3"
LWL	29'6"
Beam	11'7"
Draft	
standard	5'6"
Scheel keel	4'3"
Displacement	15,602 lbs
Ballast	6500 lbs
Sail area	627 sq ft

Morris Yachts
Clark Point Road
Southwest Harbor,
Maine 04679
(207) 244-5866

The Morris 36:
A 'Semi-Custom' Yacht

THE BOAT AND THE BUILDER

A few decades ago, when you wanted a new boat, you chose a designer, commissioned a design, selected a builder, and nursed your dream through to completion. Not many people could afford boats in those days, and not many people could afford to have a boat built in this fashion today. Today, most sailors are more likely to go to a boat show, look at a lot of boats, and pick one off a dealer's "lot"—just like buying a car.

Unless one is in the market for a very large, and very expensive boat, most of the options you will be offered are simply "add-ons"—like bigger winches, perhaps; a different rig; or more electronics.

Want a bigger nav station? Find another boat. A bigger icebox? Ditto. A non-teak interior? Just keep looking ...

Few things are more frustrating than finding a boat that has 90% of the characteristics you're looking for, and 10% that you really can't stand. You can grit your teeth and grin and bear it, or you can just keep looking.

Most of today's sailboats are marvels of production line efficiency, but with production lines comes standardization, and with standardization comes a numbing sameness that can remove a lot of the pleasure of owning a boat.

Morris Yachts can hardly be accused of running a production line operation. In his 15 years in the boatbuilding business, Tom Morris has built just 100 boats. Catalina probably turns out more boats than that every month.

But Morris's boats fall into that intriguing category called the "semi-custom yacht," boats based on a standard hull and interior that can be modified to the desires of individual owners. This isn't a cheap way to build a boat. Imagine going into the Chevrolet plant (or to Mercedes, for that matter) and asking to have the dashboard rearranged, or the interior layout changed.

For most people, the semi-custom boat doesn't make sense. If you're satisfied with what you can find in a production boat, you should by all means buy it. If you're looking for the most amount of boat for the least amount of money, the semi-custom boat isn't for you. If you're an experienced boatowner, have definite ideas about what you want, and are willing to pay significantly more to get it, the semi-custom boat may be the answer.

The Morris 36 Justine is the largest boat built by Tom Morris and his crew of 16 in Southwest Harbor, Maine. Southwest Harbor is a tiny village that supports an astonishing number of boatbuilders, including the prestigious Hinckley company. Fortunately, this means that there is a reasonable pool of skilled labor in the area, between native Mainers and boatbuilders from further south who have migrated north for the more bucolic downeast lifestyle.

Morris' reputation was built on smaller boats: Frances (26 feet), Linda (28 feet), Leigh (30 feet), and Annie (30 feet). All are Chuck Paine designs, and all share the Paine characteristics of a moderately long keel, nearly symmetrical waterlines, moderate displacement, and a lovely, lively sheer. Justine and the new Fleet 32 are the first Morris boats with "modern" underbodies, having longish fin keels and skeg-mounted rudders. The 32 will be equipped with the patented Scheel shoal-draft keel, which is an option chosen by about three-quarters of Morris 36 owners.

CONSTRUCTION

Despite their traditional appearance, Morris yachts utilize materials as up to date as any builder, including biaxial fabrics, isophthalic gelcoat, and vinyl-ester resin in the mat layers immediately beneath the gelcoat. The primary laminating resin is the more typical orthophthalic resin.

Morris is convinced that the answer to hull blistering lies not just in the choice of materials, but in the care with which the hulls are laid up. With most production builders, the glass shop receives a low priority. No one likes working in the intense styrene atmosphere of a molding room, and many builders use their less-skilled labor there.

This, according to Morris, is a serious mistake. He believes that the more care that is taken in the molding process, the less likely problems are to develop with the laminate. He is fanatical about the removal of air and excess resin from the laminate. Excess resin adds weight while reducing structural properties, and Morris believes that air in the laminate is a breeding ground for blisters.

A core sample we examined, removed for installation of a through-hull fitting, had been burn-tested. It showed a near-perfect 56/44 resin/glass ratio.

At the same time, no special care is taken in storing fiberglass materials in the shop, and the molding room lacks any sophisticated environmental controls for temperature and humidity—factors which other builders believe are important.

The hull of a Morris 36 takes two to three men about a week to lay up. The hull stays in the mold at least an additional week while interior structural components such as bulkheads, floor timbers, and supports for the hull ceiling are installed. Leaving the boat in the mold at this stage prevents any distortion of the hull, making sure that the interior furniture modules and the deck will later fit without complication.

For an extra $1750, Morris will core the hull with Airex foam. If you're going to live aboard the boat in a cold climate, the extra insulation of the Airex hull would both make the boat warmer and reduce condensation. From a pure hull performance and strength point of view, it is unnecessary.

There are no interior molded fiberglass liners in Morris boats. The interiors are built of plywood, which is glassed to the hull. This method of construction allows substantial latitude in interior design.

Between the major and minor bulkheads, each area of furniture is self-contained, and can be changed to suit the owner's desires. In Justine #14, for example, the standard arrangement of navigation station and quarterberth on the port side aft was replaced with lockers, drawers, a huge refrigerator-deepfreeze, and a big standup chart table, while the layout of forward section of the main cabin remained unchanged.

The hull to deck joint of the Morris 36 is made with an inward-turning flange at the sheer, which is actually raised well above the deck level to form a bulwark. The edge of the deck molding turns upward, then outward, overlapping the hull flange, creating the inner surface of the bulwark. Hull and deck are bolted together, with the joint bedded in 3M 5200 polyurethane.

The keel is an external lead casting, bolted to the hull. Just aft of the ballast,

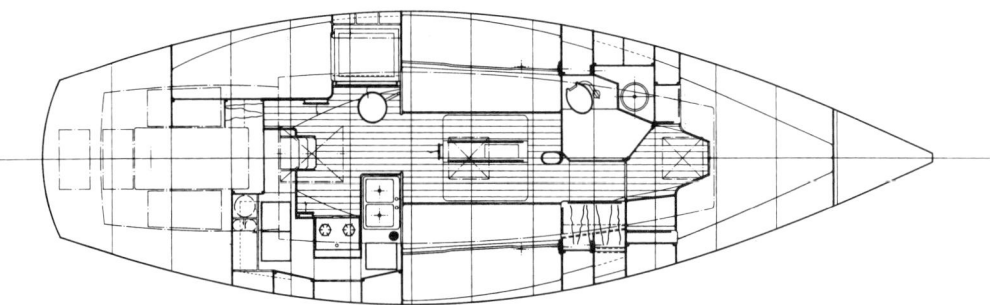

there is a deep, molded fiberglass bilge sump, which should do a good job of keeping water out of the bilges and the lockers that are low in the hull.

Glasswork and gelcoat are to very high standards, although the two-tone deck gelcoat on the new boat we sailed had some variations in color which gave a slightly splotchy appearance. A year-old boat we examined had several minor gelcoat cracks in various locations on deck. These were not stress-related. They had probably been in the deck since it was removed from the mold, but showed up over time as dirt worked into the tiny cracks. We do not consider them significant. All glass surfaces exposed inside the hull are finished with grey gelcoat.

Chainplates and through hull fittings are electrically tied to a copper strap grounding system, which is glassed over to prevent oxidation and the resultant reduction in conductivity. The strapping is then tied to a keelbolt.

While there are substantial backing plates on deck hardware such as stanchions, there are no backing plates under the foredeck cleats, two of the most heavily-loaded items of hardware on the boat. Hoses on hull fittings below the waterline are not double-clamped. In some cases this is because Spartan seacocks—which do not require double clamps—are used, but in other areas it simply appears to be an oversight.

PERFORMANCE

Handling Under Power

The hull of the Morris 36 is easily driven. The engine is the three-cylinder Volvo 2003, rated at 28 horsepower at 3000 RPM. At a more normal cruising RPM of 2000 this will give a speed of about 5-1/2 knots.

The boat handles well under power. There is little vibration or noise, although only the forward portion of the engine box is insulated for sound reduction. The boat we sailed was equipped with a feathering Max-Prop, which is probably the single best investment that any cruising sailor could make to improve performance under both sail and power. Max-Props aren't cheap, but they're worth every penny if you're concerned about performance and have an extra $1000 or so to spend.

Access to the front of the engine for service of filters and belts is good, although it does require removing the companionway ladder and engine box. Access for checking the oil is more difficult—you have to remove the lid to the engine box, which is a tight fit with the ladder in place. This could be easily solved with a small access hatch on the side of the engine box. Oil checks should be a routine part of engine operation.

There is no oil drip pan under the engine. Having never seen an engine that didn't eventually leak a little lubrication and fuel oil, or have spills at oil changes, we think a drip pan is a must, despite Justine's deep bilge sump.

Handling Under Sail

Chuck Paine likes fast boats. Although the standard rig is a sloop with a fairly conservative single-spreader rig by Metalmast, there is an optional taller,

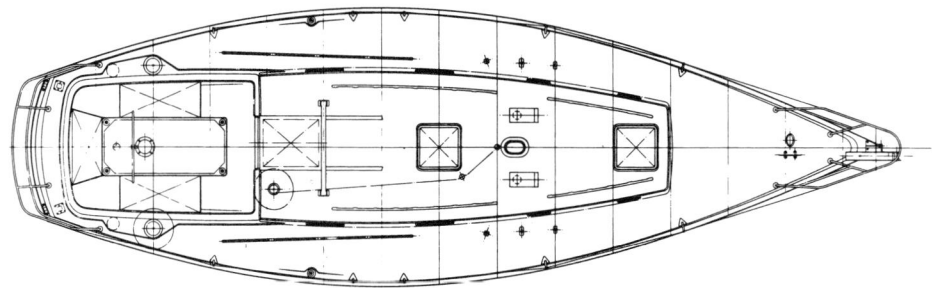

lighter, double-spreader rig with the chainplates set well inboard. No one has yet ordered this rig, but both Paine and Morris would like to talk an owner into the hotter rig, flush through-hulls, and other little goodies that would make the boat faster. The double-spreader rig adds $950 to the base price of the boat. With the standard deep keel, a Justine set up this way should be a formidable IMS racer for an event such as the Marion-Bermuda Race.

Thus far, however, all the owners are cruisers. Most have opted for the shoal-draft Scheel keel rather than the more conventional long fin, which adds a foot of draft. The Scheel keel is by all reports very slightly less efficient upwind, but about the same speed on other points of sail. The Scheel keel adds $1200 to the price of the boat. Unless shoal draft is crucial, we'd stick with the normal keel.

With a half-load displacement of only 15,600 pounds on a 29' 6" waterline, the Morris 36 has a lot of speed potential, particularly when you consider her 42-percent ballast to displacement ratio. The boat we sailed was equipped with a rig 2 feet taller than standard, a Doyle fully-battened main, and a roller-furling Doyle Quicksilver genoa. Despite a slight hook in the leech of the genoa, the boat pointed and accelerated as well as any fast cruiser of her size, and a lot better than most.

LIVABILITY

Deck Layout

The deck layout of the Morris 36 is simple and clean. The shrouds are set a few inches inboard of the bulwarks—just far enough to be in the way when going forward along the deck, so that it's easier to go forward over the deckhouse.

The helmsman's seat is a little low for looking over the cabin house, but the cockpit coamings are wide enough to sit on in reasonable comfort in order to see the jib telltales.

Sail handling hardware is excellent, with a Harken traveler and mainsheet blocks. The other deck hardware comes from a variety of sources: stainless steel genoa track from Hinckley, Lewmar winches, Bomar hatches, and other suppliers for bits and pieces.

The combination of the bulwarks and lifelines that are 27" tall give a great feeling of security on deck. Yet the bulwarks are not high enough to be visually obtrusive—you don't even notice they're there, you just feel more secure.

The stemhead fitting includes a substantial roller for a CQR anchor. A chafe pad should be fitted on the deck at the inboard end of the anchor shank, or a hole will quickly be worn in the deck from the anchor shackle. There is no anchor well on deck, and the forepeak locker for anchor rode storage is so far forward in the hull that we would not suggest storing large amounts of chain there.

We can't imagine a much more secure cockpit for offshore sailing. There are four large cockpit drains, although the actual low point in the cockpit sole requires a quirky little fifth drain to get the last bit of water out with the boat sitting at anchor. The upper parts of the cockpit coamings are angled comfortably outward.

With the optional cutter rig, two staysail sheet winches are fitted to the aft end of the coachroof. With the dodger in place, you can't swing the starboard winch handle in a full circle without fetching up on the dodger frame, an inconvenience. The mainsail sheet winch is also mounted on the coachroof, but there are no obstacles in the way of its operation.

Access to the rudder head for installing the emergency steering requires opening a bronze deckplate and inserting the welded stainless steel tiller. With the tiller in position, you will have a good-sized opening in the cockpit sole, which can allow water below in heavy weather. Some sort of boot over the opening would be a plus. Large cockpit lockers port and starboard will hold all the extra sails, anchors, and other assorted junk you care to load in them. Merriman pedestal wheel steering with Ritchie compass are standard.

Belowdecks
If you're looking for acres of varnished teak and complex joinerwork, the interior of the Morris 36 won't be your cup of tea. If you appreciate honest, solid workmanship to a high grade, and interior finish that is traditional in the best sense of the word, you're going to like this boat.

There are two standard, no-extra-cost interior finishes: oiled teak, or white Formica trimmed in oiled teak. We don't like oiled teak interiors—they're drab. An oiled teak interior is not in any sense traditional. Builders like them because they're cheap to finish. Teak plywood costs just a little more than regular marine plywood. One worker can completely oil the interior joinerwork of a boat the size of the Morris 36 in a couple of days. Varnishing or painting, on the other hand, would take weeks.

If you find that hard to believe, consider the fact that you can get all that interior teak varnished if you want, but it is an option that costs $6,250. At the Morris standard labor rate of $26 per hour, that means that they spend 240 hours—six man-weeks—varnishing the interior.

The interior of white Formica with oiled teak trim is a practical combination that is airy, light, and attractive. It is so superior to the drab varnished or oiled teak interiors of most boats as to defy comparison, although it will appear stark to those with little grounding in traditional yacht interiors. If it were our boat, we would get the Formica interior with teak trim, but we would not have the

The Morris 36
301

teak trim oiled. We would either have Morris varnish it, or do it ourselves at our leisure. Varnishing just the trim should cut the extra finishing cost by about half, and give you a truly elegant interior. You cannot put varnish over an oil finish, so you have to make a conscious decision about what you're going to do before you start.

Given the cost of domestic labor, there's no way that a U.S. builder can turn out a boat with the exquisite, labor-intensive interior details of the best Taiwan-built boats, such as the Little Harbors, and still deliver a boat at a price much less than that of the space shuttle. You won't find every locker of the Morris 36 lined with varnished wood ceiling, and you can see the hull structure in places that even a lot of cheaper Oriental builders cover up with wood sheathing.

At the same time, Morris refuses to line the overheads, hull, and inside of lockers with the ubiquitous foam-backed vinyl that you find glued into almost every American-built boat from Hunter to Hinckley. For insulation, Morris will line lockers with cork if you want—a practical, if not particularly elegant solution. As another option, you can get the hull above the waterline lined with non-structural foam to reduce condensation and noise.

There's nothing wrong with opening a locker and being able to see what holds a boat together, even if fiberglass construction details lack the hard-edged beauty of traditional wood structural components. But for those not used to seeing fiberglass surfaces, parts of the Morris 36 will have an unfinished appearance.

The forward cabin has V-berths port and starboard, with an insert to form a double. The forward cabin is pushed far into the bow, and the boat's fine entry angle results in a berth which narrows sharply at the foot. Because the berths are quite long, we doubt if the narrowness will be a problem unless the berths are occupied by two very tall adults. Headroom in the forward cabin is an honest 6 feet.

Aft of the forward cabin, there is a large hanging locker to port, with the head to starboard. The passage between the main and forward cabins is quite narrow, as is the door to the head. There is adequate locker space and elbow room in the head, and a six-footer can stand up without bending. The only interior fiberglass molding in the boat is the head floor pan, which only makes sense on a boat with a shower. However, this white, non-skid molding will be tough to keep clean. There is a small teak grate over the shower sump, but the drain is not actually at the lowest point in the head sole, so that you may end

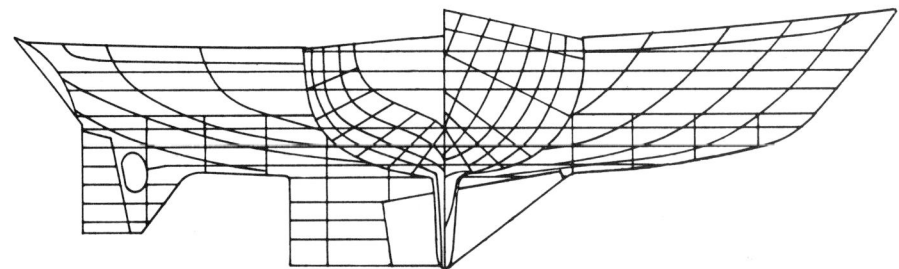

up with a small puddle in the aft corner of the head after showering. This is a problem on a lot of boats, and could be remedied in this case by changing the pan molding so that it angled upwards slightly just aft of the drain grate.

One of the big advantages of a semi-custom boat without a molded hull liner is the ability to alter the interior arrangements without breaking the bank. While the standard main cabin arrangement has settees and pilot berths both port and starboard, there are several other accommodation plans offered as reasonably-priced options. Hull #14, which had just been completed when we visited Morris, has a U-shaped dinette to starboard, and storage lockers in place of the pilot berth to port. This is fine on a boat that will not be sailed offshore, but it means that the only sea berth in the boat is the quarterberth. A more practical arrangement for occasional offshore work would be to retain either the port or starboard pilot berth. With a pilot berth to starboard and the standard port quarterberth, this would give at least one comfortable offshore berth on each side of the boat—a necessity for two-person passagemaking, when a good place to sleep can spell the difference between being rested and being dangerously fatigued.

Headroom in the main cabin varies from 6 feet, 3 inches on the centerline at the forward end, to 6 feet, 5 inches on centerline just forward of the companionway.

Aft of the settees, partial bulkheads on both sides of the boat separate the galley and navigation station from the main saloon. In the standard arrangement, there is a good wet locker just to port of the companionway ladder, and a large quarterberth outboard of the locker. Forward of the quarterberth is the nav station, which faces athwartships rather than the more common fore and aft. The chart table is big enough to accept almost any chart folded in half, and has adequate space for electronics, navigation paraphernalia, and books. The navigator's bench is a little narrow for maximum comfort, and we would miss having a back rest when trying to navigate with the boat heeled on port tack.

The electrical panels are fitted behind the companionway ladder, sheltered under the bridgedeck. While this is a good location, it is somewhat vulnerable to spray, and the panels should be protected behind an opening clear acrylic splash shield.

To starboard is a well-designed galley, which includes a three-burner Force 10 propane stove with oven. This is one of the best galley stoves made, and is typical of the quality components which go into the Morris 36. It is also one of the reasons the boat costs so much. Propane is stored in a cockpit locker holding three six-pound aluminum bottles.

The icebox and lid are well insulated, and the box itself has 4 inches of foam insulation. Sea Frost engine-driven refrigeration is an option costing $2,350. If you are planning a cruise in warm climates, a good refrigeration system is a must.

On one boat we examined, the owner wanted a larger refrigerator and freezer than would fit in the normally allocated space, so the nav station was replaced with a huge refrigerator/freezer, retaining the top for chart work.

While this arrangement wouldn't appeal to every sailor, it shows the design flexibility that is the primary advantage of the semi-custom boat.

Deep double sinks manufactured by Polar are pretty much the norm on larger boats. Instead, Morris uses a double sink with one large sink and a smaller one, shallower than usually seen. We like the idea of sinks of unequal size, since there always seems to be one pot on board that won't fit into the relatively small Polar sinks. At the same time, we'd like the sinks to be at least 9" deep. We wish some sink manufacturer would put out deep double sinks of these proportions, but we haven't seen them yet. Hot and cold pressure water are standard.

Designer Paine has also drawn a tri-cabin interior for those who want an aft stateroom, although none of the first 14 owners selected this extra-cost option.

CONCLUSIONS

The Morris 36 is an expensive boat. It is also a well-built, very attractive boat. The builder is flexible enough to alter the interior in almost any way possible, as long as the main structural bulkheads stay in the same place. This flexibility comes at a price, of course.

The base price of the Morris 36 in 1987 is $119,500. This includes commissioning and sea trials in Southwest Harbor. The sea trials take about a week, during which the inevitable little problems of a new boat are easily remedied. There's no dealer to go through—everything's done on the spot by the builder.

There's no written warranty on the boat. Morris shrugs, and says if something is wrong, he'll fix it. We believe him.

It's very difficult when comparing boat prices to avoid comparing apples with oranges, since things that are standard on some boats are options on others. To put things in a bit of perspective, we've compared the base price of the Morris 36 with other boats of approximately the same length overall, waterline length, displacement, type, and general quality. We've adjusted as much as possible for differences in standard equipment and specifications, to make the comparisons as reasonable as possible. In some cases the prices given may be lower than the actual current (1987) base price of a boat, since we've removed the value of standard equipment that is not standard on the Morris 36. Here they are: Dickerson 37, $133,000; Passport 37, $125,000; Crealock 37, $115,000; Tartan 37, $115,000; Cape Dory 36, $110,000. In all cases, the price you will finally pay for the boat will be higher depending on the optional equipment selected.

This puts the base price of the Morris 36 square in the middle of good boats similar in size and type, but substantially higher than a boat the same size of only average quality.

If you take full advantage of Morris's ability to customize your boat, the final price will be a lot higher than the base price. Hull #14, for example, has a custom interior plus such niceties as radar, central heat, and Alpha Marine autopilot. If you want to go all out, you can increase the price of the boat by 40 percent without difficulty.

Beside the price, the only disadvantage of a semi-custom boat is that you may, in creating the boat of your dreams, be building a boat that's a nightmare for anyone else—a boat that no one else is willing to buy when the inevitable time comes to sell. Thus far, that hasn't been a problem with the Morris 36. At the time of this writing, only one of the boats had come on the resale market, and it was sold before the broker even received the listing. The buyer had only been interested in one other boat, a *new* Morris 36.

Obviously, the primary advantage of a semi-custom boat is to create a boat you'll keep for years. We suspect that most Morris 36 owners will do just that.

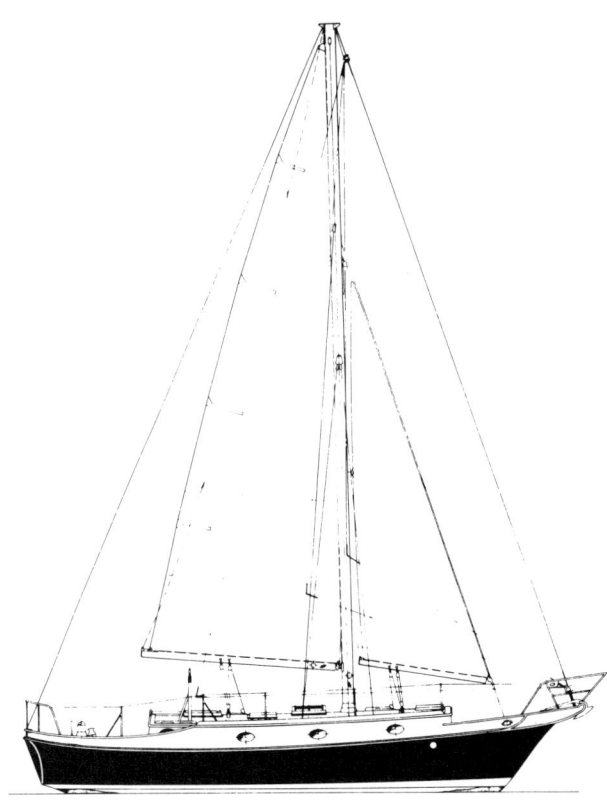

Specifications
CSY 37

LOA	37'3"
LWL	29'2"
Beam	12'0"
Draft	
deep	6'0"
shoal	4'8"
Displacement*	21,000 lbs
Ballast	8000 lbs
Sail area	610 sq ft
* approximate	

The CSY 37:
Ersatz Traditional Charter Boat

THE BOAT AND THE BUILDER

The CSY 37, designed by Peter Schmitt, was the mid-sized boat in the CSY line. Primarily designed for the Caribbean bareboat charter trade, 87 of the raised-deck cutters were built.

Schmitt combined some features most often found in "traditional" boats—the oval stern, raised deck, and semi-clipper bow—with a relatively modern underbody featuring a fairly long fin keel and a skeg-mounted rudder. On paper, the boat looks pretty good. In person, she is rather tubby and high-sided.

The CSY 37 most closely resembles the Ericson Cruising 36. The styling of both these boats can best be termed "ersatz traditional."

With the short standard rig and shoal keel, she is no performance cruiser, and with her huge cockpit she is not really a seaboat. Rather, she is a boat designed for a specific purpose, bareboat chartering, a purpose which she serves admirably. To expand her appeal to the general sailing public would be difficult, as CSY discovered. The company went out of business in 1981.

Most CSY 37's went into charter service, usually on lease-back arrangements. These boats had to be strong and reliable, for a week out of service for repairs means $1,300 in lost revenue to the charter operator. That the boats can stand up to this constant use and abuse is a credit to both designer and builder. Few other boats could, as CSY's charter experience has shown.

CONSTRUCTION

There are really only two words to describe the construction of the CSY 37: *massive overkill*. This is a mixed blessing. It means you have a strong, heavy hull. It often also means that you end up with a boat that is undercanvassed in light air. Very often it also means a boat that has a fairly low ballast to displacement ratio.

Forty percent of the CSY 37's advertised displacement is in the ballast keel. With a 29-foot waterline, the displacement of about 20,000 pounds is about average by traditional standards, heavy by modern standards.

The hull is an extraordinarily heavy solid glass layup, as is the deck. No core materials are used anywhere. Without coring such as balsa or Airex, a glass hull can sweat in a cold climate and can be excessively warm in a hot, humid climate.

The hull to deck joint is simple and effective. The hull and deck flanges, which overlap to form a molded rail, are bedded in 3M 5200 and through-bolted with stainless steel machine screws on 4-inch centers. 3M 5200 is about the most effective and tenacious adhesive sealant on the market.

The keel construction is unusual. The cast lead ballast is glassed into the hollow keel molding, with any voids being filled with fiberglass slurry. This is then glassed over to form a double bottom and to keep the ballast in place. This ballast arrangement is identical in both the shoal and deep draft versions. The deep draft boat, however, has a 16-inch deep keel extension filled with about 600 pounds of cast concrete. If a shoal draft boat is desired, this extension can simply be cut off. The shoal draft boat therefore, may be slightly faster off the wind, but will make more leeway.

The hull is molded in two pieces, then joined in the middle with heavy overlapping layers of mat and roving. This provides some flexibility in hull design, allowing such features as a molded-in rubbing strake and a stern with substantial tumblehome.

The installation of hardware is excellent. This is one of the few boats seen with through-bolted bronze seacocks. Backing plates are used on deck hardware, such as cleats and winches.

The rudder stock is a solid 2-foot round bronze rod. The cast bronze rudder heel fitting would look more at home on a 60-foot boat than on a 37-footer.

The stemhead fitting is a massive stainless steel weldment, incorporating an anchor roller, a welded chock, and the headstay chainplate. The edges of the bow chock are not rounded, and could easily chafe an unprotected anchor rode. This bow fitting could double as an effective battering ram. We suspect that the dock boys in the West Indies are wary anytime an inexperienced charterer brings one of the CSY boats into a slip.

Chainplates are heavy stainless steel flat bars with load-bearing, welded webs, through-bolted to the hull. The hull layup is reinforced in the way of the chainplates, an almost superfluous precaution, given the heaviness of the regular hull layup.

Interior bulkheads are heavy waterproof plywood, attached to the hull with solid and neatly made fillets. Airex pads along the outboard edges of the bulkheads distribute the bulkhead stresses on the inside of the hull, preventing hard spots. Cabin sole supports are clear fir. The teak-faced cabin sole is screwed to these floors, with only limited access openings to the bilge. We'd prefer that most of the cabin sole be removable, giving emergency access to the bilge spaces. CSY appears to be counting on the massiveness of the hull construction to prevent holing. This conceit could backfire. Remember the Titanic?

Hatches are molded fiberglass with translucent panels. They have good gaskets and good dogs, but a short person will have trouble reaching overhead to open the hatches due to the tremendous headroom.

Exterior finish is of good production-boat quality. Joinerwork is clean, with a few exceptions. The molded fiberglass trailboards are now shielded below the bow by a somewhat awkward, molded glass panel. This was installed after a number of CSY boats blew off their trailboards in heavy seas. We would have preferred that they just omitted the trailboards.

Construction of the CSY 37 is heavy and strong. It is doubtful if there is a stronger hull of this size in production anywhere. Unfortunately, this greatly increases the price of the boat. With OPEC's quantum leaps in oil prices in the early '70s, and the subsequent increase in the price of resins and fiberglass cloth, it is difficult to see how CSY could continue to use them so lavishly and remain competitive. A little creative engineering, reducing the shell thickness by incorporating a stringer system, could have produced a hull that was just as strong, but less extravagant in consuming materials.

PERFORMANCE

Handling Under Sail

The CSY 37 is available in two keel configurations, and with two rigs. The four possible combinations produce very different performance characteristics.

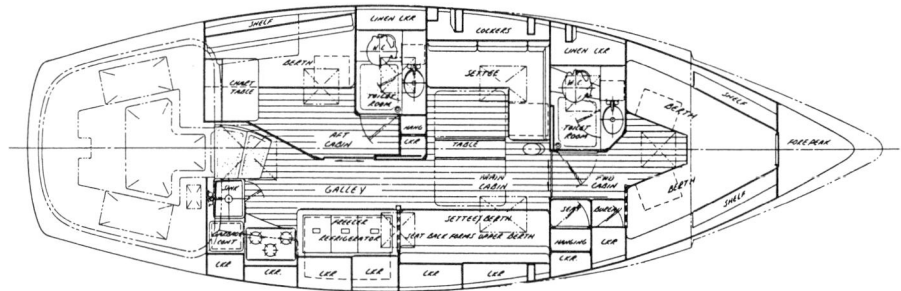

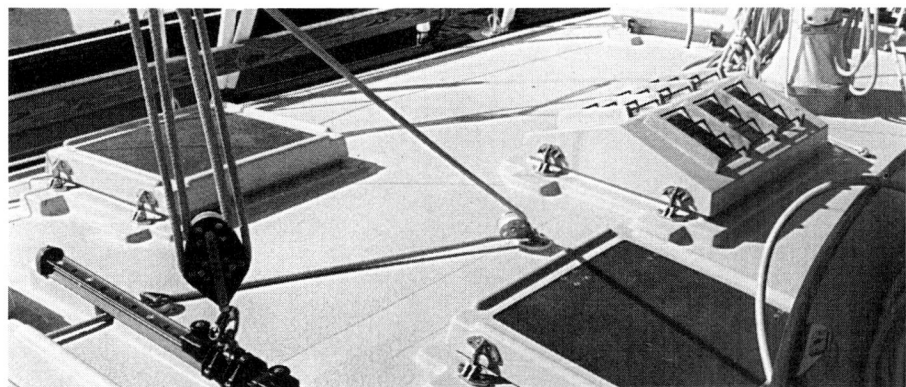

Most boats were delivered with the standard short rig. In areas of normally heavy air, such as the West Indies in winter, the normal rig is adequate. In light air with the short rig, the boat is a slug. The engine will come in handy under these circumstances. Performance is greatly enhanced by the tall rig, which is about 8 feet taller than the standard rig, and incorporates two sets of spreaders.

With the chainplates set at the outboard edge of the hull, the sheeting base is excessively wide. Sheeting a genoa in tight enough to go effectively to windward would be difficult. To avoid the necessity for running backstays, the intermediate and aft shrouds are attached to the deck, several feet aft of the mast and the attachment of the upper shrouds. Unfortunately, when broad reaching, the boom and main fetch up against these shrouds. This is a less than ideal situation for a boat whose best point of sail is off the wind.

Our test boat had the tall rig and the shoal-draft keel—not a combination we would ordinarily choose. The higher sail plan does, however, make the boat more tender, and with the cutdown keel, combines to produce a boat that makes excessive leeway when heeled more than about 20 degrees. We would prefer to combine the tall rig with the deep-draft keel.

Our test boat was overpowered in gusts of little more than 15 knots (with full main, staysail and large jib topsail), sailing hard on the wind. With a reef in, and the main eased, she stood up better, and with less leeway.

Off the wind, the CSY 37 comes into her own. She is stable as a church and visions of long tradewind passages come to mind. Under those conditions she would shine if you had plenty of chafe protection on those aft-leading shrouds.

Halyard winches are mounted on the keel-stepped, painted aluminum mast. The boom does not overhang the cockpit, and has a well-made boom gallows which also provides a good handhold on deck.

Performance under sail is not sparkling, but with the tall rig, both the 37 and the cutter-rigged CSY 44 begin to outgrow their "Tampa Tub" reputation.

Handling Under Power
With such high topsides, the Perkins 4-108 is the smallest engine we would want in the boat. As it is, handling at slow speeds in a crosswind can be tricky.

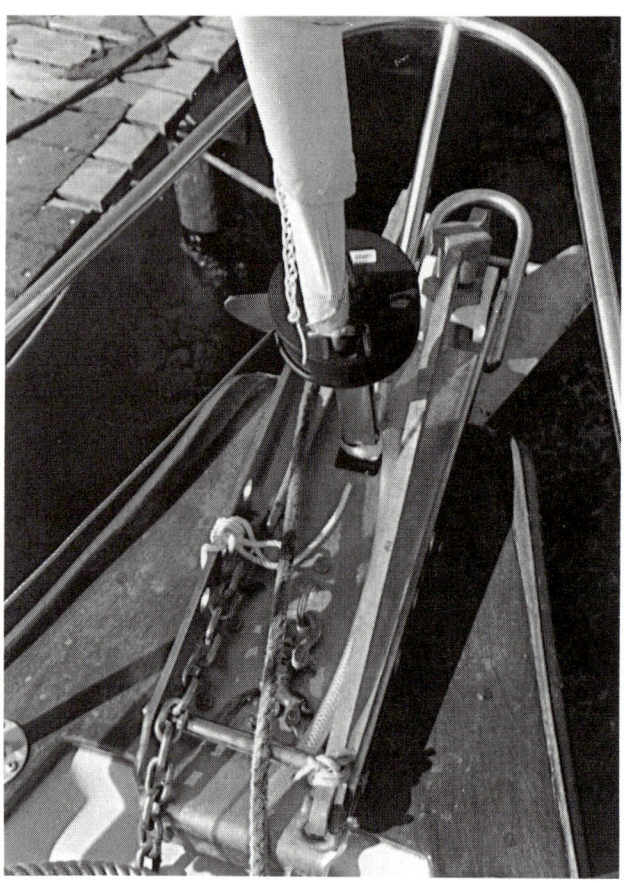

A great deal of practice is required to handle such a high-sided boat under power in a breeze.

The turning radius of the CSY 37 is substantially larger than with a shorter-keeled boat. With her heavy displacement, acceleration is not exactly neck-snapping. She should have enough power to get her out of tight spots, however.

Handling in reverse is tricky. The boat does not go where you aim it until you learn to use a combination of rudder and bursts of throttle.

Designer Peter Schmitt easily handles the boat going astern, but as it often

The massive bow fitting could double as a battering ram.

happens with tightrope walking and figure skating, the expert always makes it look easy.

Engine access through the large cockpit hatch is good, but the heavy hatch should have a more positive means of holding it open. If it fell on your head, you'd remember it (if you were lucky enough to remember anything).

To those who have been spoiled by the handling under power of some modern boats, the CSY 37 may be a disappointment. It handles like a boat, rather than a compact car, requiring some patience and planning.

LIVABILITY

Deck Layout

With her raised deck amidships, the CSY 37 has an amazing amount of deck space, giving the impression of a small ship. There is plenty of room on deck to carry a rigid dinghy. Schmitt's own CSY 37 carries a beautiful little dory with a varnished transom as a tender. She fits neatly on the starboard side and serves as a catchall for fenders and lines.

Deck space is important in boats used extensively in the charter trade. Lounging on deck is the primary charter boat activity and in this category, the CSY 37 gets five stars.

Anchor handling is fairly easy with the stubby bowsprit. There is, however, only a single bow cleat. This is one of our pet peeves, for it greatly complicates anchoring with two anchors—a common practice for cruising boats. The optional "anchoring package" included a length of stainless steel chain, which is miserable stuff to handle by hand. Use galvanized instead. We also do not care for the optional electrical anchor windlass.

Heavy travelers for both the main and the staysail are located on the main deck. Athwartships control lines should really be used with these to get optimum performance from the sails—essential on a boat which must be tweaked to get a reasonable level of performance on the wind.

The cockpit of the CSY 37 is huge—too big for an offshore boat but perfect for the charter trade. The large cockpit lockers are well divided and are partitioned from the engine space under the cockpit.

The starboard cockpit locker contains the best battery box installation we have seen on a stock boat. The port locker contains the optional 110-volt AC refrigeration compressor.

The sound-insulated engine room hatch occupies much of the cockpit sole. There are four large cockpit scuppers, which are imperative to have with the huge cockpit. The companionway sill should be higher if the boat is to be used offshore. A fiberglass seahood protects the forward end of the companionway hatch.

Belowdecks

Two interior arrangements were available: a two-stateroom, two-head plan; and a single-stateroom, single-head plan. The two-stateroom plan was used primarily in the charter trade. It is really too much interior to try to cram in a 29-foot waterline and designer Schmitt is not particularly proud of it.

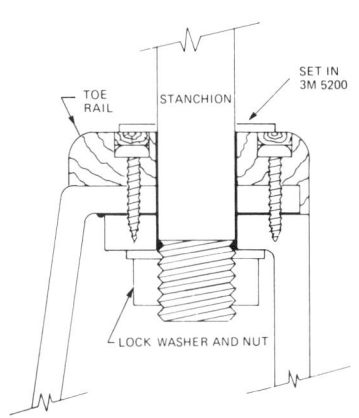

Stanchion is unique, very strong.

The single-stateroom layout is also unconventional. It gives over the forward 40 percent of the interior space to a large cabin with built-in double berth, and a huge head compartment in the forepeak. The problem with this arrangement is that with guests aboard, they must pass through the owner's cabin in order to use the head—a major inconvenience.

The space given over to the head in the single-stateroom model is almost exactly the same space occupied by the forward cabin in the two-stateroom model. With a single-stateroom layout, interior space might have been better utilized with a "conventional" layout of sleeping quarters forward with the head and hanging lockers dividing the forward cabin from the main cabin. Unfortunately, the "conventional" layout was not an option.

The interior volume of the CSY 37 is huge, thanks to the raised deck. There are many well-thought-out interior details, too many, unfortunately, to catalog here. The ice box, for example, is divided into two compartments with separate opening traps. The icebox has a minimum of 4 inches of urethane foam insulation, probably more than any other stock boat on the market. It also has a good toespace underneath, greatly facilitating reaching into depths of the box.

There are, however, lapses in this good design. Galley counter tops in our test boat were covered with a slate-like laminate, difficult to clean and too bumpy for a good work surface. Head counters and some shelves were covered with marble-grained plastic, looking more like a slice out of a multi-colored bowling ball than real marble.

The mixture of excellent design details, strange lapses in taste, and execution which ranges from fair to excellent, is difficult to evaluate reasonably. It was pleasing to see, after years of using teak-grained mica-covered bulkheads, that CSY switched to real oak-faced bulkheads in newer production boats.

The ventilation of the interior is one aspect that can only be described as excellent. There are six opening hatches or skylights in addition to the companionway. Some dorade boxes, however, might be welcome in steamy climates with frequent rain.

One could spend a great deal of time analyzing the interior details, primarily because a lot of thought has gone into them. Both of the interior layouts are unusual, and each will have adherents and detractors.

CONCLUSIONS

CSY was an unusual company, and the CSY 37 is certainly an unconventional boat. The boat is strongly built—overly built, in fact. The 1980 base price of $91,670 seemed high unless you considered that this was a 20,000-pound boat, and very well equipped one at that. Hot and cold pressure water, Edson pedestal steering, and gimballed propane stove were all standard, for example.

CSY boats were probably the strongest production boats ever marketed. They may be ungainly in appearance, and not the hottest performers under sail, but they are tough. That should be an important consideration if you're trying to get the most for your money. Recent (1987) prices on used 1979 to 1981 CSY 37s would indicate that it will cost from $60,000 to $90,000 to put one of these sturdy boats at your mooring.

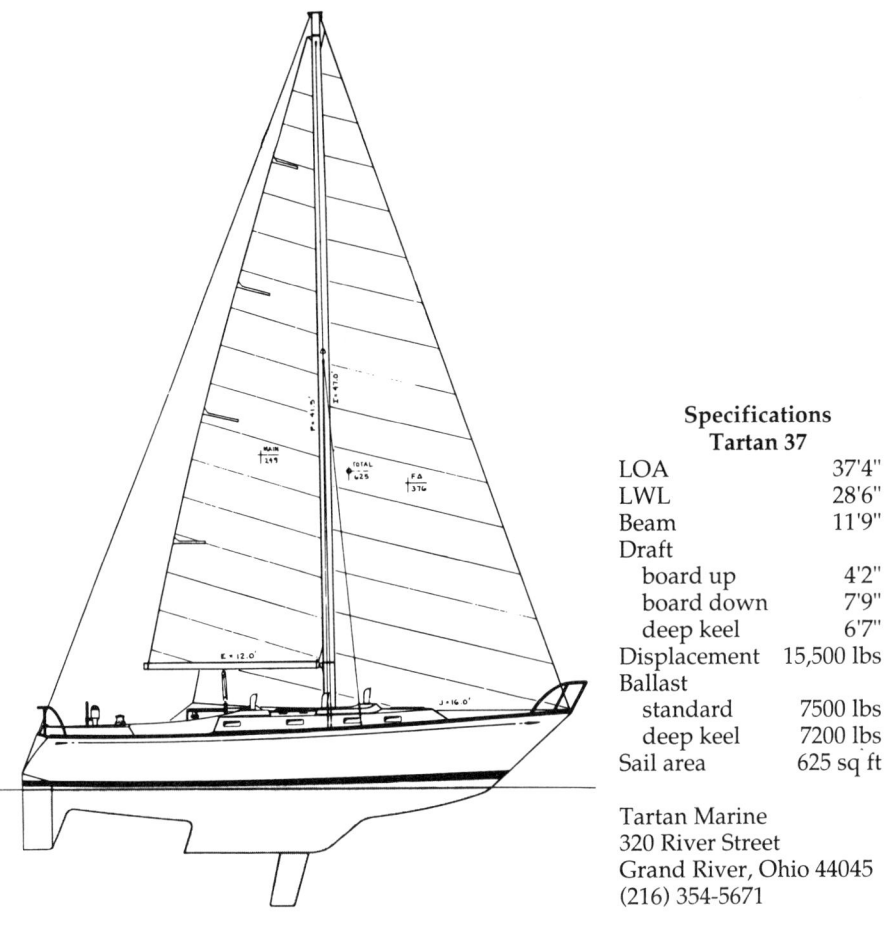

Specifications
Tartan 37

LOA	37'4"
LWL	28'6"
Beam	11'9"
Draft	
board up	4'2"
board down	7'9"
deep keel	6'7"
Displacement	15,500 lbs
Ballast	
standard	7500 lbs
deep keel	7200 lbs
Sail area	625 sq ft

Tartan Marine
320 River Street
Grand River, Ohio 44045
(216) 354-5671

The Tartan 37:
A Grey-Flannel Yacht

THE BOAT AND THE BUILDER

The Tartan 37 is a moderately high performance, shoal-draft cruiser built by Tartan Marine, with headquarters in Grand River, Ohio, and primary construction facilities in Hamlet, North Carolina. High labor costs in the Great Lakes area relative to those in other parts of the country have forced a number of boatbuilding firms to seek greener pastures with friendlier labor markets.

Over the years, Tartan has specialized in the production of well-finished boats geared toward the upper income cruising sailor. Most of these boats have been Sparkman & Stephens designs, and many have been keel-centerboarders. Tartans of the past were also geared toward "civilized" racing, with boats such as the Tartan 41 and Tartan 46. With their Sparkman & Stephens designs and high quality joinerwork, Tartans have provided a lower-priced alternative to lines of boats such as the expensive Nautor Swans.

By 1987, almost 500 Tartan 37s had been built and the demand for the boat has continued to be strong. The longevity of the 37 in production is a remarkable testament to the inherent quality of both her design and her construction. Until the early 1980s, most of the 37s were ordered with the original keel-centerboard configuration and only a few with a deep fin keel. In the 1980s, Tartan became a fan of the Scheel keel, a shoal-keel configuration designed by Henry Scheel that predated the era of winged keels. By enlarging the bottom of the keel with an end-plate, the Scheel keel helps to improve lift and to keep the weight of ballast low, in part at least overcoming two of the noted drawbacks of shoal keels. By 1985, the 37 was available with all three keel shapes.

Tartan-built boats have proved exceptionally good values over the years. On the used-boat market they are among the most sought-after boats and have tended to maintain their owners' equity. At the same time, new Tartans have never been "cheap." Over the years the Tartan 37 has been built, her base price has almost doubled, reaching $100,000. Fully equipped, her price had risen to over $120,000 by 1987. By then even 10-year-old 37s were commanding over $70,000 as used boats. A crucial question for prospective buyers enamored with the 37 is thus whether to consider a new 37, or undertake what may be a protracted search for a used 37 in top condition.

The Tartan 37 is attractively modern in appearance. She has a gentle sheer and a straight raked stem profile, with moderate overhangs at both bow and stern. Underwater, the boat has a fairly long, low-aspect-ratio fin keel, and a high-aspect rudder faired into the hull with a substantial skeg. Freeboard is moderate. The boat is balanced and pleasant in appearance. She is not a character boat, but is attractive, fairly racy, and functional—a typical modern Sparkman & Stephens design.

CONSTRUCTION

The Tartan 37 is a well-built boat. Tartan makes use of both unidirectional roving and balsa coring in stress areas. This yields a stiff, fairly light hull that is less likely to "oil can" than the relatively thin solid layup used in many production boats. Some roving print-through is evident. There are also some visible hard spots on the outside of the hull. Gelcoat quality is very good. The

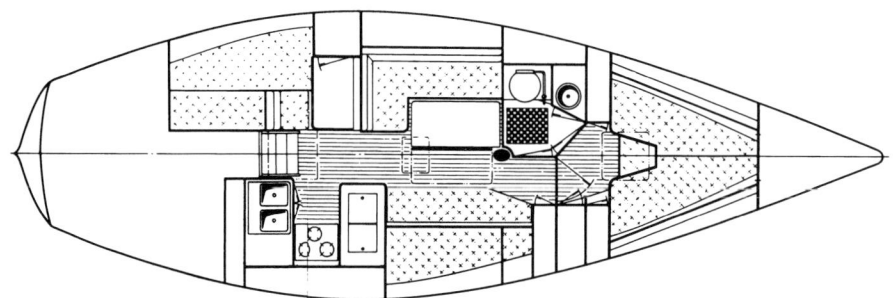

rudder is faired into the skeg with flaps to minimize turbulence. All through-hull fittings are recessed flush with the hull skin. For a cruising boat, remarkable attention is given to reducing skin friction and improving water flow.

Tartan's hull to deck joint is simple and strong. The wide internal hull flange is bedded with butyl and polysulphide, the deck dropped on, and the two bolted together via the stainless steel bolts which hold on the teak toerail. This toerail is not always properly bedded. We were able to easily insert a thick knife blade under the toerail in several areas near the bow where the rail is subject to the most twist. Water will lie in this joint if it is at all open, making it impossible to keep varnish on the toerail.

Most deck hardware is backed with thick aluminum plates. Pulpits are through-bolted but lack backing plates. The hull to deck joint is through-bolted across the transom—one of few boats so built.

Interior glasswork is some of the best we have seen. Fillet bonding is absolutely neat and clean. There are no raw fiberglass edges visible anywhere in the hull.

To keep the interior of the boat neat, the centerboard pennant comes up on deck through the center of the mast. This necessitates a complex mast step with transverse floors and a massive beam under the mast step to absorb compression.

If price is not a concern, perhaps this complexity is little ground for complaint. However, the more complex a piece of construction is, the more subject it may be to failure, and the more expensive to repair or replace.

Tartan uses bronze ball valves on through-hull fittings below the waterline. Exhaust line, cockpit scuppers, and bilge pump outlets are above the waterline, and have no shutoffs. The cockpit scuppers, which would be submerged while the boat is underway, should have provision for shutoff.

PERFORMANCE

Handling Under Sail

Owners report that the Tartan 37 is a well-mannered boat under sail. The boat will not perform at the grand prix level, but she is no sluggard, either. Several Tartan 37's have participated in the Marion-Bermuda race and regularly in the Off-Sounding series and performed respectably.

A large percentage of the boats are purchased for family cruising. On these boats, headsail roller-furling systems are usually installed. Almost inevitably, there will be some sacrifice in windward performance with roller-furling headsails.

The optional inboard genoa track should be considered essential to those concerned with optimum windward performance. Coupled with the standard outboard track, this will allow versatility in sheeting angles.

Headsail sheets and winches are within reach of the helmsman. This feature is vital for shorthanded cruising and can help make the difference between a boat that is easy for two people to handle and one that is difficult. However, no real provision has been made for the installation of secondary headsail winches, should you wish to carry staysails. Small winches could be mounted on the cockpit coamings forward, but they could interfere with the installation of a dodger.

With good sails, the performance of the Tartan 37 will not be disappointing on any point of sail. Tartan brochures show the 37 happily romping along on a beam reach in a 15-knot breeze. We suspect that under those conditions her owner is likely to be as happy as any sailor afloat.

Handling Under Power

The standard Universal 40 auxiliary diesel engine is more than adequate power for the Tartan 37. The tendency in many production boats today is toward smaller, lighter, lower-powered diesels—the opposite of the past American boatbuilding practice, which, like our automobiles, tended toward excessive horsepower.

The engine box of the Tartan 37 is only partially sound insulated. Access to the front end of the engine is good by removing the companionway ladder.

LIVABILITY

Deck Layout

With wide decks, inboard chainplates, and a relatively narrow cabin trunk, fore and aft movement on the deck of the Tartan 37 is relatively easy. It would be easier if the lifeline stanchions had been positioned further outboard, rather than about three inches inboard of the toerail.

There are proper bow chocks, and two well-mounted cleats forward. However, a line led through the chocks to the cleats bears against the bow pulpit. Shifting the cleats further inboard would provide a better lead.

Surprisingly, there is no foredeck anchor well. This means that an anchor must be stowed in chocks on deck if one is to be readily available. Then, you must face the problem of storing the anchor-rode. Molded foredeck anchor wells are becoming almost universal in modern boats. While the weight of anchor and rode (about 65 pounds in a boat this size) might be objectionable stowed all the way forward, the convenience of such a system generally outweighs the increase in pitching moment that might result. Removing the ground tackle from the deck also reduces clutter and simplifies foredeck work.

There are strong, well-mounted teak grabrails on top of the cabin trunk, although the reasoning for using two short rails on each side rather than a single long rail escapes us. The molded breakwater/cockpit coaming is a common Sparkman & Stephens feature and greatly facilitates the mounting of a dodger—almost standard equipment on a cruising boat.

The T-shaped cockpit of the Tartan 37 is comfortable for five while sailing. It has several unusual features. Rather than the usual unyielding fiberglass, there are teak duckboards on all cockpit seats. This means that you won't sit in a puddle when it rains, or when heavy spray comes aboard. These duckboards are comfortable, but they are held in place only by wooden cleats, with the

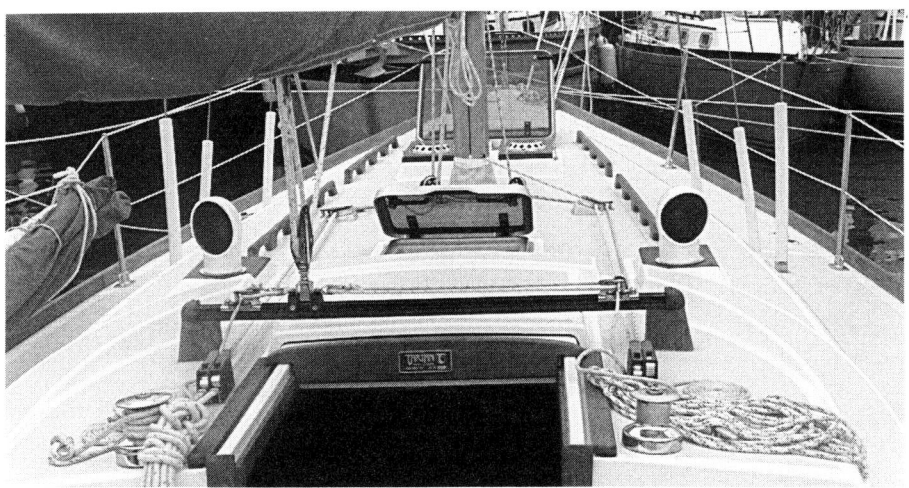

exception of the starboard seat. A more secure arrangement should be provided for offshore sailing.

There is a teak-grated cockpit sump under the helmsman's feet. This shifts the cockpit drains inboard from the edge of the cockpit. The result is that a puddle can collect in the leeward corner of the cockpit when the boat is well-heeled in a blow with heavy spray coming aboard.

Access to the steering gear is via the lazarette hatch. There is good provision for an emergency tiller, but the lazarette hatch must be held open in some way to use the emergency steering. There is a drop-in shelf in the lazarette which allows using the locker with less risk of damage to the steering system, but we would be reluctant to store anything small there that might possibly jam in the steering gear.

With a low cabin trunk, visibility from the helm is excellent. We suspect that many helmsmen would prefer a contoured seat to the flat bench provided, however. The relatively wide, flat top of the cockpit coaming provides reasonably comfortable seating for the helmsman who prefers to sit well to leeward or well to windward.

The main companionway is narrow and almost parallel-sided—features we like—but the sill is much lower than we prefer for offshore sailing. The low sill facilitates passage of the crew below. Unfortunately, it also greatly facilitates passage of water below should the cockpit fill. Coupled with the thin plywood dropboards, we feel this is a potential weakness in watertight integrity, compromising the boat as an offshore cruiser.

Belowdecks
Due to an abundance of teak and teak plywood, the interior of the Tartan 37 is dark and cave-like. This is much the same criticism we have made of the other well-finished boats. Mind you, it's a rather elegant cave, with excellent joiner-work throughout. Somehow, boat designers and builders have convinced most

of the consuming public that teak is the only wood to use belowdecks. The fact
is that there are many wonderful woods—ash and butternut, for example—
that yield interiors that are lighter in both weight and color than teak.

The forward cabin of the Tartan 37 is truly comfortable for a boat of this size,
with drawers, hanging lockers, separate access to the head, and enough room
to dress in relative comfort. The completely louvered door separating the forward cabin from the main cabin looks nice, and does assist in ventilating the
forward cabin. It limits privacy, however, and one good blow from a crew
member caught off balance in a seaway would probably reduce it to a pile of
teak kindling.

The head is quite comfortable, and it is possible to brace adequately for use
offshore. The shower drains into a separate sump, not into the bilge.

Layout of the main cabin is conventional, with settee and pilot berth to
starboard, dinette to port. The original design had a pilot berth to starboard
necessitating a complex chainplate arrangement as well as a berth of dubious
comfort and convenience. By 1986, the pilot berth was eliminated in favor of
shelves and gone, too, was the need for the cantilevered chainplate support.

While there is excellent storage space in the galley, one must reach across the
stove to reach much of it—and it's a long reach for a short person. The stove is
securely mounted and has a grab bar across its well to protect the cook, but this
grab bar also inhibits the stove's gimballing function. There is no on-deck
provision for storage for propane bottles, should you wish propane rather than
the standard alcohol stove. There is room for CNG bottles to be stowed in the
starboard cockpit locker, but CNG has never really impressed us because of its
bulkiness compared to propane.

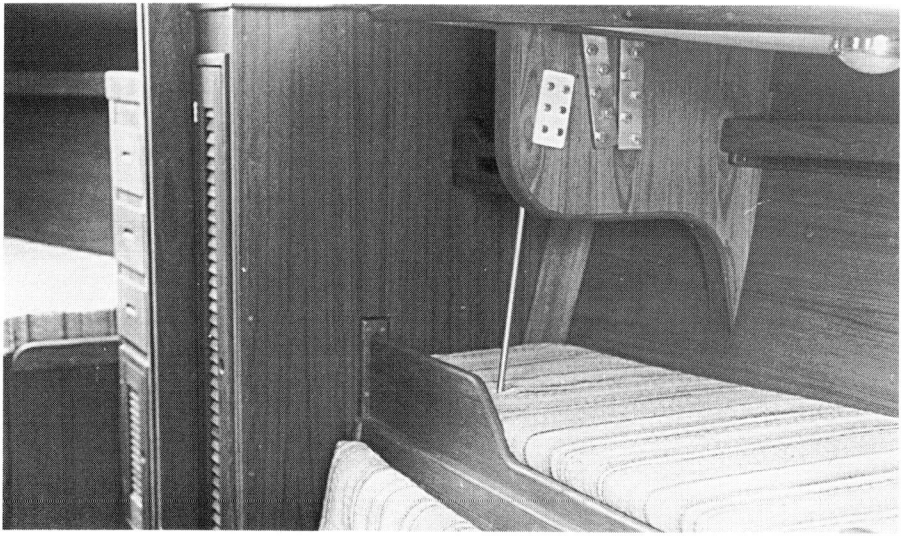

**Complex engineering of the chainplates is necessitated by the presence of the pilot
berth on the starboard side.**

The icebox appears to be well insulated. Why Tartan, like many other builders, fails to insulate and carefully fit the tops of their iceboxes totally escapes us. We have found this shortcoming on every variety of boat, from the cheapest to the most expensive.

The Tartan 37 has a large, well-designed navigation station. The quarterberth above it converts to a double berth.

Ventilation is excellent, with eight opening ports and three hatches. There are also four ventilators for the accommodations areas—two exhaust type and two low plastic cowls in dorade boxes. We think four taller cowls in the dorades would be more effective, or better still, the five tall cowls shown in the original plans for the boat. The vertical deckhouse bulkhead also allows a dropboard to be left out when it rains, further improving ventilation.

Despite our complaints about the darkness of the interior, joinerwork is of excellent production-boat quality throughout. The degree of enclosure of the interior of the hull can complicate access to deck hardware, and certainly does not facilitate survey of the vessel. In traditional wooden yacht construction, structural members are often left exposed for their intrinsic beauty, as well as for ventilation and preservation. In fiberglass boats, it is rather difficult to find intrinsic beauty in the structural material. Perhaps we are better off with it all hidden—as long as we know what holds the boat together. We certainly have confidence in what holds the Tartan together, even if we do pay a premium for that confidence.

CONCLUSIONS

The Tartan 37, like other Tartan Marine boats, is a well-built, well-mannered, fast cruising boat. The length of time she has been in production and the number of 37s sold attests to the success of her concept; their value on the used boat market attests to the degree to which that concept has been realized. Like Sabre Yachts, Tartan has remained a medium-sized builder keeping its focus strictly on a line of conservative, proven boats built and priced above the average for the production boat market.

For the boat buyer who wants a boat from a builder whose reputation he can depend on and a boat that is modern without being racy, fashionable without being faddish, and good performing without being demanding, the 37 then is worthy of strong consideration. Better still, there should always be a market for the 37 no matter how soft the sales of used boats become.

The 37 may never appreciate in the manner of some better finished (and more expensive) cruising boats such as Hinckleys that have practically become cult objects. Instead, the Tartan 37 is a Buick: popular for justifiable reasons with the likes of bankers, stockbrokers, and doctors looking for a solid, conservative grey-flannel yacht. She is neither ostentatious nor plain. She is neither cheaply designed nor cheaply built. One pays for good breeding.

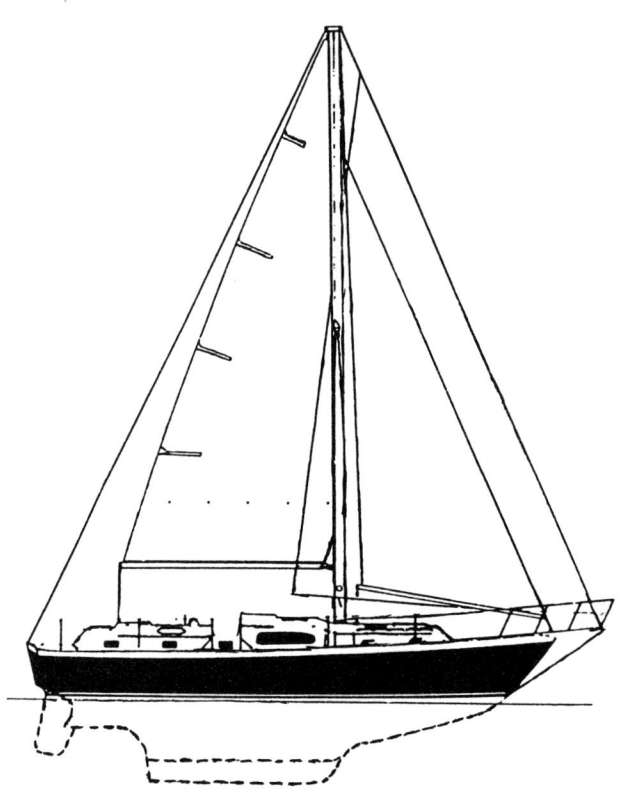

Specifications
Irwin 37

LOA	37'0"
LWL	30'0"
Beam	11'6"
Draft	
full keel	5'6"
shoal keel	4'0"
Displacement	20,000 lbs
Ballast	7800 lbs
Sail area	625 sq ft

Irwin Yacht
& Marine Corp.
13055 49th Street
Clearwater, Florida 33520
(813) 577-4581

The Irwin 37:
A Production Cruising Boat

THE BOAT AND THE BUILDER

An evaluation of the Irwin 37 threatens to expose all our prejudices about boatbuilders and cruising boats. In general we like sturdily built, finely finished, boats that perform well and reflect traditional standards (if not design) and lasting value.

Irwin Yachts, one of the two or three largest production builders, builds boats of mediocre quality and finish and markets them to buyers looking for as much boat as possible for the price. In every sense of the word, Irwin Boats, of which the Irwin 37 is archetypal, are *production* boats. They are mass produced, carefully priced, simply advertised, and widely sold to a broad spectrum of customers.

More than 600 Irwin 37s were sold during the 11 years of its production. Introduced in 1979, it had various incarnations, documented by the company as models Mark I through Mark V. We will specifically discuss a Mark V.

From the outset, the Irwin 37 has been a roomy, appealing cruising boat that has been described as the Chevrolet Belair of the boat market. Her greatest appeal has been to the owner who is not beholden to tradition, sailing performance, elegance, construction details, or investment value.

Designer/Owner/President Ted Irwin *is* Irwin Yachts. He is involved in all aspects of his independent firm (in contrast to the subsidiaries of conglomerates that many other major boat builders have become). From all reports he is one tough fellow to work for. He delegates little responsibility of authority, and turnover (at least at the executive level) is considerable. In this respect, Ted Irwin is a Florida counterpart of an equally powerful and successful independent builder, Frank Butler of Catalina Yachts in California.

Irwin has sailed all the boats he has designed, from his stock cruising boats (such as the 37) to state-of-the-art SORC racers. The Irwin line has always been a blend of out-and-out cruising boats and *almost* out-and-out racing boats.

Ted Irwin has his eyes firmly fixed on his business, with one eye glued to production costs. Irwin Yachts has perhaps the most meticulously priced-out boats in the industry. Virtually everything except hardware and sails are produced in-house. This includes the tooling for the boats, spars, rigging, and woodwork. That way, Irwin can control the design and the price. Unfortunately, he has never seemed to be able to match quality control with price control.

Irwin Yachts is considered by some to have the most notoriously slipshod quality control among the larger boatbuilders. No other boats have as poor a reputation for warranty claims, delays in commissioning, missing or incorrect parts, and mislocated hardware as Irwin's. Similarly an examination of virtually any Irwin-built boat reveals details that reflect cost savings, some, in our opinion, serious (gate valves on all through-hull fittings) and some trivial (through hull-fittings not installed flush with the hull).

Irwin's other eye is perhaps the keenest in the industry in seeing what the buying public wants, what it will buy, and what it is willing to pay. Irwin Yachts makes what it heralds ambiguously as the "value yacht." It is a boat that makes compromises to keep the price under those of the major competition.

And make no mistake, the firm has for 15 years been a remarkable success story. There has never been any question that it has been profitable for Ted Irwin, a rare exception in an industry rife with tales of economic brinksmanship.

CONSTRUCTION

There are no basic industry standards for fiberglass construction; the primary criterion for adequate hull laminate strength seems largely a matter of in-use durability. Some builders, in the absence of such standards, overbuild their products (CSY, for example). Irwin Yachts, on the other hand, molds hulls and decks to specifications that are, by industry comparison, light. As with everything else, Irwin maintains a tight control over tooling costs and the amounts of resin, glass fiber, and labor that goes into each hull. By our standards, the

Irwin fiberglass layup is minimal; that is one reason the boats have a low price. Yet basic laminate is not where cost savings are most apparent.

More conspicuous are cosmetic flaws. In two of the new 37s we looked at, there are obvious deep (up to 1/2-inch) hollows in the bottom. These are evidently the result of pulling a still "green" hull from the mold and setting it in a four-point building cradle. The supports dished the laminate, probably permanently.

For years Irwin Yachts have suffered from print-through, whereby the pattern of the underlying roving in the laminate was visible in the topside gelcoat. Recently, this has been considerably reduced with the use of Coremat between the roving and the gelcoat. In the new 37s we examined, print-though was negligible. This print-through remains an unsightly feature of older 37s, especially in the dark paint of the sheer stripe.

In our examination of the 37s, we also noted sloppy underwater fairing around the rudder gudgeon, and where the "Adapt-A-Draft" keel is attached. These types of flaws, coupled as they are with such details as protruding through-hull fittings and squared off trailing edges, produce needless drag on a boat whose performance under sail is already suspect.

The earliest Irwin 37s did not have bowsprits. The result was a boxy gracelessness that was accentuated by obvious unevenness in the sheerline, an unrelieved topside expanse, and Clorox-bottle styling, not to mention dimples and gelcoat blemishes. To improve performance with more sail area, Irwin added a molded fiberglass bowsprit. Serendipitously, the extension did wonders for the aesthetics. Less fortuitously, the glass sprit also became a source of warranty claims when, if tightening the rigging caused it to flex, the gelcoat then crazed.

The Mark V's bowsprit is of welded aluminum. On a year-old boat we examined, the bobstay is a threaded stainless steel rod with jaw terminals at each end. Newer boats have the rod welded between two plates on each end, a less costly fitting. As the lower end will be continually awash and thus vulnerable to corrosion, we think the welded construction is a mistake. Similarly we are concerned about the stainless steel rudder gudgeon; in the year-old boat we already found evidence of stress corrosion.

The Irwin 37 has a history of warranty claims against defective gelcoat—too thin (or missing), too thick, discolored, crazed, or covering voids. Where this

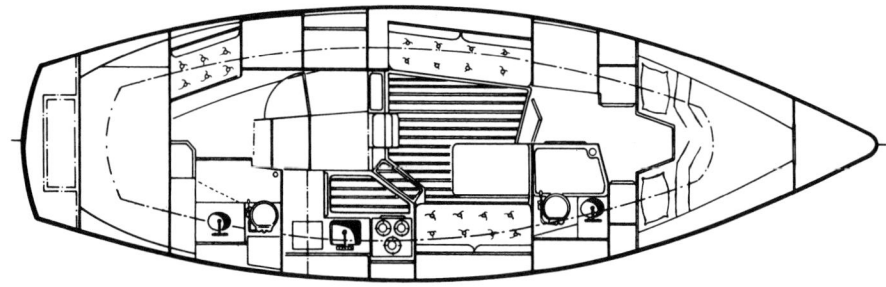

happened in the earlier diamond pattern non-skid deck surfaces, inconspicu-
ous repair was all but impossible. The problem drove Irwin dealers and new
owners to distraction and fueled much of the scuttlebutt about Irwin's poor
handling of warranty claims. Now Irwin is putting on a random non-skid
pattern, easier to repair. We also understand that Irwin has gone to a better
quality gelcoat.

Another common question about Irwin Yachts has been its hull to deck joint.
Contrary to common industry practice, the joint in the Irwin 37 consists of
overlapping flanges joined with a polyester slurry, and fastened on about 6-
inch centers with stainless steel self-tapping screws. Most builders now use a
semi-rigid adhesive and bolts, a technique we favor. We believe this more
positive attachment is called for on boats going to sea.

The chainplates of the 37 are stainless steel webs laminated into the topsides
during the hull layup. This technique was developed by Irwin and is imitated
by a number of builders whose chainplates are at the outer edge of the deck. It
seems to be a satisfactory installation and indeed preferable to early Irwin 37s,
which had the chainplates through-bolted to the topsides.

PERFORMANCE

Handling Under Power
Virtually everyone from whom we received information on the Irwin 37 either
dismissed as unimportant or derided her performance under sail. She seems a
classic example of the all-too-common cruising boat that does everything well,
except handle as a sailboat. A number of owners we talked to do not seem
bothered by this shortcoming. We, again with our aforementioned prejudice,
would be.

The Irwin 37 comes standard with a sloop rig; the roller furling genoa was an
almost unanimously specified option at a cost of $2150. A cutter rig (with a
club jib package at $1835) and a ketch rig ($2695 additional) were two other
options. In any configuration, she is a boat that seems ideally suited for a
couple to sail. The sail area is modest with the ketch carrying about 60 square
feet more sail than the sloop, just about enough to compensate for the windage
of the mizzen mast. We think the cutter rig is the best alternative of the three;
the staysail providing a handy headsail in hefty conditions and doing away
with the clutter, expense and windage of the mizzen.

Plainly, the standard shoal-draft keel (without a centerboard) is inadequate
for sailing to windward. Buyers wanting shoal draft should have considered
the centerboard option for $1300. This board does thunk in the trunk when
down, a harmless (if annoying) distraction. Fully raised it remains quiet, a
blessed relief in the middle of the night at anchor.

For optimum performance we prefer the draft keel. What bothers us is that
the tab ran to $1500 for this 18-inch add-on. Still, scintillating windward per-
formance did not result. For better performance, the wise buyer will consider a
host of boats other than the Irwin 37.

Owners have indicated to us their willingness to accept indifferent performance under sail. However, we have heard complaints about the amount of attention the helm needs and some difficulty in steering the boat, both under sail and power ("Steering is stiff and my wife ... has difficulty at times"). We suspect some of this problem is the result of an unbalanced semi-spade rudder, driven by a relatively small diameter steering wheel, through an aft-cabin layout that requires considerable routing of the steering linkage.

Handling Under Power

The Irwin 37 has a 40-horsepower Perkins 4-108 diesel engine driving a three-bladed propeller with a 2:1 reduction, through the after edge of the keel. This is a combination that bespeaks of performance under auxiliary power. In fact, with the standard shoal keel and this combination for power, the Irwin 37 might reasonably be labeled a motorsailer, if that term had not fallen into such disrepute in recent years.

The combination also suggests that the Irwin 37 should appeal to the power-boat owner looking to sail as a way of reducing fuel consumption, without sacrificing the room and amenities of the moderate sized powerboat. Certainly we think it is a worthwhile alternative to the ad hoc conversions of sailboat hulls and rigs to sailing powerboats with their high deckhouses, awkward sailhandling systems, and sundry other hermaphroditic compromises.

LIVABILITY

Deck Layout

The Irwin 37 is a handy boat to sail. The sidedecks are wide, the rail rises to a low bulwark forward to give a sense of security, and the cockpit coaming has an opening to starboard (but is low enough to climb out of anywhere.) The bowsprit is designed to carry a 30-pound plow anchor housed in a roller chock. Hawseholes (of polished aluminum, replacing the line-chafing fiberglass on older boats) are mounted in the bulwark for docklines. Oddly enough, neither the hawseholes nor the roller chock allow a fair lead to the pair of deck cleats.

The stanchions are mounted through the deck, into blocks drilled to fit—a system that we think gives rugged support. In early 37s, the stanchions went into fiberglass tubes glassed under the deck. Now they go into wood blocks (saving cost and complexity). It remains to be seen if the wood rots out in time. In contrast to this sturdy structure, the bow and stern pulpits are screwed on the teak rail cap. We hardly recommend that attachment.

The cockpit is small, accommodating (at the most) four adults at a time. Yet the seats are long enough to stretch out on and access below is easy. We are not bothered by the absence of a bridgedeck or companionway sill for safety because the cockpit is high and amidships, hence dry. Besides (Irwin's advertising notwithstanding) we doubt if many owners would consider offshore passages, given all the limitations the 37 would have at sea.

We like the number, design, and placement of the "smoked glass" opening hatches/skylights. Like many designs that have tropical cruising and charter-ing as part of their destiny, the Irwin 37 has a well ventilated interior.

On-deck stowage is limited to one gigantic locker, the lazarette. The trouble is that for storing fenders, docklines, sheets, snorkeling gear, and so forth (as well as an odd sail or two), it would leave everything hard to get at. You can't reach the bottom from the deck and without some owner-installed shelves, hooks and bins, the contents would be in chaos.

Belowdecks

If performance is not a priority in the design of the Irwin 37, livability is. The Irwin 37 is a coastal cruiser for two couples or a family of four. She has the most practical aft cabin layout we have seen on a stock boat under 40 feet. The layout has remained essentially unchanged since the 37 was introduced and features a spacious aft cabin, a step-down galley, a more than adequate walk-through passageway, and a forward cabin that should not make its occupants feel like they are in steerage.

Fundamental to the Irwin design and marketing philosophy is that the inte-rior should instantly appeal to women. The decor is "Production Boat Contem-porary;" tufted velour cushions, plenty of teak, and "color coordinated" car-peting. We are not impressed with the so-so craftsmanship and unsanded finish of the joinerwork, nor with the antiseptic molded hull liner, but these are details that do not immediately affect the illusion of quality, comfort, and spaciousness.

Thus the interior of the 37 minimizes seagoing machismo. There are no handrails, sea berths, navigation sanctum, or sailbag stowage. Below, with the possible exception of the gimballed stove, one can easily forget that under certain circumstances a sailboat may not always be upright.

It would be hard to imagine being aboard an Irwin 37 at sea. There is no berth one could sleep in comfortably. The settee berth to port is too narrow, and the settee to starboard is too short. One owner remarked that even when the settee berth is to leeward, a nap-taker is rolled out of it during a gentle afternoon sail.

But what the 37 may lack at sea she more than makes up for at bedtime at anchor. Both the athwartships aft cabin berth and the forward V-berth are queen size with 4-inch mattresses. The two cabins are separated by 30 feet of boat, and closed doors. Each has a private head.

There are good hanging lockers, lots of drawers, a few scuttles, and assorted nooks and crannies. Yet someone forgot to include places to store dry, warm food. For cold food there are (now get this) one front opening Norcold refrig-erator (standard) and two (yes, two) large top-opening iceboxes. In fact, both iceboxes are so sizable that their bottoms are difficult to reach. One of them (under the rudimentary chart table) might be better used for dry food storage, except that getting at its contents would be at best inconvenient. The alterna-tive is to use the galley icebox as a dry well and rely on the Norcold, despite our longtime prejudice against using front opening boxes (which depend on electrical power) away from a dock. Perhaps this refrigerator is the best indication of the type of cruising for which the 37 is best suited.

Two other points about the interior deserve comment, one favorable and one not so. Engine access and sound insulation are among the best we have seen in a production boat, helped by removable panels on the sides of the walk-through. To check the dipstick and heat exchanger water, there is no need to move the companionway ladder. In short, if the engine of the 37 seizes from lack of oil or overheats for lack of water, the owner has only himself to blame.

On the other side, the bulkhead-mounted, fold-up, drop-leaf cabin table will not survive the first fall against it when a powerboat leaves a wake. It might not even withstand the weight of a rib roast. The first thing we would do after buying an Irwin 37 is find ourselves a rugged, attractive fixed cabin table. (The next thing we would do is make the seats comfortable).

CONCLUSIONS

Having exposed our prejudices, we hasten to add that the more than 600 Irwin 37s sold, conclusively prove that many sailors do not share those prejudices. The all-up price of an Irwin 37 was $75,000 with the options we mentioned as desirable, plus a flow-through/holding tank head system, commissioning, and freight. This price included working sails (made by Johnson Sails), fresh water pressure system, 110-volt AC system, and basic electronics. We also would add a Bimini top if we expected to sail in a warm climate.

At this price the Irwin 37 was $15,000 less expensive than, say, the Tartan 37 or the Pearson 365. A Hunter 37, by contrast, could be sailed away for about $10,000 less than the Irwin 37.

Ironically, considering the persistent badmouthing of the Irwin 37 around the waterfront, older models have retained their value. A five-year-old 37 is still bringing up to $75,000 on the used boat market, having appreciated at about half the inflation rate in the intervening years. The reason is simple: the Irwin 37 offers many buyers what they are looking for in a boat, new or used.

And, for the dollars, the Irwin 37 is a lot of boat. Many owners report looking seriously at smaller boats and settling on the 37 when they (and their wives) saw the spacious 37 for the same price as the smaller boat. For that price, they get what they see as a summer home afloat. Deep water cruising may be a distant dream, but the immediate desire is a comfortable and impressive boat for weekending and trips to the Bahamas, the Eastern Shore, or the like.

We'd plan systematic and regular upgrading. Expect to replace the standard through-hull gate valves with seacocks or ball valves. Divide the awesome lazarette. Run the halyards aft to the cockpit when they need replacing. Build some pitch into the seats of the settees. Rebuild the "navigation station" into handy food storage. Mount a large diameter steering wheel so you will no longer have to steer standing up or perched on the edge of your seat. Smooth the rough texture of the interior teak trim.

Finally, take a sail on some boat meant to sail effectively to windward—just so you'll see what you're missing.

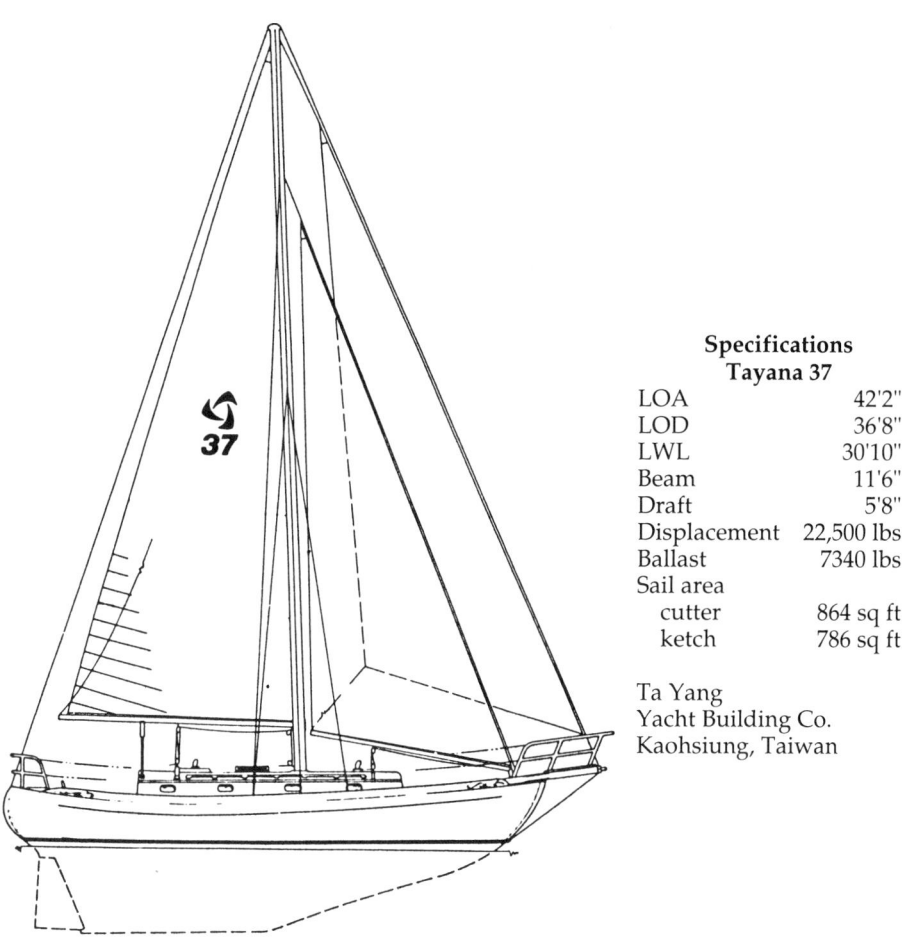

LOA	42'2"
LOD	36'8"
LWL	30'10"
Beam	11'6"
Draft	5'8"
Displacement	22,500 lbs
Ballast	7340 lbs
Sail area	
cutter	864 sq ft
ketch	786 sq ft

Ta Yang
Yacht Building Co.
Kaohsiung, Taiwan

The Tayana 37:
For Experienced Cruisers

THE BOAT AND THE BUILDER

With over 560 boats sailing the seas of the world, the Tayana 37 has been one of the most successful products of the Taiwan-built boat invasion that began in the early 1970s. Her shapely Baltic stern, scribed planking seams molded into the glass hull, and lavish use of teak above and below decks have come to epitomize the image that immediately comes to mind when Oriental boats are mentioned.

Not all thoughts of Far Eastern boats are pleasant, however. To some, Taiwan-built boats mean poor workmanship, overly heavy hulls, unbedded hardware of dubious heritage, wooden spars that delaminate, and builder-modified boats light years removed from the plans provided by the designer. Add to that a serious language barrier and the inevitable logistical problems of dealing with a boatyard halfway round the world, and you have a situation ready-made to generate potential nightmares for the boat buyer. To the credit of the builder, the designer, the primary importer, and a powerful owners' association, the Tayana 37 has weathered 10 years of production—a lifetime in the world of boatbuilding—while making steady improvements and maintaining an average output of over 50 boats per year.

Washington-based designer Bob Perry had just hung out his own shingle when the Tayana 37 was designed in the early 70's. The Westsail 32 had just come lumbering onto the scene, bringing with it a resurgence of interest in the double-ended hull form, and more people than ever before were beginning to have the dream of dropping out of the rat race and sailing away to a tropical paradise.

In the last 12 years, Bob Perry has become an enormously successful designer of cruising boats, from traditional full keel designs such as the Tayana 37, to modern fin-keel cruisers such as the Nordic 40, Golden Wave 42, and the Valiant 40. A remarkable number of his designs have been built in the Orient, in both Hong Kong and Taiwan.

Perry conceived the Tayana 37 as a cruising boat of traditional appearance above the water, with moderately heavy displacement, a long waterline, and a reasonably efficient cutter rig of modern proportions. Below the water, the forefoot of the long keel has been cut away, and a Constellation-type rudder utilized rather than the more traditional "barn door." Perry sought to cash in on the popularity of the double-ended hull while keeping displacement moderate and performance reasonable, avoiding the plight of boats such as the Westsail 32—the inability to go to windward, and sluggish performance in anything short of a moderate gale. The design of the stern of the Tayana 37 borrows heavily from the well-known Aage Neilsen-designed ketch, *Holger Danske*, winner of the 1980 Bermuda Race. It is one of the more handsome Baltic-type sterns on any production sailboat.

The Tayana 37 began life as the CT 37. In 1979, the boat became known as the Tayana 37, named for Ta Yang Yacht Building Company. While some snobbiness exists among some owners who own the CT version, Perry insists that this is illusory. According to the designer, the CT 37 and the Tayana 37 are the same boat, built by the same men in the same yard. In much the same way that

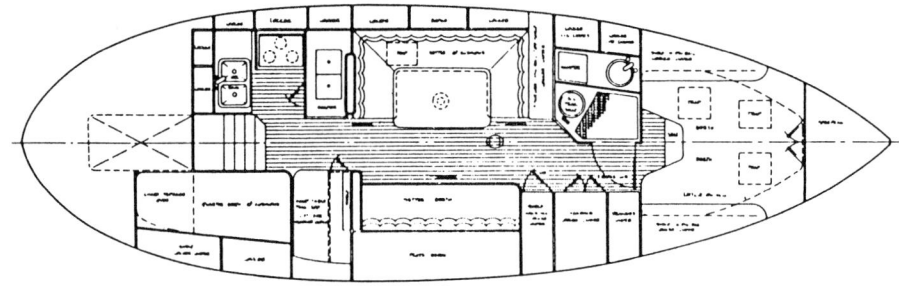

the early Swans imported by Palmer Johnson were known by the name of the importer (the names Nautor and Swan were unknown here in the late 1960's). The early Tayanas were known as CTs because the name CT had already become known in this country.

Perry, who has worked with many yards in the Far East, considers Ta Yang one of the best. The yard has been very responsive to input from both dealers and owners. Over the years the Tayana 37 has been in production, this has resulted in steady improvement in the quality of the boat.

Ta Yang also builds the Robert Harris-designed Vancouver 42, plus three larger Tayanas, the 47 and 52, both Perry designs, and the 55 from the board of Dutch designer Pieter Beeldsnijder, who also designed a boat known as the Ta Yang Surprise 35.

On the east coast of the U.S., Tayanas are imported by Southern Offshore Yachts with offices in Canada, Rhode Island and both coasts of Florida. Henshaw, Windships, and Blue Water Yachts handles Tayanas on the West Coast. Tayana buyers have been high in their praise for Southern Offshore, although somewhat less enthusiastic about other dealers elsewhere. Perhaps this is one reason why the Tayana 37 has had more success on the market on the East Coast than any other Far Eastern importer.

CONSTRUCTION

The hull of the Tayana 37 is a fairly heavy solid glass layup. Some roving print-through is evident in the topsides. The hull to deck joint has in the past occasionally been a problem with the boat. There is no doubt it is strong, but there have been numerous reports of leaking.

Part of the problem with the hull to deck joint is the fact that the hull and deck moldings form a hollow bulwark extending well above the main deck level. This bulwark is pierced by hawsepipes and several large scuppers. Careful bedding of all fittings that penetrate the bulwarks is essential to avoid leaks. On new boats, the entire hollow bulwark is glassed over from inside the hull, greatly reducing the possibility of leaks. This results in an incredibly labor-intensive joint, but labor-intensive is the name of the game in Taiwanese boatbuilding.

None of the numerous through-hull fittings is recessed flush with the exterior of the hull. The argument is frequently made that this is unnecessary on cruising boats. Nothing could be further from the truth. The cruising boat is frequently undercanvassed for her displacement and wetted surface. Add to this the drag associated with projections from the hull, and you have a boat that spends a lot of time motoring in light air when she should be sailing. While the Tayana 37 is far from undercanvassed, she could benefit from a little more bottom fairing as much as the next boat.

The rudder stock is a substantial stainless steel rod, with the rudder held on by welded arms riveted through the rudder blade. The heel fitting is a bronze casting. This is fastened to the hull with stainless steel bolts. Inevitably, there will be galvanic action between the bronze and the stainless, with the fasten-

The Tayana 37

ings coming out on the short end. There is provision for protection of the rudder straps with zincs.

All items of deck hardware, including cleats and stanchions, are through-bolted and backed with stainless steel pads. Most of the hardware is fairly accessible from belowdecks.

The ballast keel is an iron casting dropped into the hollow fiberglass keel shell. The casting is glassed over on the inside of the boat.

The glasswork of the Tayana 37 is of good quality. There are no rough edges, the fillet bonding is neat, and there is no glass or resin slopped about. Tayana warrants the hull against defects for 10 years.

The standard steering system is now a pedestal system built in Taiwan, but remarkably similar to the Edson pedestal steerer.

Seacocks are used on all through-hull fittings. The seacocks appears to be copies of U.S.-made Groco valves. The hoses to seacocks are all double clamped.

PERFORMANCE

Handling Under Power

A number of different auxiliary engines have been used in the Tayana 37 over the years. The standard engine is now the Yanmar JHE-44. The Perkins 4-108 is available as an option at $1,800, but we see no reason to choose the Perkins over the Yanmar for this boat.

While the engine box removes completely to provide good access for service, there is no provision for easy access to the oil dipstick. This means that this vital task is likely to be ignored. A simple door in the side of the engine box would solve the problem.

The placement of the fuel tank has caused substantial discussion on the part of owners. The standard 90-gallon, black-iron tank is located under the V-berth in the forward cabin. When full, the tank holds almost 650 pounds of fuel. This is about the same weight as 375 feet of 3/8-inch chain—a substantial amount to carry around in the bow of a 37-footer. A Tayana 37 with the bow tank full and a heavy load of ground tackle will show noticeable bow-down trim. The design was originally drawn with the fuel tanks under the main cabin settees, but the builder put the tank forward to create additional storage in the main cabin.

This is a good example of one of the basic recurring problems with Far East-built boats. Frequently the builders have good glass men and good joiners, but their inexperience in sailing results in strange inconsistencies which may compromise their boats.

Fortunately, thanks to the pressure from owners and from Southern Offshore Yachts, the builder offers optional tankage amidships, where it belongs. By all means select this tankage option so that the fore and aft trim of the boat will remain unchanged as fuel is consumed.

Handling Under Sail

The Tayana 37 comes as a ketch or cutter, and with aluminum or wood (spruce) spars. Understandably so few buyers specify the wooden spars that they are no longer built by Ta Yang. In this day and age it seems incredible that anyone would even consider wood spars over aluminum, but as recently as 1982, the wood spars were standard on the Tayana with aluminum as an option.

In 1987, the basic spar sections were from Isomat plus some from a Japanese sparmaker with the rigging made up by Ta Yang. Surprising as it sounds, it has been less expensive to ship the extrusions to Taiwan, assemble and afix the standard rigging, and ship the package back with the boat, than it has been to supply made-up rigs in this country as is done with a number of other Far East-built boats.

We see no reason to select the ketch rig. Both performance and balance with the cutter rig will be better. The cutter's mainsail is 342 square feet. Any couple healthy enough to go world cruising should be able to cope with a sail of this moderate size.

The cutter rig is tall and well proportioned. Perry has drawn an unusually high aspect rig for a cruising boat, and the result is a boat with good perform-ance on all points of sail. With the aluminum spars, the optional Nicro Fico ball bearing mainsheet traveler, and a good suit of sails, the Tayana 37 will be surprisingly fast. Her working sail area of 864 square feet is generous.

Despite a ballast to displacement ratio of 33 percent, the Tayana 37 is not a stiff boat. This is due in part to the tall, heavy rig and the substantial amount of other weight above the boat's vertical center of gravity. Much of the boat's heavy joinerwork and glass work is well above the waterline, raising the center of gravity and reducing initial stability. Perry believes the initial tenderness to be an asset, reducing the snappiness of the boat's roll and making her a more comfortable sea boat. We agree.

Many owners report that the boat carries substantial weather helm. The sail plan is drawn with significant rake to the mast. This creates just enough shift in the center of effort of the sail plan to create a lot of weather helm. Bringing the mast back toward the vertical by tightening the headstay and forestay while loosening the backstay should cure much of the problem, according to reports from other owners. If may be necessary to shorten the headstay to do this, so take this possibility into consideration when ordering a roller-furling system.

Sails (mainsail, staysail, and jib, plus mizzen for the ketch rig) are included as standard equipment and are made by Neil Pryde of Hong Kong. In ordering boats of this size and type, many owners might opt to work with a local sailmaker especially on selection of a roller furling system, an inventory of headsails, and mainsail reefing. Unfortunately, the allowance should a buyer not want the standard Pryde sails is only $900. It would be tough for a buyer to want his own sailmaker's equivalent inventory to the tune of $5000 and only get credit for enough to maybe pay for the staysail. Such, however, are the facts of boat buying from the Orient; the relatively modest cost of the boat is for a package and any buyer will have to decide whether he wants to add to that cost with upgraded equipment and sails. Certainly we would recommend supplementing the inventory with a good genoa.

LIVABILITY

Deck Layout

With her bulwarks, high double lifelines, and substantial bow and stern pulpits, the Tayana 37 gives the sailor a sense of security on those cold, windy nights when he's called out for sail changes. A teak platform grating atop the bowsprit coupled with the strong pulpit relieves that appendage of its "widow-maker" reputation.

The bowsprit platform incorporates double anchor rollers which will house CQR anchors. Unfortunately, there is no good lead from the rollers to any place to secure the anchor rode. Line or chain led to the heavy bowsprit bitts would chafe on the platform. An anchor windlass mounted to port or starboard of the bowsprit would provide a good lead and is an available option.

There are hawsepipes through the bulwarks port and starboard well aft of the stern. These will be fine for dock lines, but are too far aft to serve as good leads for anchoring. There is room at deck level outboard of the bowsprit to install a set of heavy chocks for anchoring, although anchor rode led to this point will chafe on the bobstay as the boat swings to her anchor.

This is a classic problem of the boat with bowsprit. The anchor rode must really lead well out the bowsprit to avoid the bobstay, yet the long lead complicates securing the inboard end of the rode.

The long staysail boom makes it difficult to cross from one side of the foredeck to the other. The standard staysail traveler is merely a stainless steel rod on which a block can slide on its shackle. Under load, this can bind when tacking, so that it may be necessary to go forward and kick the block over after every tack. By all means get the optional travelers with their roller-bearing cars. Complaints about the standard travelers are frequent.

The standard winches on the 37 are Barient. Buyers should look at the standard winch package carefully. Most Tayana dealers offer alternatives not only with winches, but numerous other items as well. Those dealer-offered options not only increase the commission the dealer gets for his sale of the boat, but allow Tayana buyers many choices worth considering, albeit at added expense. One reason why the Tayana 37 is best bought by someone with at least a modicum of experience is so he can make some good decisions on what to add or replace. As a starter, we'd go for a heftier winch selection and make most of them self-tailing.

Although the sidedecks are relatively narrow due to the wide cabin trunk, there is reasonable access fore and aft. A full-length handrail on either side of the cabin trunk provides a good handhold.

The cockpit of the Tayana 37 is small, as befits an oceangoing sailboat. There are cockpit scuppers at each of the four corners of the cockpit well, with seacocks on the through-hull outlets.

With the now-standard pedestal steering, the cockpit seems to have shrunk.

Only three can be seated in real comfort. Although this is no real problem for the cruising couple, it is not a cockpit for extensive entertaining in port. The elimination of the coaming around the stern of the boat has made the cockpit seats long enough for sleeping on deck, but at the expense of exposing the helmsman to a wet seat in a following sea. The coaming can optionally be continued around the rear of the cockpit. The configuration of the cockpit lockers varies with the interior options chosen, but the lockers are large enough to provide reasonable storage.

Belowdecks
The interior of the Tayana sells more boats than any other feature. There is a "standard" interior, but almost all 37s have to some extent an interior custom-designed for each buyer in conjunction with the importer. Indeed, a "blank" accommodation plan to scale is included with brochure material so that prospective owners can doodle their variations on the interior scheme. Better still, the added cost of the customized layout ranges only up to an added $2,500 or thereabouts.

The cost of producing these interiors is not prohibitive. Interior joinerwork is labor intensive, and labor in the Orient is still far cheaper than it is in this country.

Like other Taiwanese boats, the interior of the Tayana 37 is all teak. This results in an interior that can be oppressively dark to some people, exquisitely cool to others. To keep it looking good, someone is going to have to do a lot of oiling or a lot of varnishing.

The interior joinerwork is some of the best we have seen on any boat, whether it is built in the U.S., Taiwan, or Finland. Joints are just about flawless, panelled doors beautifully joined, drawers dovetailed from solid stock. There were no fillers making up for poorly fitted joints, no trim fitted with grinders, no slop anywhere. The men who put the interior in the new boat we examined were real craftsmen. Older boats we have looked at did not boast quite this caliber of workmanship, but their joinerwork was certainly of good quality.

With such an array of interior options it is difficult to really evaluate the boat's interior. This may be a mixed blessing to the buyer. For the couple who have owned other boats, have kept copious notes about what they want and don't want in their next boat, and who are experienced, well read, and knowledgeable, the ability to plan their own interior offers an opportunity that is probably unequaled in a boat in this price range.

If you have only vague ideas of what you want in the interior of a cruising boat, one of the real advantages of owning the Tayana 37 may be lost. Do you want a pilot berth or storage? Drawers or bins? Propane or kerosene for cooking? Quarterberth or wet locker? Fold-up or drop-leaf table? To the inexperienced, the choices may be bewildering. To those who know what they want, the opportunity is a gold mine.

In all fairness, there is a "standard" interior. It is prosaic but good, with a V-berth forward, followed by head and lockers just aft. The main cabin has a U-shaped settee to port, straight settee and pilot berth to starboard. Aft is a good U-shaped galley to port, navigation station and quarterberth to starboard. For not much more money, you can have pretty much what you want, from a "standard" array of interior options to a fully custom interior. You're missing a good bet if you don't spend some time creating your own dream interior.

CONCLUSIONS

The Tayana 37 has been both typical and atypical of Taiwanese-built boats imported into the U.S. She has the abundance of teak, heavy construction, locally replicated hardware and "traditional" design that have so marked the Far Eastern product. The 37 had a history of early problems, a boat built by those who have little experience with offshore yachts, plus a dealer network of varied talents and concerns. Further, the boat is built in a faraway location with its difficulties in communication and understanding. In these ways the boat is typical.

The 37 is different in that with almost 600 boats already in the hands of U.S. sailors, the Tayana 37 is a proven product. In the 10 years since production began, there has been steady improvement in the boat and in the way the customers are treated. All but gone are the clumsy wooden spars, the fittings of questionable quality, and the massive amounts of teak seemingly just for the sake of using that wood.

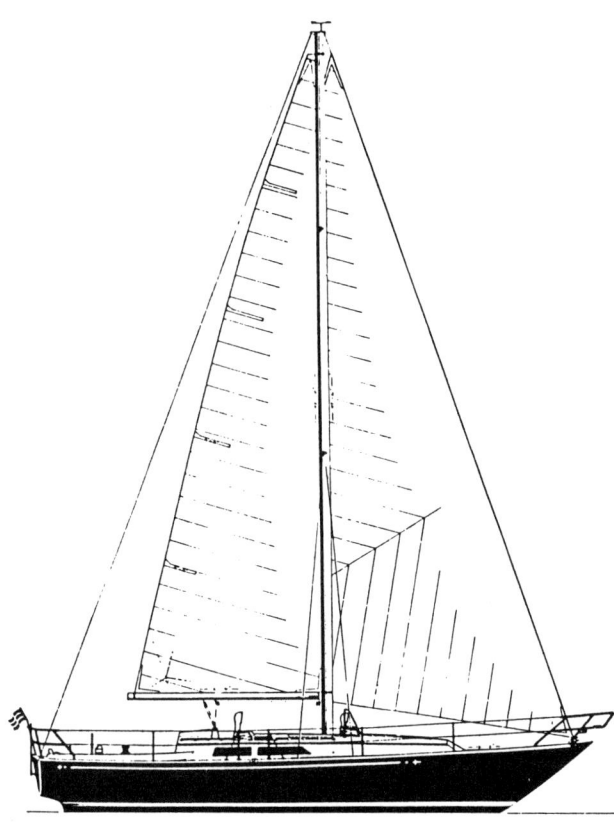

Specifications
C&C Landfall 38

LOA	37'7"
LWL	30'2"
Beam	12'0"
Draft	5'0"
Displacement	16,700 lbs
Ballast	6500 lbs
Sail area	649 sq ft

C&C Yachts
526 Regent Street
Niagara-on-the-Lake
Ontario, Canada L0S 1J0
(416) 468-2101

The C&C Landfall 38:
A Stylish Cruiser

THE BOAT AND THE BUILDER

The C&C Landfall 38 is the midsize boat in the Canadian company's three-boat Landfall range, which also includes a 35-footer and a 43-footer. Unlike other C&Cs, whose interior and deck layouts are designed for racing as well as cruising, the Landfalls are geared toward cruising, with more amenities, a slightly higher degree of finish detail, and deck layout concessions to the cruising couple.

These are performance cruisers, however. Despite more wetted surface, more displacement, and a slightly smaller rig than the original C&C 38, the Landfall 38 is a fast boat, designed for cruisers who want to get there quickly, as well as in style.

The Landfall 38 is a direct descendant of the old C&C 38, the older hull design having been modified with slightly fuller sections forward, a slightly raked transom (rather than IOR reverse transom), a longer, shallower keel, and a longer deckhouse for increased interior volume.

Nevertheless, the hull is more that of a sleek racer rather than a fat cruiser. To gain the additional performance that makes a true performance cruiser, you trade off a hull volume that is slightly smaller than you would expect in a pure cruiser of the same waterline length. This is most apparent in the ends of the boat. The V-berth forward narrows sharply, and the hull rises so quickly aft that C&C's normal gas bottle stowage at the aft end of the cockpit is completely eliminated.

C&C was a pioneer in composite fiberglass construction. Balsa coring has just about become synonymous with the company name over the years. In addition to production boat facilities in the U.S. and Canada, C&C maintains a custom division which turns out both high-tech IOR racing boats and custom cruisers, such as the huge schooner *Archangel*.

The builder has an excellent reputation for warranty service. The company's dealer network also has an excellent reputation.

CONSTRUCTION

The construction of the Landfall 38 is typical of the C&C line. Hulls are a one-piece, balsa-cored molding. The deck and the top of the cabin trunk are also balsa-cored. Hull and deck are through-bolted with stainless steel bolts on 6-inch centers. The hull to deck bolts also serve as fasteners for the teak toerail, which replaces the familiar and business-like slotted aluminum toerail used on other boats in the C&C line.

C&C uses butyl tape as the bedding compound in the hull to deck joint. Although this is a good, resilient compound, it has no real structural properties. We would rather see an adhesive compound such as 3M 5200 used in the joint to provide a chemical backup to the strong mechanical fastening.

The keel is an external lead casting, bolted to an integral keel sump. The keel is a fairly low aspect ratio fin, keeping the draft of the Landfall 38 confined to 5 feet. The keel is flat on the bottom, and the boat will stand on its keel, something that can't be said for a lot of fin keel boats.

All deck hardware is through-bolted, and is equipped with either backup plates or oversize washers. The relatively narrow hull to deck flange, however, means that some of the backup plates do not lie flat on the underside of the deck, as they bridge the narrow flange. This can result in uneven local stresses

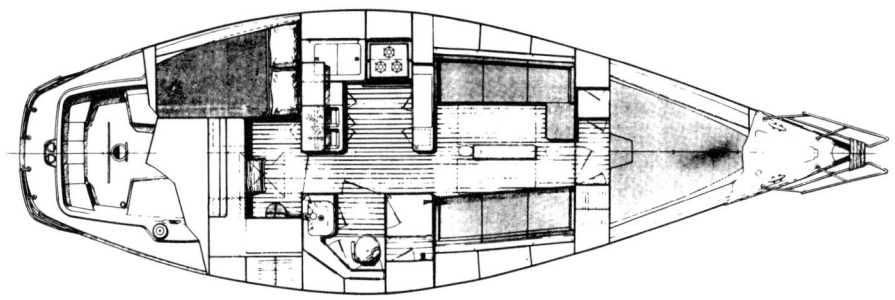

which can lead to gelcoat cracks in the vicinity of hardware such as lifeline stanchion bases.

The Landfall 38 uses bronze seacocks on all underwater through-hull fittings. These are properly bolted to the hull, and their hoses are double clamped. The skin fittings are neither recessed flush to the hull nor faired in, however. This would be a fairly easy task for the owner.

In contrast to many boats, the mast step does not sit in the depths of the bilge where it can slowly turn to mush, taking the bottom of the mast with it. Rather, the mast step spans two deep floor timbers in the bilge sump, keeping the heel of the mast out of the water and providing stiffness in an area which is frequently too weak in fin keel boats.

Although most construction details are excellent, there are some shortcomings surprising on a boat of this quality. The engine compartment has no sound-proofing, despite the fact that the engine sits a few feet from the owner's berth.

C&C construction is light but strong. The Landfall 38 is heavier than the old C&C 38 because of extra ballast, more interior joinerwork and molding, and a longer deck.

PERFORMANCE

Handling Under Sail

Although the Landfall 38 is a cruising boat, her performance approaches or exceeds that of many production racer-cruisers. Her hull is basically an undistorted IOR shape, and the rig is a slightly shorter version of the old C&C 38 rig.

The Landfall is a full 2,000 pounds heavier than the original C&C 38. Nevertheless, there is relatively little difference in the performance of the two boats.

In typical C&C fashion, the rig is aerodynamically clean, with airfoil spreaders and Navtec rod rigging. The chainplates, also Navtec, are set inboard for good upwind performance. The large rig and big headsails of the Landfall may be intimidating to some cruising couples. The 100-percent foretriangle area of 385 square feet is daunting because it means that the 150-percent genoa has an area of almost 580 square feet. Because of the large foretriangle, the boat is a natural candidate for a good roller furling headsail system if it is to be cruised by a couple.

The main halyard, reefing, and cunningham lines are all led aft to the cockpit. Headsail halyards, however, lead to winches atop the cabin trunk just aft of the mast. This prevents the helmsman from assisting with headsails when the boat is sailed by a couple. This may or may not be a problem, depending on how agile the foredeck crew is. Since you can get two headsail halyards and two headsail halyard winches, a better solution might be to relocate one of the headsail winches aft, leaving the other near the mast. Then, headsail hoisting and dropping can be tailored to the particular crew's needs.

Surprisingly, the self-tailing winches are not standard on the boat, except for the mainsheet winch. On a $100,000 boat which has hot and cold water as standard items, we'd certainly expect to see self-tailing genoa sheet winches,

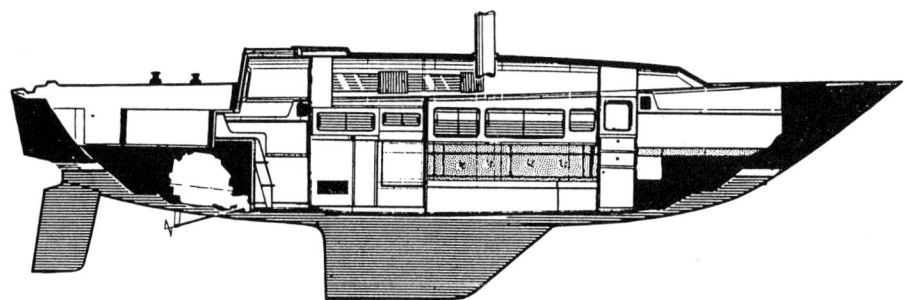

particularly if the boat is to be used for short-handed sailing. Self-tailers make sailhandling so much easier when cruising, that they are just about the first thing we'd add to any cruising boat (they would be the biggest self-tailers we could fit on the winch islands).

The Landfall 38 is stiff and well-balanced under sail. Owners report that she is as fast or faster than similar boats of the same size. The Landfall 38's PHRF rating, for example, is 120, squarely between the 114 of the Cal 39 and the 126 of the Tartan 37—two boats to which the Landfall 38 will inevitably be compared in size, type, and price.

To our way of thinking, performance cruising is what it's all about. It's all well and good to have a heavy, underrigged boat if you're cruising around the world. Most people's cruising, however, is limited to a few weeks a year, with moderate distances between ports, and schedules that have to be met. A boat that will get your there fast, safely, and in comfort is a highly desirable type of boat for this kind of cruising. From a performance viewpoint, the Landfall 38 meets those requirements.

Handling Under Power

C&C was one of the first boatbuilding firms to introduce Yanmar diesels into the U.S. market, and they have stuck with Yanmar through thick and thin. Yanmar engines have been a paragon of reliability, but they have had the reputation for vibration and noise. Vibration has at times been so bad that engine mounts have broken and shafts have refused to stay in their couplings.

It is always difficult to say, in an engine problem, whether the engine, the design of the installation, or the person doing the installation is at fault. One Landfall 38 owner has had three prop shafts in his boat. Now, after careful matching of the shaft flanges and careful alignment of the engine, he reports satisfaction with the installation. C&C picked up a hefty bill on that one, but they did it without hesitation.

When buying a new boat, be sure to align the engine after the boat is launched, and before you use it. Don't just blithely hook up the coupling. Careful engine and shaft alignment is a key to good engine performance, particularly in a modern boat with a short shaft and a flex-mounted diesel engine.

The 30-horsepower Yanmar, 3HM, which has replaced the 3QM in the Landfall 38, is perfectly adequate power for the boat, easily achieving hull speed. The boat handles well under power in either forward or reverse.

Engine access for service is a mixed bag. The engine is tucked well aft, under the cockpit, and drives the prop through a V-drive. The oil is checked by removing a panel in the quarterberth in the owner's cabin. The companionway ladder, and a bureau next to it, remove fairly easy for access to the back of the engine—although it will probably be necessary to empty the drawers before the bureau can be lifted out. The oil filter is reached by climbing down into the starboard cockpit locker. Once again, emptying the locker may be necessary.

Since there is no engine drip pan, you must exercise great care when changing oil and oil filters to keep the bilge clean. The engine is wedged so tightly under the cockpit sole that a funnel with a long hose is required to add either oil or engine coolant. A partial plywood bulkhead that hangs over the engine complicates this, and could easily be cut away to give slightly better access.

Battery access is poor. A mirror is required to check electrolyte levels, and filling the batteries just about requires removing them from the battery boxes.

The standard prop is a solid two-bladed wheel. To reduce the considerable drag of this installation, we'd change to either a folding prop such as a Martec, or a feathering prop such as the Maxprop.

LIVABILITY

Deck Layout
Although the deck layout of the Landfall 38 is similar to that of other boats in the C&C line—performance oriented—some changes have been made to make the boat more suited to cruising. The stern rail incorporates a fold-down swimming ladder, and the bow pulpit is the walk-through European type, suited to tying up bow-to at the dock. The bow pulpit also incorporates international-style running lights, rather than the running lights mounted in the topsides that were a C&C trademark for years.

Unfortunately, the wiring for the running lights is relatively unprotected inside the anchor locker, and the electrical connections there are simple butt splices with no weathersealing.

The anchor locker has strong hinges but lacks a positive latch. There is also no means of securing the bitter end of the anchor rode. Prudent owners will install an eyebolt or through-bolted padeye.

A new stainless steel stemhead fitting incorporates bow rollers for both chain and rope. There is no provision for a keeper pin in the bow roller, however, and the cheeks of the fitting do not extend high enough to guarantee that the rode will not jump out of the roller when the boat pitches at anchor.

With the shrouds set well inboard, fore and aft access is excellent. There are handrails along the cabintop, and a stainless steel guardrail over the forward dorade boxes to keep headsail sheets from fouling.

Two Landfall 38's have been built with teak decks. This is a $10,000 option that really makes the boat elegant, and is practical underfoot. However, you could also buy a whole suit of first-class sails with that $10,000, or go cruising for a year.

Although this is a cruising boat, there is no molded coaming for the attachment of a cockpit dodger, except for a small lip around the companionway hatch. Admittedly, leading all sail controls aft along the cabintop complicates the installation of a dodger, but it can be done. Of course, the dodger can be installed without a breakwater, but it won't be as effective in keeping water out of the cockpit.

The cockpit is a fairly typical T-shaped C&C design. A large-diameter Edson wheel makes it possible for the helmsman to sit to weather or to leeward, but requires making the cockpit seats too short to lie on. On some C&C models, molded seats in the aft corners of the cockpit serve both to support the helmsman's seat, and as storage for propane bottles. On the Landfall 38, the cockpit has been pushed so far aft because of the longer deckhouse, that the hull is too shallow under the aft end of the cockpit for the traditional gas locker. A separate molded bottle locker under the helmsman's seat is installed when a gas stove is used. Unfortunately, this eliminates the normal life raft shortage position. Owners who want both propane and a life raft are going to have to figure out another place to stow the life raft.

A shallow locker under the port cockpit seat is handy for small items, and there is a deep locker under the starboard seat. Changing oil filters requires climbing down into this locker, as does adjusting the stuffing box.

The forward end of the cockpit is protected by a good bridgedeck. Although the companionway is slightly off center, it is not enough to be concerned about in heavy weather. The companionway has other problems, however. Since the bulkhead slopes forward, the dropboard must be left in place when it rains. Also, since the bottom of the companionway is below the top of the cockpit coamings, ORC requirements demand that the dropboard be left in place when racing offshore. Although this isn't a racing boat, the ORC requirements make good guidelines for offshore cruising practices. Because the dropboard is a single teak-faced plyboard, the companionway must be all the way closed, or left all the way open.

The companionway sill has no lip, so water can enter the cabin under the dropboard. This is a simple fix for owner or factory. The prudent owner will also install a barrel bolt to secure the dropboard in place when sailing offshore.

Belowdecks

C&C's interior design is usually among the best in the business, and the interior of the Landfall 38 is no exception. The preponderance of teak is a little overwhelming, but it is varnished, rather than oiled, making it slightly lighter than you might expect. An optional light pine hull ceiling will make the interior even lighter.

It takes quite a bit of ingenuity to cram a three-cabin interior, and huge head with separate shower stall, into a 38-foot boat. In the Landfall 38, this has been accomplished with a reasonable amount of success.

The forward cabin has the usual V-berth, drawers, several lockers, and a cedar-lined hanging locker. This hanging locker is the only really usable hanging space on the entire boat, despite the existence of a rudimentary hanging locker in the aft cabin.

A large hatch over the forward cabin can be used as an escape hatch; a single step is mounted on the bulkhead to make it possible to climb out the hatch. There is solid 6 feet of headroom in the forward cabin, and enough standing room for comfortable dressing. The V-berth, however, is too pointed at the foot for reasonable comfort for two tall people. There are reading lights over each side of the berth, and a light in the hanging locker—a welcome feature.

The main saloon begins immediately aft of the forward cabin, with no intervening head compartment.

Light and ventilation of the Landfall 38 is about the best we've seen in a production boat. Both fluorescent and incandescent fixtures are located throughout the main cabin. Remember that you should not use fluorescent lights when you are operating the Loran, as the RF noise of fluorescent lights may interfere with signal acquisition.

The main cabin, galley, and head are ventilated by four large cowl vents in dorade boxes, plus small opening hatches in head and galley. C&C gets an A-plus for ventilation in this boat.

Water tanks are located under the main cabin settees—right where they belong. Unfortunately, these tanks vent to the outside of the hull, risking contamination of the water supply. This is a common fault in American production boats, and with no real justification. We'd rather risk spilling a little water in the inside of the boat by overfilling the tanks, than risk salt water in our fresh water supply from water siphoning into the tanks in heavy weather through vents mounted in the topsides.

The Landfall 38 uses molded polyethylene water tanks. Occasionally, these tanks are "overcooked" during manufacture, imparting an unpleasant taste to the water than can't be removed. We've seen it on more than one boat, including C&C's.

Freshwater plumbing is butyl tubing rather than the more commonly seen clear PVC. Butyl is far less likely to impart any taste to your water, and is highly desirable. It is easily recognized by its battleship grey color and relative rigidity. A manifold under the sink allows switching between the three water tanks, which have a total capacity of 99 gallons. In addition, the 30-gallon holding tank could easily be replumbed as a fresh water tank, giving a very respectable water capacity properly distributed throughout the boat.

In typical C&C fashion, the galley is well laid out and well executed, with deep centerline sinks, kickspace under the counters, and a large icebox. The icebox lid is insulated but ungasketed, and the icebox meltwater is pumped overboard rather than draining into the bilge.

Counter space is excellent. In an attempt to get more, a fold-down counter is fitted over the stove. Unfortunately, it must be folded up when the stove is in use, making the locker behind the stove inaccessible. Since the boat already has good counterspace, we'd eliminate this folding nuisance.

The standard stove is a large gimballed alcohol affair. Don't even consider it. Get either the optional propane installation, or the optional CNG stove. Alcohol has no business as a cooking fuel on any boat to be used as a serious cruising boat. The stove recess is protected by a stainless steel grabrail, which gives the cook a handhold and prevents him or her from being thrown against the stove in a seaway. A counter with built-in bottle storage separates the galley from the main cabin.

Generally, the galley is usable at sea or at anchor, with excellent storage, usable spaces, and functional appliances. Hot and cold pressure water is standard and a backup fresh water foot pump is provided at the galley sink.

The main cabin table is strongly mounted to both cabin sole and mast, and easily serves six at dinnertime. Port and starboard settees can be used for sleeping, although the backrests at the head and foot of each settee will have to be removed for anyone over five and a half feet tall. Storage is provided outboard of each settee. The handy owner will install shelves in these lockers to better utilize the space.

Opposite the galley is a huge head complete with separate shower stall. The sink and counter are a single fiberglass molding. The sink is large and has a high protective lip—making this part of the head infinitely more usable than the usual tiny oval sink.

Although at first glance there appears to be a great deal of storage in the head, much of the locker space is occupied by plumbing. The only locker really suited for linens is located in the shower stall, and is equipped with a latch which must be reached through a finger hole in the locker door. Water will inevitably find its way into this locker. The locker could easily be fitted with another type of catch, and ventilation holes could be bored through to the head compartment to help prevent mildew. The separate shower stall will make those unaccustomed to boat living far more comfortable, although some might prefer the additional storage space the boat had before the separate stall appeared.

Oddly, the water closet is tucked so far under the side deck that it's impossible to sit upright on it. While you may argue that few people sit upright on

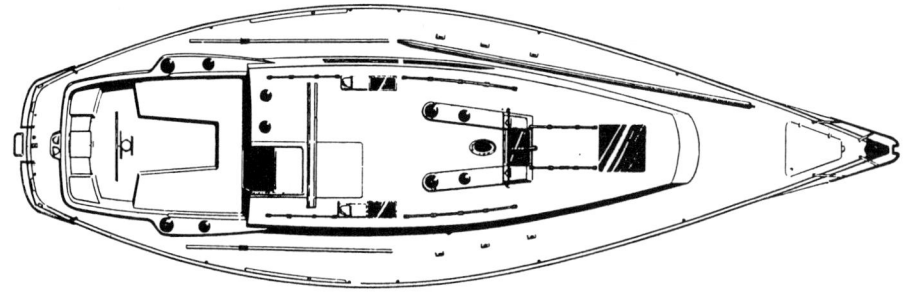

the toilet, there will be plenty of cracked heads before you get used to the required position.

Another oddity is that the head door is louvered. Admittedly, there is little privacy in the head on any boat. Since the Landfall's head is well vented by a cowl vent and an opening hatch, we'd eliminate the louvered head door to restore at least a modicum of privacy.

The aft cabin makes a good owner's stateroom, with a large double quarter-berth to port and chart table to starboard. Unfortunately, the chart table makes a better dressing table than chart table. There is no provision for the installation of instruments (such as radio or Loran) in the navigation area. A shallow hanging locker occupies the space outboard of the chart table, where these instruments would normally be mounted. It is unusable as a wet locker, since you'd have to drag your wet foul weather gear over the chart table.

For serious cruising, we'd eliminate this hanging locker, using the space to mount radios, Loran, repeaters, and provide a bookcase for our navigation books. This has the serendipitous side effect of allowing the shallow chart table to be made deeper, which it sorely needs.

What about hanging space? Well, here goes. Make the linen locker in the shower stall a hanging locker by eliminating, or reducing, the size of the holding tank under it. Or (and we can see marketing people putting guns to their heads), eliminate the separate shower stall and create more storage space. So much for redesign.

In the way of modifications, however, the nice double quarterberth is going to get soaking wet the first time a big one comes over the weather rail and water pours through the companionway when the boat is on starboard tack. In the same situation on port tack, the chart table will get soaked. A set of plexi-glass screens on either side of the companionway should solve that one, and should be considered if the boat is to be used offshore. For shorthanded cruis-ing, that quarterberth is the ideal place for the offwatch, provided it can be kept dry. The necessity for keeping the navigation station and its fragile electronics out of the weather should be obvious.

The basic interior layout of the Landfall 38 is excellent for the cruising couple that likes a private cabin aft, who will sometimes entertain others for extended periods of time. As with most boats, a certain amount of fine tuning of interior spaces will be necessary to get the most from them. The boat has a fair number of complex systems: hot and cold water, electric pumps, and multiple tanks. In fact, the 16 circuits provided for in the electrical panel are almost all used up before you get to things like navigation and performance electronics. Fortu-nately, there is space for an additional electrical panel. You're probably going to need it.

CONCLUSIONS

With a typical sailaway price of about $110,000, the Landfall 38 is not a cheap way to go cruising. The price is typical of luxury performance cruisers in its class. General design and construction are excellent. The hull is a proven design, the rig is efficient and strong. There are a number of design details that should be improved for serious cruising, notably the companionway, cockpit protection, life raft storage, and provision for shorthanded handling under sail.

A serious cruising boat must function as well bashing to windward for days on end, as it does at the dock. Above all, it must keep its crew dry and comfortable. We have yet to find the perfect cruising boat, but many of the things we'd look for are found in the Landfall 38. We wish they were all there, but the fact that they aren't is what keeps designers and builders in business.

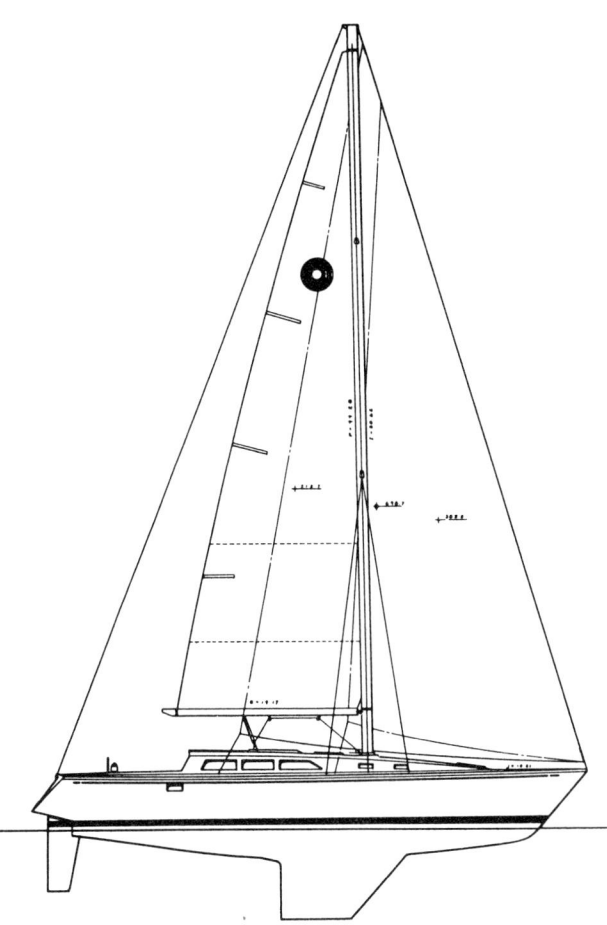

Specifications
O'Day 39/40

LOA 39	38'7"
LOA 40	39'7"
LWL	33'6"
Beam	12'8"
Draft	
shoal keel	4'1"
fin keel	6'4"
Displacement	
shoal keel	18,500 lbs
fin keel	18,000 lbs
Ballast	
shoal keel	7100 lbs
fin keel	6600 lbs
Sail area	701 sq ft

O'Day Yachts
848 Airport Road
Fall River, Mass. 02720
(617) 678-5291

The O'Day 39/40:
A Satisfactory Compromise

THE BOAT AND THE BUILDER

The "O'Day" is George O'Day, an Olympic Gold medalist in 1960 who cashed in on his success by building and selling some of the first fiberglass daysailers—particularly the O'Day Day Sailer which continues in production today.

O'Day himself has had no involvement with the company he organized since the mid-1960s when the boatbuilder, along with Jeanneau, Cal Boats, and Ranger Yachts, began a long series of ownership by conglomerates, first Bangor Punta, then Lear Seigler as part of its Starcraft Sailboat Products.

The story of O'Day as a boatbuilder has been its evolution from perhaps the foremost builder of smaller boats, when its brand name was almost synonymous with one-design and daysailing craft, to larger and larger boats as they became increasingly more profitable. In the mid-1960s, O'Day branched first into trailerable mini-cruisers and then, one by one, into larger cruising boats through the 1970s and 1980s. Yet, from its Prindle catamaran to the O'Day 40, O'Day continues to be one of the few boatbuilders (Catalina is another) that covers the market with a wide size-range of boats.

No boatbuilder has over those years had more models in its line than O'Day, in notable contrast with such builders as Hunter and Catalina. In addition to its plethora of dinghy-sized boats, O'Day, at various times has produced boats in almost every one-foot increment from 17 feet to 40 feet. Some of these have been highly successful. The O'Day 22-foot and 23-foot "trailer cruisers" set a standard in the 1970s for boats of this size and type. The O'Day 25 was one of the most successful "transition cruisers" ever built with 3000 produced in the nine years she was in production. Similarly, the O'Day 37, for years the largest boat in the O'Day line, helped popularize the midships cockpit/aft cabin in a boat under 40 feet.

The chief designer of O'Day sailboats for almost 20 years has been the design firm of C. Raymond Hunt & Associates of Boston. This long-term association with a single designer, like Ericson Yachts with Bruce King, has resulted in a close resemblance among the many O'Day models. A 10-year-old O'Day boat and the latest boat out of the O'Day plant, apart from styling details that reflect changing times and tastes, are equally identifiable as O'Day-built. This continuity has been important in the marketplace. Prospective buyers recognize the name and the style of boats, and many O'Day owners "trade up" within the O'Day line.

Over the years, O'Day also established an extensive dealer network, but not as successfully as the firm established product identity. Partly the fault of many changes in O'Day ownership, O'Day customers have given its dealers mixed reviews and O'Day's customer relations department barely passing grades.

Yet there is a possible explanation for this problem in addition to the matter of ownership. Despite the fact that O'Day boats have typically been in competition with such lower-priced boats as Hunter and Catalina—and built for that competition—O'Day is perceived as a higher quality builder. From this perception comes higher expectations. And expectations not satisfactorily met generate complaints. The fact is, however, that O'Day boats are not Sabres, Ericsons, or Tartans. Over the years, O'Days have been good values, but buyers should

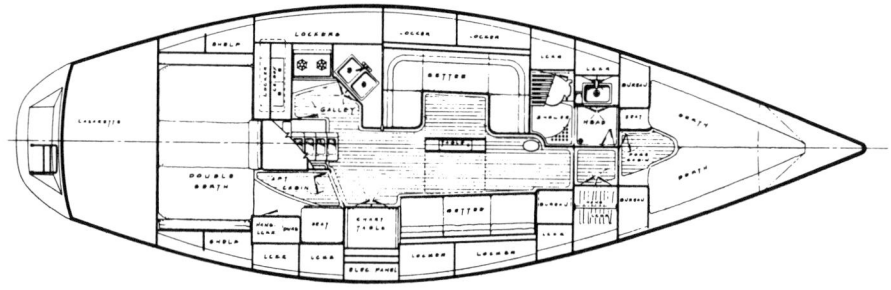

keep in mind that at lower prices, they may not get the attention and service that owners of higher priced products can more realistically expect.

In contrast to the uniformity in the O'Day line of Hunt-designed boats, the O'Day 40 began life in Europe as a 39-footer from the drawing board of French designer Phillipe Briand, and was first built by Jeanneau as the "Sun Fizz." O'Day reached an agreement with its sister company to build the boat in America and began selling her as the O'Day 39 in 1981.

After about 120 boats were built, O'Day had Hunt & Associates do a redesign, leaving the basic hull the same, but lengthening the cabin house, rearranging the interior, moving the mast aft a bit, and adding a platform extension with boarding ladder to the transom. The new version was christened the O'Day 40.

By the end of her first year, in the summer of 1986, 50 boats had been built, and two years after her introduction the number had reached 175. These numbers have made the 39/40 a successful product for her company during a period when most other American builders were not doing too well.

The 39/40 is very typical of modern racer-cruisers in design. She is moderate in displacement by current racing standards, but has a cutaway underbody with fin keel and spade rudder. The widest beam is carried far enough aft to allow for a good-sized aft cabin and a roomy galley, and the shallow bilges are compensated for by rather high topsides, to provide lots of living space below. At a distance of 200 yards, she would be nearly indistinguishable from a dozen Jeanneau and Beneteau models if she had blacked-out windows and different hull stripes.

CONSTRUCTION

The hull construction is a departure from O'Day's traditional solid fiberglass laminate since it is balsa-cored. The balsa core makes for a strong and stiff hull and has the advantage of reducing the amount of fiberglass and resin required for a given strength; consequently it reduces weight and cost. The balsa also provides insulation against heat and sound, and helps to eliminate condensation inside the cabin.

The disadvantage of the balsa-cored hull is simply that much greater skill and quality control are required in the laminating process to ensure the potential strength inherent in sandwich construction.

There are skeptics who question the longevity of the balsa-glass laminate due to potential problems with water absorption. But the technology has been used in production sailboats for the last 20 years, and a great many hull moldings have been made (particularly by C&C and J-Boats) with little evidence that there has been any more laminate failure or osmotic blistering than with conventional layups.

We extensively examined the hull of one 39 and did a quick examination of a 40, and the glasswork looked good. Unfortunately, with balsa coring, there is no way to see the quality of the laminate. Potential owners must depend on the reputation and track record of the builder.

The exteriors of both hulls we examined were fair with no evident hard spots. Gelcoat work seemed to be average production-line quality, though the 39 had a bad color flaw in the bootstripe and some peculiar "crinkles" on the transom. Overall, the glass work on the O'Day 40 appeared to be somewhat better than on the O'Day 25, 27, 28, and 32 models that we have examined in the past.

The keels are external lead, bolted to a keel stub on the hull (some early keels were iron). Two versions are available, deep and shoal. The deep keel is a better shape and much to be preferred unless the extra 17 inches of draft is a critical consideration. The one keel we examined was poorly faired; anyone thinking of racing the boat in PHRF will have to spend quite a bit of time fairing it.

The deck layup is a standard balsa-core laminate with plywood inserts under cleats and winches. Non-skid is a molded pattern which is marginally adequate when wet. The 39 we examined had a number of small voids in the cockpit gelcoat, but there was little evidence of stress cracking anywhere outside the cockpit—a sign of decent workmanship.

In the hull to deck joint, O'Day has adopted the European practice. There's a standard inward-turning flange on the hull on which the deck molding rests with polyurethane compound serving as a sealer. Stainless bolts are then inserted through the hull flange, the deck, and an exterior aluminum toerail. A

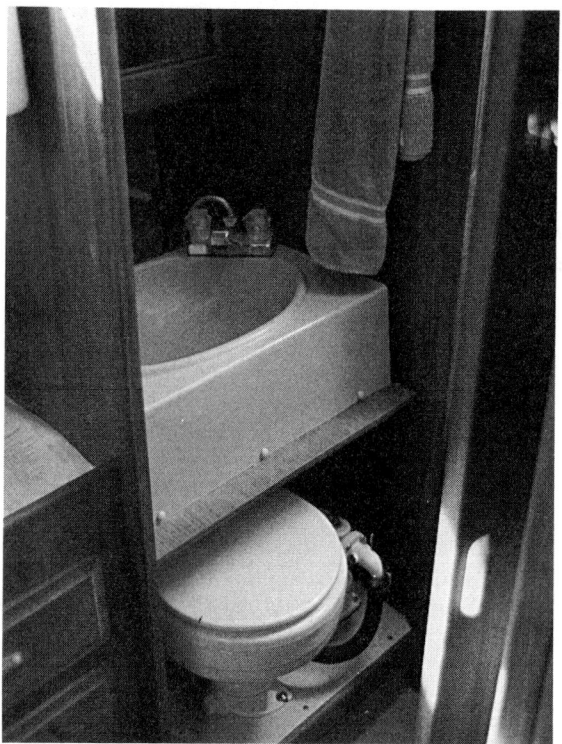

thick layer of fiberglass is laid over the interior of the joint, bonding the hull to the deck. It's a good strong joint, the only concerns being the difficulty of tracing any leaks that develop and the problems of repairing them.

Inside, a fiberglass pan forms the foundation for interior cabinetry and is bonded to the hull for additional stiffening. The chainplates are also anchored to this fiberglass pan with Navtec rod between the pan and the deck. Early on, O'Day 39 brochures claimed that this construction resulted in "quite possibly the strongest production sailboat of its size built in the United

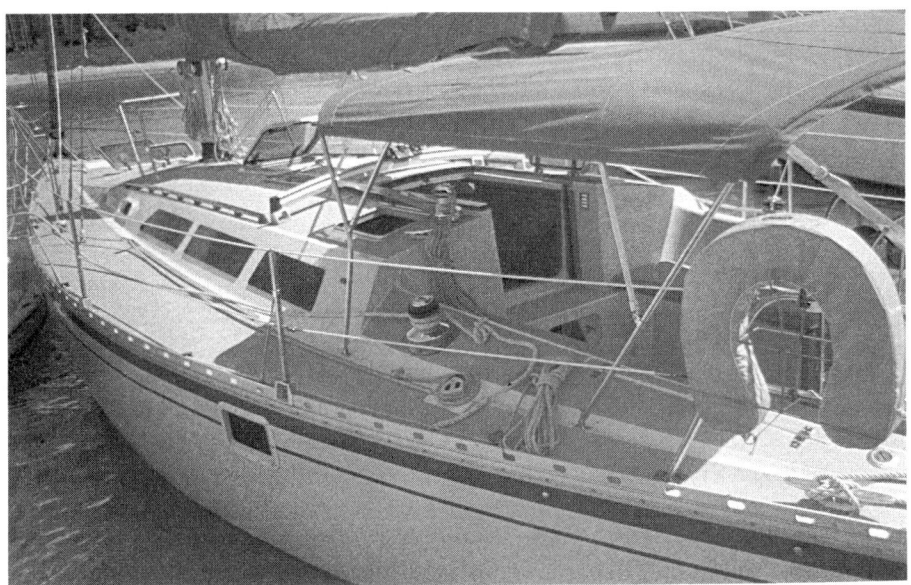

States." Clearly, this is a case of the advertising department conquering both common sense and reason.

Bulkheads are conventional teak-faced plywood, and the overhead is a fiberglass headliner. For ceiling, cabinetry is used in some spots, carpeting in some spots, and wood strips on a plastic fabric in others.

There's nothing very distinctive about the mechanical systems, but the boat comes pretty completely equipped with shore power, propane stove, a 110-gallon pressurized water system and water heater, and twin batteries.

Undoubtedly the best part of the mechanicals is the engine compartment, enormous in the 39 and roomy in the 40, to provide plenty of room for add-ons such as engine-driven refrigeration or multiple alternators. Access is good on the 39—the companionway steps hinge upward—and excellent on the 40, where additional access is provided through the aft cabin.

All the interior woodwork is standard-issue pre-fab; decent looking from a distance, but with a number of sloppy joints, rough cabinet interiors, cheap hinges and latches, and loose drawer and door fits when examined closed up.

PERFORMANCE

Handling Under Power
The 39 was fitted with a Universal 44 diesel, and the 40 has a Westerbeke 46, both fresh-water cooled. The four-cylinder engines run smoothly with minimal vibration. The noise from the engine compartment is muffled by insulation, but if we cruised the boat much, we would want to add a better lead/foam sandwich to quiet things down a bit more.

Both engines provide more than enough power to drive the boat at hull speed in strong headwinds and seas; in fact, the horsepower to weight ratio is closer to that of a motorsailer than a typical racer-cruiser. With a 42-gallon aluminum fuel tank, powering range will be well over 200 miles.

We chartered the 39 for a week in the Virgin Islands and found in about 10 hours of powering that the boat handled well with the two-bladed solid prop, backing where she was told to and powering forward in a good straight line. There should be no problem fitting a folder or a feathering prop which would improve sailing performance while retaining ample powering ability.

One bad design detail is that the engine's key and instrument panel is at the front end of the cockpit, well out of reach of the helmsman.

Handling Under Sail

During our week in the Virgin Islands, the boat proved to be a good sailer. The shallow-draft keel keeps her from pointing well, but she sailed fast on every point off the wind. With the deep-draft keel, she should be a good all around performer. The sail area is divided a bit unevenly with a smaller high-aspect mainsail and a larger jib, on a double-spreader Isomat mast.

The small main and large foretriangle undoubtedly reflect the designer's racing background and mean that, for high performance off the wind, a spinnaker will be required. However, the mast is tall enough and the sail area great enough that satisfactory performance can be obtained in most conditions with the standard roller-furling 150-percent genoa and a main with two reefs. A Hood Stoway mast and mainsail are options, but the main is small enough and easily enough handled that the added expense is probably not a reasonable investment.

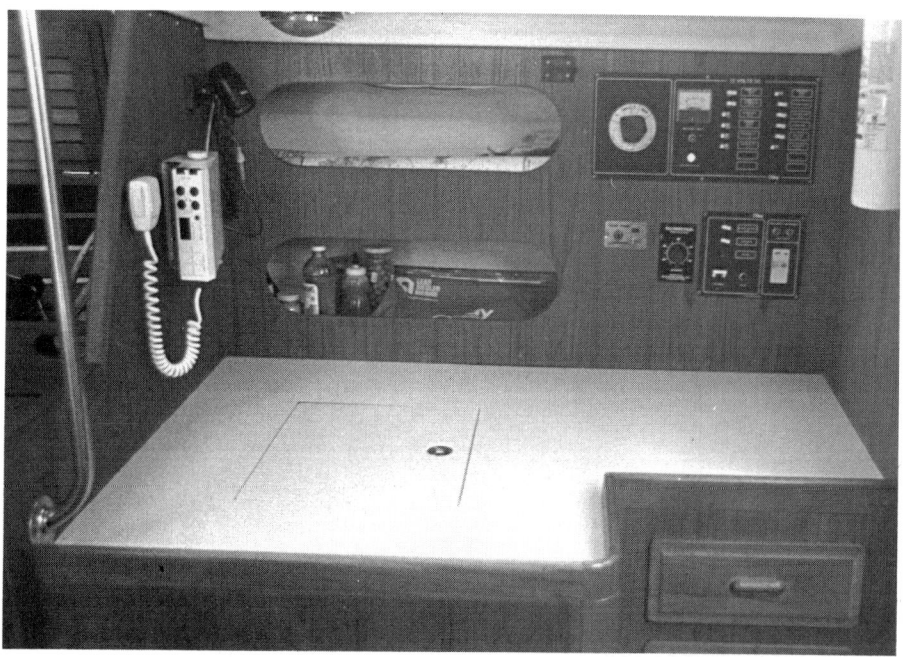

The spade rudder far aft makes for quick response to the helm, and the boat demonstrated no serious bad habits in a wide variety of conditions, although she does pound a bit going to windward in a chop. Some might find her a bit tender, and an early reef in the main is necessary to keep the boat upright and sailing well. But, overall she is definitely on the performance end of the cruising boat spectrum, rapid enough to make owners at least think of entering a Wednesday-night race. With a PHRF rating of around 114 for the deep draft version, she has the same speed as all-out racing boats in that size range did only 10 years ago.

Standard equipment on the latest 40 includes a Hood furler but only one pair of Barlow 27 self-tailing winches. The winches are absolutely minimal for easy handling of a 150-percent genoa. To make for more reasonable jib trimming we would want to upgrade to Barlow 32s or their equivalent. The cockpit coaming has built-in recesses for an extra set of winches—only necessary for the serious racer.

The short boom is sheeted to a traveler forward of the companionway. With the mainsheet so far forward, hand trimming of the main is impossible, but the standard self-tailing winch is adequate. The traveler has only mechanical stops, so adjustment under load is impossible. With the traveler, as well as most other sail controls, anyone wanting to race the boat will have to add a number of fine-tuning devices.

LIVABILITY

Deck Layout

As you might expect on a 40-foot boat, there is plenty of deck space all around. The sidedecks are wide enough that the inboard shrouds can be smack in the middle of them and still allow sufficient walk-around room. The design of the hull means that the foredeck is relatively pinched, but still there's enough room for sail and anchor handling.

The 39 had a stainless "pulpit" around the mast as standard equipment—a very good feature for heavy weather work—but the pulpit was made an option on the 40.

The stanchions, set in aluminum toerail sockets, the bow pulpit, and the stern pulpit are substantial enough, and there are double lifelines all around. The stern pulpit opens up to a transom-mounted ladder on the 39, and to a foot-wide swim platform and off-center ladder on the 40.

The cockpit is long and roomy but has a couple of irritating flaws. The main one is that the wheel is just wide enough that you have to squeeze between it and the cockpit seats. Unfortunately, the hasp for the cockpit lockers is exactly opposite the wheel, and anyone using the boat extensively will have permanent bruises on the shins at hasp level.

The lazarette hatches are outboard of the wheel. The lids are not only part of the seat but also part of the coaming. This makes for a cavernous opening, but the lid is big and heavy enough to also be an effective guillotine.

The lazarette compartment itself is huge, but in practice too deep for the bottom to be usable. An owner will want to divide up the compartment with partitions or netting to provide reasonable access to frequently used gear.

In the 39, a large storage compartment under the cockpit sole offered space for a life raft or other gear, but the compartment was eliminated to provide more aft cabin room in the 40. Propane tanks fit under the helmsman's seat.

Belowdecks

The principal difference between the 39 and 40 interiors is that the 39 had two after cabins—one port, one starboard. While this is ideal for charter work, both aft cabins are quite a squeeze for double occupancy.

On the 40, the port-side aft cabin has been eliminated, the starboard aft cabin was expanded with a huge athwartship double berth, and the galley was enlarged to occupy what was left of the former port cabin. The 40's arrangements are clearly preferable for an owner or family using the boat.

The galley is good-sized and convenient, the only shortcoming being the minimal dry storage areas. The chart table opposite is adequate, with a cute little swing-out seat that looks to be unusable in heavy weather. On the 39, a second icebox frequently replaced the chart table for charter work. Unlike many earlier O'Days, the iceboxes are well insulated.

The main saloon is comfortable and will seat a crowd, the head is adequate for family use (the 39 had a second toilet and washbasin in the after cabin), and the forward cabin is big enough for an adult couple to use on a two-week cruise. Throughout, the dead spaces are used pretty well to provide storage bins and bureaus as well as two small hanging lockers. The bilges are shallow, so there's no storage there, and any water taken on will make a real mess.

There are numerous hatches and opening ports, and in fair weather and calm sailing, ventilation is excellent. With the hatches and ports closed, however, there are only two dorades on the 40 and there was nothing on the 39. Opening ports into the cockpit footwell alleviate the problem a bit, but additional dorades or other waterproof vents would be mandatory for wet weather cruising.

The opening ports in the topsides are likely to be a concern for some buyers. Sailing, we found it hard to put the ports under water, and when we did, leaking was minimal. If we ever went offshore in the boat, we would install storm shutters.

Other than the potential ventilation problems, the interior is well thought out, and the balsa-cored hull provides good insulation.

CONCLUSIONS

In general, the O'Day 39/40 is a wholesome boat that fits a definite niche in the American cruising-boat market. It would be inappropriate to think of her as finished like a high quality yacht—she is definitely mid-line production quality—or to consider her as an offshore or world cruiser.

Rather, she is a contemporary coastal cruiser, the sort of boat to be used mostly for weekends, occasional casual races, and a two- or three-week cruise each season. For those purposes, we can only conclude that her design and production have been well executed. She will be no one's ideal boat, but a moderate and satisfactory compromise for a great many.

More notably, she is about the only American-made boat her size which is a reasonable alternative to the host of foreign imports that have invaded the American market. There are American-built boats in her price and size range (like the Hunter 40 or Morgan 38), but we think she is somewhat better built and an overall better value than those.

There are many boats available that are higher quality, especially in finish details, but with a base price of around $91,000, the O'Day can be fully outfitted with good gear and sails for well under a hundred grand. That's a lot of money, but any quality 40-footer will cost you $150,000 these days, and the best will be in the $200,000 range. Most sailors will have to ask themselves if they would really be getting twice as much boat as the O'Day.

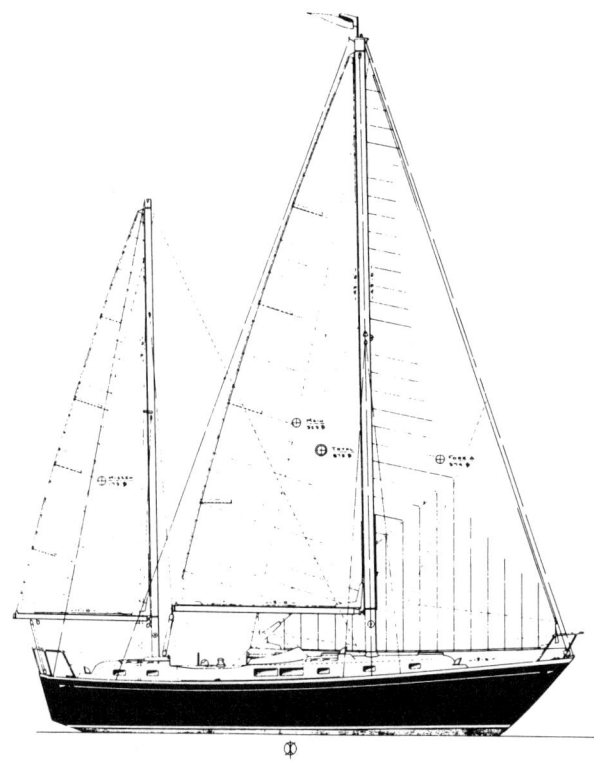

Specifications
Whitby 42

LOA	42'0"
LWL	32'8"
Beam	13'0"
Draft	5'0"
Displacement	23,500 lbs
Ballast	8500 lbs
Sail area	875 sq ft

WhitbyBoat Works Ltd.
1710 Charles St.
Whitby, Canada L1N 1C2
(416) 668-7755

The Whitby 42:
Improving with Age

THE BOAT AND THE BUILDER

The Whitby 42 is another one of the small success stories of the boatbuilding industry. Designed by Ted Brewer in 1971, the Whitby 42 has been in production since 1972. By the middle of 1987, Whitby Boat Works had built 233 42s. A similar boat called the Brewer 12.8 has been built by Fort Myers Yacht and Shipbuilding in Florida.

It is safe to say that Whitby Boat Works is a conservative boatbuilding firm. Whitby only recently ceased production of the venerable Alberg 30 that had been in continuous production since 1962, and continues to produce the Alberg 37 and C&C-designed Whitby 45, both older designs than the Whitby 42.

When the Whitby 42 was introduced in 1972, the cost of the boat, including such features as diesel auxiliary, generator, hot and cold pressure water, and refrigeration, was $42,000 including U.S. duty. In the same year, the Morgan Out Island 41 had a base price of $33,000, and the Coronado 41 was $30,000.

By 1987, the Coronado 41 has long since become a memory, an Out Island 41 will set you back about $140,000, and the Whitby 42 will cost you just shy of $125,000, with the U.S. duty paid. In other words, the Whitby 42 has good staying power, and if anything, has improved on its value in the market.

When we first saw the Whitby 42 in 1973, she seemed an ungainly whale of a boat with high topsides, white decks, white everything. Over the years, through the subtle use of color (dark sheerstripe, two-tone decks), the appearance of the boat has been quietly altered. While the Whitby 42 will never have the sleek grace of an ocean racer, she has acquired a sturdy grace of her own, the product of endless refinement and subtle improvement over the years of her production.

Much of the credit for the changes in the Whitby 42 goes to Kurt Hansen and his wife Doris, who both own Whitby and oversee most of the details of production. A large portion of the rest of the credit goes to the owners of the boats, who exhibit an extraordinary interest in improving the breed.

The Whitby 42 is a full-powered auxiliary, rather than a motorsailer. Although she won't go to windward like a light displacement fin-keeler, the boat is fully capable of good performance.

Many owners have put tens of thousands of sea miles on their boats. A fair number of owners are retired couples who purchased the boat as a cruising home. Since the boat has the elbowroom, accommodations, storage, and comforts that you would associate with a retirement home, she has proved a remarkable success in that capacity.

The Whitby 42 does not particularly look like an oceangoing boat with her center cockpit, high topsides, wide beam, and shoal draft. Nevertheless, an astounding percentage of the boats are used for serious passagemaking.

CONSTRUCTION

Construction of the Whitby 42 is sturdy, but without the dramatic overkill seen in some cruising boats. The hull is balsa-cored from just below the sheer to just below the waterline.

The hull and deck are joined with an internal flange, which is glassed together and mechanically joined with stainless steel rivets. In the way of the genoa track and some of the deck fittings, the hull and deck are also bolted together. If you prefer, the builder will use bolts throughout to join hull and deck for a slight additional charge.

On current boats, all through-hull fittings are equipped with through-bolted seacocks. Older boats may have gate valves on underwater fittings.

Deck and deckhouse are also balsa-cored. Solid glass is used in the way of deck hardware. In some older boats, owners report that the area under the mizzen-mast was not solid glass, resulting in compression of the deck in the vicinity of the mast. Owners of older boats also report that the underdeck support for the mizzen was marginal. In later boats the problem appears to have been solved.

For those accustomed to looking at the massive construction of some cruising boats, notably those built in the Far East, some of the construction details of the Whitby 42 may look light. The success of these boats as cruisers indicates that proper proportioning in design and construction are more important than massive scantlings.

PERFORMANCE

Handling Under Power

With a fuel capacity of 210 gallons, the Whitby 42 has a range under power of about 1500 miles. The Volvo Penta MD30 now used as auxiliary power produces about 62 horsepower, enough to drive the moderate displacement hull in almost any conditions.

Fuel tanks are located amidships. This means that the trim and balance of the boat will not change significantly as fuel is consumed. Although a three-bladed prop in an aperture is standard, light air performance would be significantly improved by replacing it with a feathering prop. With a feathering or folding prop there would be little sacrifice in performance under power, but there could easily be an increase in speed of a half knot or more under sail in winds under 10 knots. If you're off cruising in the South Pacific, just carry along the standard prop as a spare. Amazingly, none of the Whitby 42 owners we talked to had added a feathering prop. It would be one of our first major changes if we owned the boat.

Because of her windage and fairly long keel, the boat does not handle like a sports car under power. One owner says that his boat "turns like the Queen Mary" so give yourself plenty of room and take your time when docking.

Like most center-cockpit boats, the Whitby 42's engine is located under the cockpit. The result is a huge engine room with stopping headroom. The entire cockpit sole is the engine-room hatch cover, and it can be unbolted in an hour or so to allow removal of the engine without tearing the interior of the boat apart. For a cruising boat that puts a lot of hours on the engine, this is a real plus.

The engine room has enough space for a small auxiliary generator. A generator was standard when the boat was first built but is now an option. If you intend to do extensive cruising in the boat, a generator of about 3.5 kilowatts would be worth installing. Unfortunately, the weight of the generator, which is mounted on the portside, may give the boat a slight port list.

Access to the stuffing box is good through hatches in the cabin sole in the aft cabin. General access to the engine is excellent.

Handling Under Sail

Owners characterize the Whitby 42 as slightly faster than other boats of the

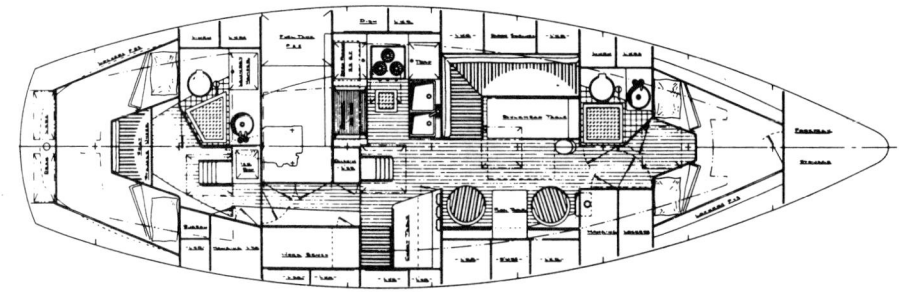

same size and type. When equipped with a mizzen staysail and a spinnaker—a very reasonable combination for offwind sailing in this boat—the boat is quite fast. One West Coast owner has raced his boat with success, but racing is certainly not the boat's strong suit.

In the past, there have been problems with the mizzenmast. Since the main boom ends fairly close to the mizzen, the mizzen forestays do not have an effective angle for forward support. The mizzen spreaders are now swept back enough to provide after support without the use of running backstays, although we would probably still rig them in heavy weather or sloppy seas. Forward support of the mizzen is improved by the addition of a triatic stay between the main and mizzen mastheads.

The mainsail is equipped with slab reefing, a great improvement over the roller reefing found on older models of the Whitby 42. A separate track on the mainmast for a storm trysail is an option we'd go for if the boat is to be used offshore.

Another highly desirable rig option is the double-head rig, which comes in a package with a platform bowsprit and a removable inner forestay. Owners report that the extra sail area forward improves the balance of the boat. The vast majority of Whitby 42s in recent years have been delivered with this double-head rig—in effect, cutter ketches. An attempt to give the 42 a sloop or cutter rig, eliminating the mizzen and lengthening the boom, was not successful; the mast is stepped so far forward that any such modification requires too long a main boom and becomes ungainly even with a bowsprit. The Whitby 42 is clearly intended for buyers looking for a ketch. For cruising boats over 40 feet or so, especially those commonly sailed shorthanded, the ketch rig certainly makes more sense than it does in smaller boats.

Despite the great beam of the boat, her midships hull section is almost round. This means that the boat picks up very little form stability as it heels. Coupled with a ballast to displacement ratio of about 35 percent, this yields a boat that is not particularly stiff under sail, according to owners.

Although the boat comes with hydraulic steering, it is also possible to use an Edson pull-pull system. Since this is a less powerful steering system than the hydraulic steerer, you should go with the maximum size steering wheel that will fit in the cockpit—about a 40-inch diameter wheel. In addition to providing the extra leverage for the pull-pull system, a larger wheel lets you sit further outboard, an absolute necessity on a center cockpit boat when using a large genoa.

We prefer the pull-pull steerer because it gives the helmsman feedback about the balance of the boat. In the long run, the steering feedback will make you a better sailor. When the boat steers hard, it is out of balance and not being sailed with maximum efficiency.

With a high aspect rig and a generous sailplan for her moderate displacement, there is no excuse for the Whitby 42 to be a dog under sail. If you have the boat heavily loaded, you'll just have to add more sail to maintain perform-

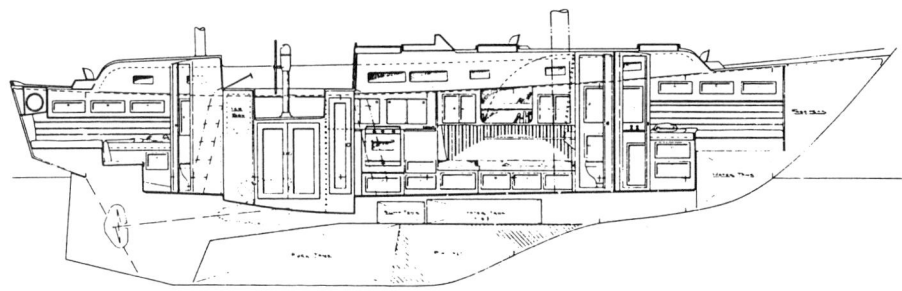

ance. Fairing in the through-hull fittings and adding a feathering prop will also help performance, particularly in light air.

Finally, by all means spring for the bowsprit and the extra sail area it gives you. According to one owner, designer Ted Brewer said the addition of the bowsprit is the single greatest improvement in the boat over the years.

LIVABILITY

Deck Layout

The deck layout of the Whitby 42 is about as simple as the deck on a boat can be. There are sturdy Skene chocks and large cleats forward, and chocks plus big cleats aft. With the platform bowsprit, anchors can be made self-stowing. Large urethane bow rollers would be preferable to the small stainless steel rollers found on the boat we examined.

The foredeck has plenty of space for an anchor windlass, an absolute must if the boat is used for extended cruising. The forepeak locker could be used to hold anchor chain, but we'd be reluctant to add another 500 pounds of ground tackle in the bow of the boat, since there's already a large water tank under the forward berths.

Despite a wide cabin trunk, access forward along the deck is good. To go from the cockpit aft, however, it is necessary to go over the top of the aft cabin, as the mizzen standing rigging takes up much of the sidedecks aft.

The stanchions and the bow and stern rails are tall and sturdy. There are two lockers on the afterdeck, one useful for lines and fenders, the other containing the propane bottles. There is also a larger locker on the port side of the cockpit. This locker, too, lacks a good set of hatch dogs, and since it opens into the engine room, we'd give high priority to making it secure despite its location well above the waterline.

The cockpit is huge, however, it is not particularly vulnerable since it is fairly high. We've seen few cockpits which would be better in port. There's even a big icebox next to the helmsman, making it unnecessary to truck down to the galley for a cold one.

A sturdy molded breakwater protects the front of the cockpit. We'd add a dodger for offshore use. The original drawings of the boat also show a permanent windshield, which would be a good feature on a boat used primarily in northern latitudes.

One Whitby 42 we've seen has a permanent shelter over the front end of the cockpit, which both improves the look of the boat (the shelter was designed by someone with a good eye) and gives a remarkable protection to the front of the cockpit, allowing the companionway hatch to be left open in all but the worst weather offshore.

For offshore use, the louvered companionway drop boards should be replaced with solid boards, since a remarkable amount of water can get below in heavy weather. This is particularly important in the companionway to the aft cabin, which faces forward.

The companionway to the aft cabin makes it impossible to fit a mainsheet traveler. Therefore, a good boom vang is a must.

We strongly recommend the two-tone deck option. Not only will it break up an otherwise overwhelming amount of deckspace visually, it will be much easier on the helmsman's eyes. Although it's not listed as an option, you could probably also get the deckhouse top in a color other than white. This would visually lower the height of the deckhouse as well as reducing glare.

Belowdecks

Down below, the Whitby 42 really shines. The boat has one of the more livable interiors we've seen.

The owner's cabin aft has two large berths. If they are to be used as sea berths, they must be fitted with lee cloths. Since the berths are not parallel to the centerline of the boat, they do not make particularly good sea berths. The person sleeping in the leeward berth will find his head lower than his feet, while the occupant of the weather berth will be in the opposite situation.

Although there are a fair number of storage bins and a good hanging locker, the aft cabin has only a few drawers. Although drawers are not a particularly efficient way to use space, they are extremely convenient, particularly for those who have lived their lives in houses.

The aft head is huge. A few handrails would make it more comfortable offshore. A passageway with stooping headroom joins the aft cabin to the rest of the boat. Getting full headroom in this passage would unnecessarily complicate the cockpit layout.

A workbench which can be converted to a berth is on the starboard side of the passage. The space below the bench is filled by a fuel tank, some storage space, and a big chart locker.

Outboard of the workbench is the electrical panel. Despite the stooping headroom, this is just about the ideal location for the electrical panel since it is completely protected from spray.

On the port side of the passage, just aft of the companionway, there is a large locker for foul weather gear. Little touches like the chart storage and the wet gear locker make the difference between a floating condominium which is miserable at sea and a true cruising boat.

The main cabin is roomy, light, and well-ventilated. The galley to port has a large refrigerator and deep freeze, a three-burner propane stove, and deep double sinks. The only weak point in the galley is the mounting of the stove. On starboard tack, it fetches up against the back of the stove well when the boat heels much over 15 degrees. On port tack, the stove blocks access to the drawers under the sink counter. Although the boat is meant to be sailed at slight angles of heel, the stove should be free to gimbal, through at least 90 degrees without inconvenience. Except for the stove limitation, the galley deserves high marks.

To starboard is the navigation table with adequate room for the mounting of instruments and a good chart table. The chart table slopes toward the navigator, making it easier to work on from a seated position, but it is equipped with a folding support which allows the table to be leveled for use in port, making a handy desk.

Originally, there was no settee on the starboard side of the boat. Rather, the boat had two swivel chairs, a familiar touch to those accustomed to life ashore. However, if the boat is to be used offshore, it should be ordered with the optional starboard settee, since the main-cabin settees are the only good sea berths on the boat. There is plenty of storage space outboard the settees on both sides, including an excellent liquor locker with a folding cocktail table.

The cabin table folds up against the port forward bulkhead. On a boat of this size, a fixed cabin table makes more sense. If we owned a Whitby 42, we'd build a narrow dropleaf table with deep fiddles, incorporating a pipe to the cabin overhead for a handhold when sailing offshore. While this would intrude into the main cabin space, it would reduce the chance of a bad fall in rough conditions, would free up the bulkhead for other uses, and would create

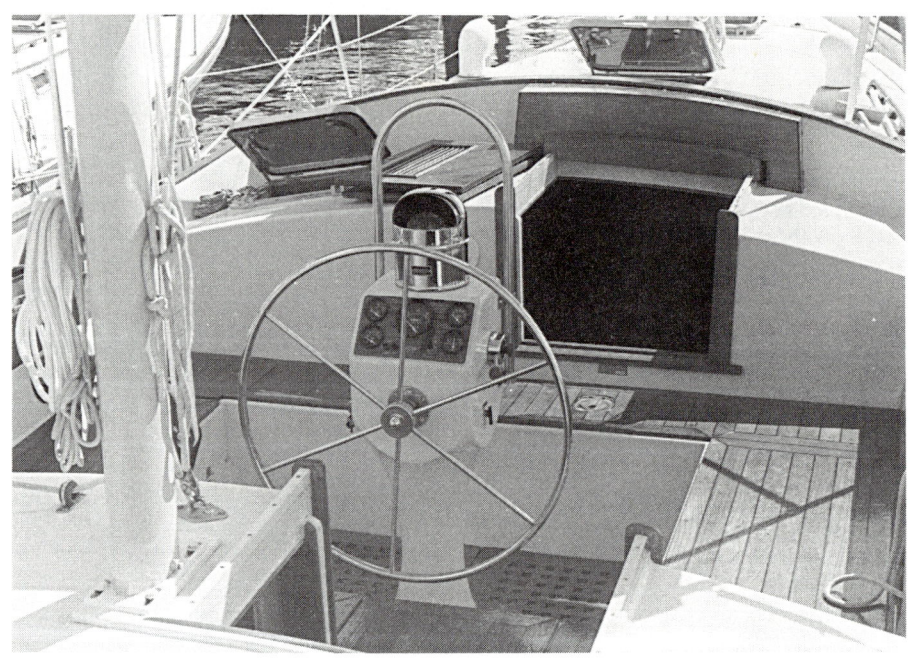

a storage space on the cabin sole where bulky objects like spare sails could be stowed offshore.

The forward cabin and head are almost as roomy as the after cabin. In port, the occupants of the forward cabin are not second class citizens. Except for light air sailing downwind, the forward cabin will probably not be used for sleeping offshore.

All in all, the interior of the Whitby 42 is an excellent compromise between the needs of the long-term liveaboard and the long-distance cruiser.

CONCLUSIONS

In these days of astronomical prices, the Whitby 42 represents a good value for living aboard or cruising. While finish details are not particularly fancy, the boat is solidly built, and should be easy to maintain.

The boat comes with a rather remarkable list of standard equipment included in the base price of just under $120,000, with such items as hot and cold water, refrigeration, huge tankage, two showers, dual voltage electrical systems, and ground tackle.

The options are practical and born of experience. Many of them are highly desirable, such as the double headsail rig with bowsprit, contrasting deck color, dark sheer indent, autopilot, and windlass. Fully equipped for cruising—and we mean fully equipped—the boat will cost about $140,000, depending, of course, on current exchange rates.

You can expect reasonable sailing performance from the Whitby 42. Obviously, her best point of sail will be reaching in moderate to heavy air.

Because of the improvements that have been made in the boat over the years, we would prefer a new boat rather than a used boat. Given the fact that used boats sell for nearly as much as new boats, and given the fact that you can pretty much customize the boat any way you want when you have it built, a new Whitby 42 looks very good indeed.

Most owners are very enthusiastic about their boats. For most of them, this is not a first boat. Although most consider the boat a good boat dockside, they also consider it a boat in which to go places. We agree.

Evaluations:
Date of Original Publication

The evaluations of sailboats published herein are collected from previously published issues of *The Practical Sailor*. Because of the time required for evaluation and reporting, each evaluation may not reflect the latest models, features, options or construction methods. The main criteria for evaluation were that the boats were in production at the time of the original evaluation and had proved their popularity in the marketplace. Unfortunately, in a number of cases, the boats now may be out of production. Up-to-date information on prices, the availability of each model, or each feature, would require the kind of checking that goes well beyond *The Practical Sailor's* staff resources. However, some checks on the names and addresses of the boatbuilders, and some updating of prices and features, have been made. With or without updating, we believe the unique form of the evaluations—fashioned as they were without any influence from commercial advertisers—will make the information herein invaluable to both the new and the used boat buyer.

Model	Date of Publication	Model	Date of Publication
Starwind 19	6/1/85	Catalina 30	11/15/80
San Juan 21	5/1/84	Jeanneau Arcadia	10/1/85
Catalina 22	12/1/81	Nonsuch 30	9/15/81
O'Day 22	12/1/81	J/30	7/15/80
Tanzer 22	12/1/81	Olson 30	10/15/82
Flicka	2/15/82	Pearson 30	1/15/80
J/24	12/1/82	Cal 31	3/15/80
Cape Dory 25	5/1/82	Southern Cross 31	8/1/81
Cape Dory 25D	5/1/82	Nicholson 31	11/15/82
Ericson 25	10/15/81	Allied Seawind II	1/15/82
Freedom 25	8/15/82	Mason 33	2/1/87
O'Day 25	7/15/83	Freedom 33	12/15/80
Montego 25	7/15/83	Tartan Ten	10/1/83
Bayfield 25	1/15/84	Contest 36	3/1/86
S2 7.9 Meter	8/1/85	Morris 36	12/1/87
MacGregor 26	11/1/87	CSY 37	4/15/80
Stiletto Catamaran	6/15/82	Tartan 37	2/15/81
Hunter 27	1/15/81	Irwin 37	5/15/81
Sabre 28	4/15/81	Tayana 37	3/15/82
Laser 28	1/1/85	C&C Landfall 38	2/15/83
S2 8.5 Meter	7/15/82	O'Day 39/40	8/1/86
Bristol 29.9	9/15/84	Whitby 42	11/15/83